Behavioral Aspects of Pediatric Burns

Issues in Clinical Child Psychology

Series Editors: **Michael C. Roberts,** *University of Kansas-Lawrence, Kansas*
Lizette Peterson, *University of Missouri-Columbia, Missouri*

BEHAVIORAL ASPECTS OF PEDIATRIC BURNS
Edited by Kenneth J. Tarnowski

CHILDREN AND DISASTERS
Edited by Conway F. Saylor

HANDBOOK OF DEPRESSION IN CHILDREN AND ADOLESCENTS
Edited by William M. Reynolds and Hugh F. Johnston

INTERNATIONAL HANDBOOK OF PHOBIC AND ANXIETY DISORDERS IN CHILDREN AND ADOLESCENTS
Edited by Thomas H. Ollendick, Neville J. King, and William Yule

MENTAL HEALTH INTERVENTIONS WITH PRESCHOOL CHILDREN
Robert D. Lyman and Toni L. Hembree-Kigin

Behavioral Aspects of Pediatric Burns

Edited by
KENNETH J. TARNOWSKI
University of South Florida
Fort Myers, Florida

PLENUM PRESS • NEW YORK AND LONDON

Library of Congress Cataloging-in-Publication Data

Behavioral aspects of pediatric burns / edited by Kenneth J.
Tarnowski.
p. cm. -- (Issues in clinical child psychology)
Includes bibliographical references and index.
ISBN 0-306-44840-8
1. Burns and scalds in children--Psychological aspects.
I. Tarnowski, Kenneth J. II. Series.
[DNLM: 1. Burns--in infancy & childhood. 2. Burns--psychology.
3. Child Behavior. WO 704 B419 1994]
RD96.4.B44 1994
617.1'1'0083--dc20
DNLM/DLC
for Library of Congress 94-30884
CIP

ISBN 0-306-44840-8

A Division of Plenum Publishing Corporation
233 Spring Street, New York, N.Y. 10013

Printed in the United States of America

To my extraordinary parents, Bill and Ellen
and
wife, Pat, for their support, love, and encouragement

Contributors

F. Daniel Armstrong, Ph.D., Department of Pediatrics, University of Miami School of Medicine, Miami, Florida

Patricia Blakeney, Ph.D., Shriners Burns Institute, Galveston, Texas

Christopher P. Brandt, M.D., Department of Surgery, Case Western Reserve University School of Medicine, MetroHealth Medical Center, Cleveland, Ohio

Ronald T. Brown, Ph.D., Departments of Psychiatry and Behavioral Sciences and Pediatrics, Emory University School of Medicine, Atlanta, Georgia

Joseph P. Bush, Ph.D., Graduate School of Psychology, Fielding Institute, Santa Barbara, California

Arden D. Dingle, M.D., Departments of Psychiatry and Behavioral Sciences and Pediatrics, Emory University School of Medicine, Atlanta, Georgia

Marion Doctor, M.S.W., Children's Hospital Burn Center, University of Colorado School of Medicine, Denver, Colorado

Richard B. Fratianne, M.D., Department of Surgery, Case Western Reserve University School of Medicine, MetroHealth Medical Center, Cleveland, Ohio

Caryl L. Gay, Ph.D., Department of Pediatrics, University of Miami School of Medicine, Miami, Florida

Russell T. Jones, Ph.D., Department of Psychology, Virginia Polytechnic Institute and State University, Blacksburg, Virginia

Nadine J. Kaslow, Ph.D., Department of Psychiatry and Behavioral Sciences, Emory University School of Medicine, Grady Memorial Hospital, Atlanta, Georgia

Kamela Koon-Scott, Ph.D., Department of Psychiatry and Behavioral Sciences, Emory University School of Medicine, Grady Memorial Hospital, Atlanta, Georgia; *present address*: Department of Pediatrics, University of Florida College of Medicine, University Medical Center, Jacksonville, Florida

Jacqueline D. Levy, Ph.D., Department of Pediatrics, University of Miami School of Medicine, Miami, Florida

Marlene T. Maron, Ph.D., Otter Creek Associates, Burlington, Vermont

Thomas Pruzinsky, Ph.D., Department of Psychology, Quinnipiac College, Hampton, Connecticut

L. Kaye Rasnake, Ph.D., Department of Psychology, Denison University, Granville, Ohio

Kenneth J. Tarnowski, Ph.D., Department of Psychology, University of South Florida, Fort Meyers, Florida

Vasiliki Zaharopoulos, Department of Psychology, Virginia Polytechnic Institute and State University, Blacksburg, Virginia

Preface

In recent years, considerable professional attention has centered on the behavioral aspects of various childhood illnesses and injuries. Indeed, child health psychology has grown exponentially over the past decade. One index of this growth is found in the number of texts that have recently appeared in the area (Gross & Drabman, 1990; Karoly, 1988; Krasnegor, Arasteh, & Cataldo, 1986; Levine, Carey, Crocker, & Gross, 1982; Routh, 1988; Russo & Varni, 1982; Tuma, 1982; Varni, 1983). In general, these texts provide summaries of the psychological literature across a variety of established (e.g., oncology) and emerging (psychoneuroimmunology) areas of child health.

Until recently, many books on the psychological aspects of pediatric health provided no or minimal information about the psychosocial plight of child burn victims. In some instances, pediatric burns might be mentioned parenthetically as another example of a population for which behavioral treatment procedures (e.g., pain management) may be of value. In part, the relative inattention devoted to this population may be related to the perception that the literature in this area is sketchy and characterized by significant methodological and substantive shortcomings. In many instances, this perception is largely justified. However, it is also the case that the pediatric burn literature has evolved considerably over the past decade and that the incidence of, and morbidity associated, with severe burn injuries mandates immediate and increased attention by mental health professionals.

Several factors prompted the development of the current volume. In the process of providing inpatient and outpatient assessment, treatment, and consultation and liaison services to burned children and their families, it has been time-consuming and often disappointing to search the literature for materials of potential value in answering specific referral questions. Common referral questions often involve issues pertaining to acute psychological reactions, pain management, and long-term psychosocial sequelae. A summary of the existing literature that extends well beyond the scope and detail of a typical book chapter would be of obvious value. Another impetus for the book involved consideration of the uniqueness of burn injuries. Severe nonfatal burns by thermal, electrical, chemical, or radiation causes constitute the most serious form of human injury (McLoughlin & McGuire, 1990). Burns share characteristics with other types of acute injuries (e.g., orthopedic), as well as those of chronic illness (e.g., sickle-cell disease). As such, not only do they pose unique clinical considerations but also warrant increased attention from a developmental perspective. These injuries, and the circumstances surrounding their occurrence, have the potential to seriously disrupt a variety of important developmental processes. Indeed, the fact that severe pediatric burns do not invariably cause such devastating or lasting disruption attests to the impressive resiliency of children and families. Finally, it is important to call attention to the fact that the vast majority of pediatric burns are entirely preventable.

The purpose of the book is to survey the literature on the behavioral aspects of pediatric burns and to consider the implications for prevention, consultation, treatment, and follow-up. The book is divided into four sections. The goal of the first section is to provide a general introduction to the topic of pediatric burns including epidemiological, medical, and surgical aspects. The second section of the book considers broadly the acute reactions and long-term psychosocial sequelae associated with severe burn injury. In the third section of the book, a variety of behavioral topics are considered. The goals of the contributions in this section are to build on the information presented in earlier chapters and to acquaint the reader with the range of applied considerations that one confronts in the context of clinical work with this population. Issues relevant to consultation and liaison, pain management, body image disturbance, school reintegration, family functioning, and injury prevention are discussed in detail. The final section highlights and integrates the themes of the previous chapters and provides a general prospectus to guide future clinical and research efforts.

The book is intended for mental health professionals (psychologists, psychiatrists, social workers, and counselors), physicians (surgeons, pediatricians), nurses, and other specialists (child life workers) who are involved in the inpatient/outpatient care of burned children and their families. Wherever possible, an attempt is made to draw conclusions and establish recommendations based on review of the pediatric burn literature. For several topics, readers may be surprised at the limitations of and gaps in the primary literature. In such instances, every effort is made to examine the literature in related areas (e.g., family, chronic illness, adult burns) in the interest of establishing tentative recommendations, including those for future research. There is little doubt that research on the behavioral aspects of pediatric burns comprises an exceptionally fertile area. An enhanced appreciation of the considerable problems and prospects that exist in this area will hopefully challenge some readers to undertake further study of these children and their families.

A number of individuals contributed to the development of this volume. First, thanks are due to the contributors to this volume for their willingness to share their expertise. Second, are the series editors, Lizette Peterson and Michael C. Roberts, for their receptivity to the volume proposal and continued assistance and support. Third, we gratefully acknowledge the assistance of Mariclaire Cloutier and the Plenum staff for bringing the project to fruition. Fourth, special thanks to Ron Brown for his friendship and sage advice. Fifth, appreciation is extended to Kathleen E. Cochrane for secretarial support. Finally, we are indebted to the parents, children, and staff with whom we have worked over the years for teaching us important lessons about the tragedy of burns, the triumph of the human spirit, and for challenging us to continually examine ways in which we might broaden the scope of our applied activities.

REFERENCES

Gross, A. M., & Drabman, R. S. (Eds.). (1990). *Handbook of clincal behavioral pediatrics*. New York: Plenum Press.

Karoly, P. (Ed.). (1988). *Handbook of child health assessment*. New York: Wiley.

Krasnegor, N. A., Arasteh, J. D., & Cataldo, M. F. (Eds.). (1986). *Child health behavior: A behavioral pediatrics perspective*. New York: Wiley.

Levine, M. D., Carey, W. B., Crocker, A. C., & Gross, R. T. (Eds)., (1983). *Developmental–behavioral pediatrics*. Philadelphia: Saunders.

McLoughlin, E., & McGuire, A. (1990). The causes, cost, and prevention of childhood burn injuries. *American Journal of Diseases of Children, 144*, 677–683.

Routh, D. K. (Ed.). (1988). *Handbook of pediatric psychology*. New York: Guilford Press.

Russo, D. C., & Varni, J. W. (Eds.). (1982). *Behavioral pediatrics: Research and practice*. New York: Plenum Press.

Tuma, J. M. (Ed.). (1982). *Handbook for the practice of pediatric psychology*. New York: Wiley.

Varni, J. W. (1983). *Clinical behavioral pediatrics: An interdisciplinary biobehavioral approach*. New York: Pergamon Press.

Contents

1

Overview

KENNETH J. TARNOWSKI

INTRODUCTION

Virtually all children and parents have experience with common childhood afflictions such as viral infections, stomachaches, headaches, and minor injuries. Unfortunately, many children and their families encounter more threatening forms of acute and chronic childhood illness and injury. By age 18, approximately 10–31% of children and adolescents experience one or more chronic medical conditions (Hobbs & Perrin, 1985; Newachek, Stoddard, & McManus, 1993; Pless & Douglas, 1972). Based on national survey data, it has been estimated that childhood chronic illnesses result in 35 million bed days and 40 million school absences annually (Newachek & Taylor, 1992).

Chronic illnesses involve a protracted course, may be fatal or result in compromised mental/physical functioning, and are often characterized by acute exacerbations that require hospitalization or other forms of intensive treatment. There is significant mortality associated with several childhood disorders and injuries. In addition, many disorders and injuries result in marked medical (e.g., residual physical disability) and psychological morbidity (e.g., disruption of normal developmental processes) (Tarnowski & Brown, in press). Not only do children and families experience negative psychosocial sequelae (e.g., depression, disrupted social relations) in response to specific pediatric conditions, but behavioral factors

KENNETH J. TARNOWSKI • Department of Psychology, University of South Florida, Fort Myers, Florida 33919.

Behavioral Aspects of Pediatric Burns, edited by Kenneth J. Tarnowski. Plenum Press, New York, 1994.

have been demonstrated to be integral in determining the onset, course, prognosis, and prevention of many illnesses and injuries (Gross & Drabman, 1990; Krasnegor, Arasteh, & Cataldo, 1986; Routh, 1988; Russo & Varni, 1982).

In the past two decades, we have gained tremendous insight into the role of psychological factors involved in childhood illness, injury, and health. The importance of such variables in understanding and improving children's well-being has been highlighted repeatedly in the results of empirical work emanating from the fields of psychology, psychiatry, pediatrics, social work, nursing, and education. Indeed, the focus on behavioral aspects of various childhood disorders has proven to be a ubiquitous multidisciplinary shared interest (Breslau, 1985; Levine, Carey, Crocker, & Gross, 1983; Tarnowski, 1991; Varni, 1983).

Current pediatric health texts almost invariably include material on the behavioral aspects of cardiology, oncology, hematology, endocrinology, neurology, pulmonology, neonatology, gastroenterology, and dentistry. General topics that cut across disorder-specific areas (e.g., adherence, pain management, prevention) routinely receive enhanced coverage in the primary and secondary research literatures.

A review of recent texts in the area (Gross & Drabman, 1990; Karoly, 1988; Krasnegor *et al.*, 1986; Levine *et al.*, 1983; Routh, 1988; Russo & Varni, 1982) also reveals other emphases. Given the number of children affected and the primacy of behavioral factors in understanding injury and illness, a major focus of recent work has been on increasing our knowledge of health-related developmental variables (Burbach & Peterson, 1986). Models of cognitive development, such as that described by Piaget (Piaget & Inhelder, 1969), have been invoked frequently to conceptualize children's understanding of illness and health (Bibace & Walsh, 1980; Brewster, 1982). In addition to children's cognitive developmental status, increased attention has been devoted to understanding the socioemotional development of ill and injured children (Ferrari, 1990; Spirito, DeLawyer, & Stark, 1991). Programmatic research has also enhanced our understanding of the environmental context of injury and illness. This later emphasis includes not only an interest in how basic utilitarian (e.g., financial) and psychological (e.g., parental support, stress, caring) risks and resources affect child well-being (Daniels, Moos, Billings, & Miller, 1987; Tarnowski, King, Green, & Pease, 1991; Wallander, Varni, Babani, Banis, & Wilcox, 1989) but also an analysis of variables broadly related to family functioning (Kazak, 1989; Melamed & Bush, 1985; Rape, Bush, & Slavin, 1992) and an analysis of the specific behavioral contingencies in effect for children in hospital, home, and school settings (Linscheid, Rasnake, Tarnowski, & Mulick, 1989; Russo, Bird, & Masek, 1980; Tarnowski & Kaufman, 1988). Of course, considerable effort has also been devoted to assessing the interaction of medical-biologic and psychological variables as they mediate disease onset, expression, course, and prognosis (Baum, Grunberg, & Singer, 1982; Epstein, 1992; Herbert & Cohen, 1993; Kaplan, 1990). Finally, there has been an increased emphasis on practice issues including assessment, intervention, consultation, and prevention (Peterson & Mori, 1985; Roberts & Wright, 1982; Russo & Varni, 1982).

The development of this relatively new field of scientific inquiry (alternatively labeled child health psychology, pediatric psychology, or behavioral pediatrics) (Gross & Drabman, 1990; Russo & Tarbell, 1984; Varni & Dietrich, 1981) has been most welcome from the perspective of those involved in the clinical practice of psychology, psychiatry, pediatrics, social work, nursing, and related allied health fields. Indeed, as noted above, we now have an extensive behavioral data base on several serious diseases and injuries of childhood including cancer, asthma, diabetes, epilepsy, and traumatic brain injury. Applied researchers have also begun to focus on other pediatric conditions including sickle-cell disease, AIDS, renal disease, and rheumatoid arthritis.

The major impetus for undertaking the current volume stems from the relative lack of attention devoted to pediatric burn victims and their families. Despite the fact that burns are a relatively common phenomenon (see section below on epidemiological aspects), are considered the most serious of all human injuries (McLoughlin & McGuire, 1990), share many characteristics with those of chronic diseases (e.g., compromised functioning, protracted course of treatment) (Hobbs & Perrin, 1985), and can result in serious long-term physical and psychological morbidity (Patterson *et al.*, 1993; Tarnowski, Rasnake, Gavaghan-Jones, & Smith, 1991), it appears that other childhood maladies have garnered more attention.

Serious attempts to study the behavioral aspects of pediatric burns date back to the late 1950s and early 1960s (Long & Cope, 1961; Watson & Johnson, 1958; Woodward, 1959; Woodward & Jackson, 1961). Early studies consisted largely of uncontrolled case reports. Conclusions concerning patient and family adjustment were based on anecdotal reports and subjective clinical impression. As is the case for much pediatric health psychology research, the majority of work in this area has occurred over the past 15 years. However, unlike many areas of child health psychology, the relative dearth of basic and applied interest in the psychological aspects of pediatric burns has continued. For example, a recent review of the behavioral assessment and treatment literature with pediatric burn victims revealed only 14 investigations (Tarnowski, Rasnake, & Drabman, 1987). The emergence of a specialty journal (*Journal of Burn Care and Rehabilitation*) has helped to call attention to the population of burn survivors. However, as in many areas of behavioral health research, most efforts are devoted to the adult patient.

The relative inattention devoted to pediatric burn victims is unfortunate for a variety of reasons. In many ways, burns are unique injuries and present novel opportunities to study child and family adaptation. The relative uniqueness of burns is readily apparent when one considers that such injuries often: (1) share characteristics of acute disorders as well as those of chronic illness; (2) simultaneously affect several members of the same family; (3) result in losses not typically associated with other forms of injury (e.g., parents, siblings, home, possessions, pets); (4) result in characteristic forms of permanent disfigurement (i.e., burn scarring); (5) are related to premorbid parent/child psychopathology; (6) are associated with the emergence of negative psychosocial sequelae that are disproportionate to the extent of physical injury; (7) result in protracted periods of severe pain that is frequently recalcitrant to pharmacological management; and (8) present challenges that severely tax and frequently exceed the coping capabilities of children, families, and staff.

Many professionals are typically involved in the provision of services to pediatric burn victims and their families. Medical specialists include surgeons, intensivists, nurses, respiratory therapists, physical therapists, and nutritionists. Mental health professionals include psychologists, psychiatrists, and social workers. A variety of other individuals, including child life specialists and educators, are also likely to be involved in the care of these children. During inpatient treatment, mental health professionals are often consulted concerning emergent child and family problems (e.g., pain management, cooperation with staff, affective disturbance, abuse as potential etiology) (Hurt & Tarnowski, 1990). Mental health professionals are also likely to interact with these children and families on an outpatient basis where typical referral problems include posttraumatic stress symptomatology, depression, externalizing problems, body image disturbances, dysfunctional peer relations, academic decline, school refusal, career planning, sexuality issues, marital and family discord, and long-term follow-up. Many children treated for serious pediatric burn injuries will receive such treatment in the context of a regional burn treatment center. Staff at such centers tend to be highly specialized and most facilities are located in major metropolitan areas. However, because of the limited number of specialists (e.g., pediatric psychologists) available to consult with these children and their families, on many occasions, assessment and treatment will be conducted by individuals in the community who may not be well acquainted with the behavioral aspects of pediatric burns.

In summary, the goals of the book are to call attention to the psychosocial plight of pediatric burn victims and their families, provide a reference for professionals involved in the day-to-day care and consultation with this population, and acquaint the nonspecialist with some of the central issues involved in community aftercare and follow-up.

The present chapter presents a historical overview of burn treatment, provides a general epidemiological perspective on pediatric burn injuries, outlines the difficulties and challenges experienced by burned children and their families, and concludes with an orientation to the organization of the book and chapter contents.

NATURE AND SCOPE OF THE PROBLEM

Overview of Burn Injuries

Burn injuries are categorized as thermal, radiation, chemical, or electrical and are typically described in percent of total body surface area (TBSA) affected and burn type (degree). Percent TBSA is calculated using standard charts displaying dorsal and ventral views of the body divided into discrete areas of known percent body surface area (Lund & Browder, 1944).

Heat intensity and duration of skin contact determine the extent and depth of skin damage. Damage restricted to the epidermis is labeled a first-degree burn. The epidermis consists of multiple layers of epidermal cells. Injuries to the dermis are called second-degree or partial-thickness burns. The dermis or corium is composed of a vascular plexus containing arterioles, venules, and capillaries. Epidermal appendages (sweat glands, sebaceous glands, and hair follicles) are found in the dermis, as are nerve endings and connecting tissue. Under this structural base is found the fatty tissue of the subcutaneous fascia, muscle, and bone. Full-thickness (third-degree) burns are extensive injuries involving multiple skin layers, possible damage of subcutaneous tissue and peripheral nerve fibers.

In general, burns are classified as minor, moderate, or severe according to American Burn Association (ABA) criteria (American Burn Association, 1984). Moderate and severe burns require intensive treatment at a specialized burn facility or hospital with staff trained and experienced in the management of burn injuries (Dyer & Roberts, 1990).

Major burns are partial-thickness burns involving (1) more than 25% TBSA for adults and 20% for children, (2) full-thickness burns of 10% TBSA or greater, (3) the majority of deep partial-thickness or full-thickness burns involving the hands, face, eyes, ears, feet, or perineum, (4) burns complicated by smoke inhalation, (5) the majority of electrical and chemical burns and those complicated by fractures or other major trauma, and (6) poor-risk patients (those at extremes of age range or with existing disease). Moderate uncomplicated burns are partial-thickness burns that involve 15–25% TBSA for adults and 10–20% for children, with less than 10% full-thickness burns and those not involving the conditions described above for severe injuries. Minor burns are partial-thickness less than 15% TBSA for adults and 10% for children with less than 2% of full-thickness injuries.

Early Treatments

Historically, burn victims have been subjected to a variety of treatments. Detailed discussion of the history of burns is found in Artz (1970), Artz, Moncrief, and Pruitt (1979), and Constable (1983). Early treatments by the Egyptians consisted of coating injuries with combinations of resins, fats, honey, and myrrh. During the 6th century, Chinese treatments used tinctures and tea extracts. Early Greek remedies included the use of vinegar solutions. Seventh century treatments continued to involve topical applications including those derived from brine, animal gallbladder, and dung (Constable, 1983). Around the 9th century, cold water was applied as an analgesic. This was later (1600s) followed by attempts to apply heat (e.g., hot iron) as a means to "extract" the burn and associated pain. The use of oils and similar agents with occlusive dressings followed during the 16th and 17th centuries. During the 1800s, the need for conservation of patient strength and the importance of adequate nutrition were widely recognized. Mineral baths were a common form of treatment.

A major development occurred in the early 1900s when the importance of fluid volume changes was recognized. This prompted the development of fluid resuscitation formulas, common use of topical antiseptics, and experimentation with skin grafts. Although skin grafting was used in ancient times (Hindus), widespread application of this procedure did not occur until the 20th century. The invention and subsequent refinements of the dermatome greatly enhanced the clinical viability of modern-day grafting procedures. Dyer and Roberts (1990) noted that medical and technological advances in the areas of fluid resuscitation, improved antibodies, advanced monitoring, nutritional support, surgical interventions, and understanding of human immune function led to the current focus on the treatment of the "whole patient." Increased attention to patient psychosocial needs also became a critical component of this integrated approach to patient care.

Current Treatments

The medical treatment of the burn patient consists of three overlapping phases: emergency period, acute phase, rehabilitation phase (Miller,

Elliott, Funk, & Pruitt, 1988; Wernick, 1983). The central components involved in these three treatment phases are outlined below. The discussion is based on a review by Dyer and Roberts (1990). A detailed presentation of the medical and surgical management of pediatric burns is presented in Chapter 2.

The initial at-the-scene emergency treatment involves removing the source of heat from the injured person. First aid procedures are implemented to ensure a clear airway and evaluate breathing, bleeding, and shock status. Many burns involve significant smoke inhalation. The presence of singed facial hair, coughing, hoarseness, darkened oral or nasal mucous membranes, carbonaceous or bloody sputum, and burns to the face, neck, or lips suggest likely inhalation injuries. Cardiopulmonary resuscitation (CPR) may be required. A high liter flow of oxygen is administered as soon as feasible. On arrival to the emergency room, a brief account of the injury is obtained and the primary goal is to evaluate and stabilize respiration. In cases of suspected smoke inhalation, blood gases as well as routine blood work and urinalysis are conducted. Bronchoscopy may be required to assess inflammation and irritation and assess for the presence of carbonaceous materials. In cases of serious inhalation injury, placement of an endotracheal tube will be required. Injured extremities may require splinting and the patient is regularly repositioned. A tetanus toxoid injection is routinely administered. The patient's level of consciousness needs to be monitored carefully. Dyer and Roberts (1990) note that even burn patients with major injuries are typically alert and oriented and that any deterioration of sensorium needs to be treated seriously.

Burns cause diffusion of the intravascular fluid into the extravascular fluid. This process results in electrolyte imbalance and decreased blood volume (Demling, 1987). A variety of fluid resuscitation formulas are available (e.g., Parkland, modified Brooke formulas) that correct homeostatic imbalances. A central line is typically used for fluid infusion and a Foley catheter inserted into the bladder permits evaluation of output. As capillary functioning increases (within 2 days), a "fluid shift" occurs that is accompanied by marked diuresis. The fluid shift is associated with increased cardiac output and complications may arise from pulmonary edema or congestive heart failure (Rubin, Mani, & Hiebert, 1986). Monitoring is an integral component of care and involves the frequent measurement of vital signs, cardiac functions, temperature, and intravenous (IV) fluid titration. Gastrointestinal (GI) complications are often encountered as the decreased blood volume shunts fluid away from the GI tract. GI functions decrease markedly or cease entirely and abdominal distention results. Patients who are unconscious or with more than 20% TBSA may require insertion of a nasogastric tube and low suction to decrease distention, empty stomach contents, and reduce the probability of aspiration. GI hemorrhaging (Curling's ulcer) may also occur secondary to burn stress and can pose a serious hazard to survival. Within a few days, bowel sounds return and nutrition supplements are often administered as burns induce a hypermetabolic state.

Once the patient is stabilized, intensive effort is devoted to the care of the burn wound itself. The acute phase of treatment is typically the most painful as the patient is subjected to a variety of aversive procedures (e.g., IV placements, dressing changes, wound cleansing, grafting). A critical concern during this period is that of serious infection. Bacterial invasion occurs at an accelerated pace in children (O'Neil, 1979). Within 2 days, an untreated burn wound contains gram-positive organisms. Gram-negative bacteria are present by the fifth day. Burn sepsis is a major threat to patient survival and is defined as a surface bacteria count greater than 10^5 organisms per gram of tissue. Clinical indications include altered mental status, hypo- or hyperthermia, GI disturbances, deterioration of grafted burn sites, and conversion of partial-thickness to full-thickness injuries. Treatment requires aggressive parenteral administration of antibiotics, autografting (transplanting healthy skin from undamaged areas to the site of burn injury), and intensive nutritional support. If such treatments are unsuccessful, sepsis is typically fatal.

Eschar (burned tissue) must be removed surgically as it combines with edema to produce circulatory compromise. Circumferential burns (those that affect an entire limb) involving hands, arms, fingers, neck, trunk, and feet frequently require escharotomy. Regular debridement procedures that involve the removal of necrotic (devitalized) tissue are instituted. Patients are placed in a hydrotherapy tub that contains a solution of hypoclorite. Minor debridement is conducted at admission and care is taken to maintain the integrity of all intact blisters as they serve a protective function for underlying tissue. To prevent wound infection, topical antimicrobial agents must be applied. This process of daily vigorous debridement and application of topical dressings is typically the most painful procedure that patients must endure. The recurrence of such procedures daily for extended periods often contributes to serious patient management problems.

Partial-thickness wounds heal in a period ranging from 2 to 4 weeks and full-thickness injuries in a period of 3 to 5 weeks. Physiological dressings may be used during this period. These dressings consist of transplanted skin from cadavers (heterografts), animals (zenografts), or artificial preparations (Shuck, 1979). Such dressings serve as a barrier to reduce heat and fluid loss. However, these dressings are temporary and will be biologically rejected. Severe burns will require autograft procedures. Autografting is often conducted in phases because of differential rates of wound healing and inadequate donor materials. Pressure dressings and garments are worn to maintain the integrity of autografted sites.

During the rehabilitation phase, physical therapy, nutritional, medical, surgical, and specific self-care procedures (e.g., wearing pressure garments, movement exercises) and interventions continue. Repeated hospitalizations may be required for additional reconstructive surgeries.

Epidemiological Considerations

In the United States, approximately two million individuals sustain burn injuries each year (American Burn Association, 1984; Silverstein & Lack, 1987). It has been estimated that 70,000 of these injuries require hospitalization (American Burn Association, 1984; Frank, Berry, Wachtel, & Johnson, 1987) and approximately one-half of these victims are children and adolescents. Thirty-eight percent of burn patients who require hospitalization are under 15 years of age (Barrow & Herndon, 1990). Annual estimates of pediatric burn hospitalization range from 24,000 to 40,000 patients (Luther & Price, 1981; McLoughlin & McGuire, 1990).

The overall fatality rate for burns is 3.9 per 100,000 (National Safety Council, 1979). Of these deaths, approximately 1400 are children. Children younger than 15 account for two-thirds of all burn fatalities with males outnumbering females by more than 2:1 (U.S. Fire Administration, 1978). Fire and burn injuries are the third leading cause of death for all children and adolescents (to age 19 years) and second to motor vehicle accidents for children ages 1 to 4 (Guyer & Gallagher, 1985). House fires account for the greatest share (84%) of pediatric burn mortality. However, most deaths are attributable to smoke inhalation as opposed to direct burn insult.

Recent advances in the medical and surgical care of burns have resulted in increased survival for pediatric and adult burn victims (Curreri, Luterman, Braun, & Shires, 1980; Demling, 1985; Feller, Tholen, & Cornell, 1980; Jay, Bartlett, Danet, & Allyn, 1977). Children now routinely survive massive burns (e.g., greater than 80% TBSA). Data indicate that in 1968, patients with more than 35% TBSA had a 50% survival rate. Currently, the survival rate for patients with more than 70% TBSA is 50% (Burn Injury Reporting System, 1986). Concomitant with the growth in medical and surgical knowledge in this area has been a dramatic increase in the number of specialized burn care facilities. Currently, there are approximately 1800 total beds available in the burn units of 146 U.S. hospitals.

Burns account for more hospitalization days than any other form of injury (Warden, Kravitz, & Schnebly, 1981). From an epidemiological "cost" perspective, McLoughlin and McGuire (1990) estimated that in 1985 alone, pediatric burn mortality and morbidity resulted in the loss of more than 101,000 life years with a societal cost in excess of $3.5 billion. These authors estimate that more than 75% of childhood fire/burn deaths could be readily prevented through the use of residential sprinklers, smoke detectors, fire-safe cigarettes, and child-resistant lighters.

Children under 5 account for more than 50% of all pediatric burns. In approximately 80% of cases, children are injured as a result of their own behavior (Carvajal, 1990). In general, the manner in which children sustain burn injuries varies as a function of their developmental level (McLoughlin & Crawford, 1985). For example, infants often incur scald burns during bathing and from liquid spills. Scalds account for 75–80% of injuries to infants (El-Muhtaseb, Qaryoute, & Ragheb, 1984; Libber & Stayton, 1984). Ninety-five percent of burn injuries during the first 2 years of life occur indoors. With the increased mobility of toddlers, they are at heightened risk for burns from accidental liquid and food spills and hot tap water scalds. Preschool and school-aged children are often injured while playing with matches, lighters, and cooking devices (stoves and microwaves). Breslin (1975) noted that flame burns account for 20% of pediatric hospitalizations but 80% of the mortality. Scalds were found to account for about 50% of the cases and 20% of the deaths. With increasing age, the proportion of indoor to outdoor injuries shifts such that during adolescence 60% occur outdoors and only 20% are related to scalds (Green, 1984). Older children continue to be injured with matches and lighters but often expand their range of experimentation to include flammables, such as gasoline or high-voltage electrical apparatuses (McLoughlin, Joseph, & Crawford, 1976). Some evidence suggests that the gender discrepancy (approximately 2:1 male to female) increases disproportionately as a function of age such that older children may present with a ratio that approximates 4:1 (Clark & Lerner, 1978). These findings on gender differences are consistent with those for a variety of childhood injuries (Rosen & Peterson, 1990).

Other means of injury include firework injuries (McCauley *et al.*, 1991), and burns from household devices such as hair dryers (Prescott, 1990) and microwaves (Hibbard & Blevins, 1988). Although difficult to estimate, burns from child abuse account for approximately 4–25% of all pediatric burn unit admissions (Deitch & Staats, 1982; Stone, Rinaldo, Humphrey, & Brown, 1970).

Psychological Considerations

We have seen that pediatric burns are relatively common and invariably painful injuries that involve protracted and intensive medical and surgical management. It is apparent that burn injuries present numerous medical challenges to pediatric patients, their families, and the staff responsible for their care. It is also the case that the psychological challenges posed by burn injuries often serve to severely tax and overwhelm the coping resources of children and their families.

There is consensus that psychological variables are of central importance to the discussion of pediatric burn injuries. However, the breadth of potential areas of psychological interface may not be fully appreciated. It is one of the primary purposes of this volume to discuss a subset of these areas in detail. To acquaint readers with the range of these issues and present a context for the information presented in the chapters that follow, a brief overview of the psychological considerations involved in consultation, rehabilitation, and prevention is provided below. This overview is temporally organized and presents possible points of psychological interface from the time of injury to extended aftercare with consideration of preventive strategies.

Burn Injury Occurrence

In many instances, behavioral factors are directly or indirectly responsible for the occurrence of the burn injury. It was previously noted that many burns, particularly in younger children, are related to child abuse. The majority of these injuries are immersion burns which are often sustained as caretakers attempt to "quiet" or "punish" infants and toddlers (Caniano, Beaver, & Boles, 1986; Purdue, Hunt, & Prescott, 1988). However, contact burns (e.g., cigarettes, hot spoon, light bulb, hot coals) also are observed routinely (Showers & Garrison, 1988).

Child neglect is often found to be a central factor in a subset of cases. The topography of "neglect" can vary widely (e.g., lapse in parental supervision, failure to make incendiary devices inaccessible to children). Neglect is often invoked as an explanation under conditions where an adult evidences compromised caretaker judgment by permitting a child to be unsupervised with access to a source(s) of potential injury (e.g., cigarette lighter, fireplace, flammables, hot liquids). Unfortunately, an entry of "parental neglect" in the medical chart does little to further one's understanding of the actual environmental variables, setting events, and psychological processes that mediate such occurrences. For example, many children are injured during a momentary lapse in caretaker attention. However, on closer inspection, it may become apparent that specific child developmental variables (e.g., curiosity) often combine with caretaker underestimation of child developmental competencies (e.g., motor skills) to interact with environmental variables (e.g., availability of potentially dangerous items), setting factors (e.g., variables associated with economically disadvantaged living conditions), and psychological states (e.g., negative affect) which erode caretaker coping resources and contribute to the probability of accidental injury. Although the contributing factors and processes may vary, we often invoke simple descriptive labels (i.e., neglect) that offer little insight and are often simply incorrect. As one might expect, the identification and labeling of "neglect" is a subjective process and there very well may be a bias to label injuries that occur under similar circumstances as "neglect" in one case and "accidental" in another. This differential labeling may occur as a function of case differences in demographic variables (e.g., socioeconomic status) or other factors (e.g., case presentation by parents). The topic of child abuse and neglect is beyond the scope of the present volume and is not considered here in detail except to note its importance as a source of child burn injury and as part of the discussion on preventive strategies (Chapter 10).

In assessing the circumstances under which children are injured, the interplay between specific environmental factors and family variables becomes important (Tarnowski & Brown, in press). For example, we know that the probability of sustaining a serious burn injury increases as one descends in socioeconomic status (SES) (Center for Disease Control Division of Injury Epidemiology and Control, 1987). Several factors may be operative here. For example, economically disadvantaged families may not be able to afford quality housing. Substandard housing may pose specific risks of injury (e.g., crowding, faulty electrical systems). Lack of adequate basic resources also may lead parents to choose unsafe methods to meet daily living needs (e.g., heating homes with makeshift portable stoves) (Remensnyder & Gryska, 1981). Another factor to consider is that rates of certain psychological disorders are highest in lower SES populations (Belle, 1990; Neugebauer, Dohrenwend, & Dohrenwend, 1980) and that the symptoms of such disorders may contribute to increased risk of childhood burn injury. For example, parental depression or other disruptive symptomatology may result in a decreased ability to maintain the vigilance required to prevent child injuries (Davidson, Hughes, & O'Connor, 1988). Other setting events have been associated with increased probability of injury. For example, children with acute illnesses appear to be at particular risk (Wilson, Buckland, & Sully, 1988). There is also evidence that families of pediatric burn victims experience more geographic moves (Knudson-Cooper & Leuchtag, 1982). A subset of these families may be entirely unstable. Alternatively, the attendant stressors of moving coupled with the natural proclivity of young children to explore their new environments may combine to potentiate risk.

Behavioral factors contribute to injury occurrence in a variety of other ways. One area of interest concerns child characteristics (Davidson, Taylor,

Sandberg, & Thorley, 1992; Manheimer & Mellinger, 1967). Specifically, it is well known that a significant subset of children who sustain severe burn injury present with various forms of marked premorbid psychopathology (Tarnowski, Rasnake, Gavaghan-Jones, & Smith, 1991). It has been suggested that children with specific symptomatology (e.g., attention deficit–hyperactivity disorder, conduct disorder) present supervision and monitoring challenges and may be more inclined to engage in impulsive risk-taking behaviors (e.g., experimenting with gasoline and other flammables, climbing electrical tension wire towers) that lead to burn injury (Cole, Herndon, Desai, & Abston, 1986; McLoughlin *et al.*, 1976). Rarely, children and adolescents are also injured or killed via self-immolation (Hammond, Ward, & Pereira, 1988).

Parental nonadherence to specific preventive health care advice is responsible for a subset of burns, for example, those related to accidental immersion burns. Parents are routinely advised to reduce and monitor hot water tank temperatures but often fail to do so (MacKay & Rothman 1982). Other examples of nonadherence involve those related to safeguarding electric outlets, gasoline, and providing fire-retardant sleepwear (Baker & Chiaviello, 1989; Cole *et al.*, 1986; McLoughlin, Clarke, Stahly, & Crawford, 1977). Of course, judgment errors also account for a subset of injuries (e.g., use of hair dryers to dry infants, dishwasher effluent burns) and contribute to morbidity if caretakers are ill-educated about first aid treatment.

Acute Phase Considerations

From a psychological perspective, children hospitalized for burn injuries face multiple challenges including separation from family, restricted visitation, immobility, isolation procedures, extended hospitalization, repeated exposure to painful procedures, observation of other seriously ill patients, reduced sensory stimulation, disfigurement, disrupted physiological functioning, surgical interventions, treatment side-effects, and other potential losses (e.g., death of family members, destruction of home, possessions) (Tarnowski *et al.*, 1987; Tarnowski, Rasnake, Linscheid, & Mulick, 1989a; Thompson & Vernon, 1993).

Early postburn responses may include disorientation, confusion, labile affect, clouded sensorium, agitation, delusions, and hallucinations. Delirium and transient psychosis (burn psychosis) may represent functional conditions related to sensory overload, sensory deprivation, sleep deprivation, or shock reactions (Patterson, 1987). Pathophysiological and metabolic compromise underlie much of this type of symptomatology. Less serious mental status changes occur in about one-third of all burn patients (Klein & Charlton, 1980). Another serious concern are reports of patient loss of the will to live (Tempereau, Grossman, & Brones, 1989). Loss of volition may be evidenced as apathy with refusal to cooperate with required care, devaluation, and extended social isolation. Little is known of the phenomenon in the pediatric population.

More common pediatric acute behavioral reactions include anxiety and depression. Prolonged crying, clingingness, verbal and physical aggression toward staff, sleep disturbances including nightmares and disrupted sleep–wake cycle, injury/survivor guilt, mourning, regressive behavior, disrupted play, and denial of the physical consequences of the burn are commonly evidenced during the initial stages of acute rehabilitation (Goodstein, 1985; Mahaney, 1990; Roberts & Gordon, 1979; Tarnowski *et al.*, 1987; Tarnowski, Rasnake, Gavaghan-Jones, & Smith, 1991).

Common issues for which consultation may be sought often involve pain assessment and management including methods to enhance the predictability of and control over the treatment environment, monitoring drug effects, compliance with medical and physical therapy procedures, self-excoriation, emergence of posttraumatic stress disorder (PTSD) symptomatology, management of negative parent and sibling responses (e.g., depression, guilt, anger), body image disturbance, sexuality issues, and assessment of contribution of premorbid psychopathology to current functioning and adjustment (Beard, Herndon, & Desai, 1989; Cella, Perry, Poag, Amand, & Goodwin, 1988; Cromer & Tarnowski, 1989; Kavanaugh, 1983; St. Lawrence & Drabman, 1983; Stoddard, Norman, & Murphy, 1989; Tarnowski *et al.*, 1989a).

Psychological input to interdisciplinary staffings is critical and widely sought after (Goodstein, 1985; Hurt & Tarnowski, 1990). Issues frequently involve treatment planning and coordination (Sampson, 1990) including those related to psychoeducational and neuropsychological assessments, discharge planning, transitioning patient to the home environment, school reentry, educational and occupational consultation, and aftercare follow-up. Requests to assist with staff stress are also common (Powers, Maher, Helm, Cruise, & Luria, 1986).

Throughout the acute and long-term rehabilitation process, positive coping and adjustment and the design of treatments to facilitate such outcomes, will vary widely as a function of children's developmental status (Tarnowski *et al.*, 1989a; Tarnowski, Rasnake, Gavaghan-Jones, & Smith, 1991). Knowledge of the developmental underpinnings of children's understanding and conceptualization of injury and its treatment will be of central importance in addressing the constellation of symptoms exhibited by children and their families in response to the challenge of severe burn injury (Maddux, Roberts, Sledden, & Wright, 1986).

Concerning aftercare and extended follow-up, it has been noted that many burn survivors will be rehospitalized for additional surgeries and follow-up medical treatments. In addition, deleterious long-term psychosocial sequelae have been reported for pediatric burn victims (Stoddard, Norman, & Murphy, 1989; Tarnowski, Rasnake, Linscheid, & Mulick, 1989b). It is quite understandable that many would project poor adjustment for pediatric burn patients given the devastating physical and psychological trauma imposed by such injuries. However, there is little support for the contention that the *majority* of burn victims evidence poor postburn adjustment (Patterson *et al.*, 1993; Tarnowski, Rasnake, Gavaghan-Jones, & Smith, 1991). In general, it appears that adjustment outcome is a complex function of several variables including patient injury parameters, hospitalization course, premorbid adjustment, developmental status, family variables, and personal and social demographics. Such risk and resource variables may combine in novel ways to produce different outcomes. Long-term adjustment concerns frequently involve issues related to affect disorders, disrupted social functioning, family discord, disfigurement, and educational/occupational adjustment. The effects of burns on existing premorbid psychopathology in child, parent, and family deserve particularly close scrutiny (Cella *et al.*, 1988; Stoddard, Norman, Murphy, & Beardslee, 1989; Tarnowski, Rasnake, Gavaghan-Jones, & Smith, 1991). Unfortunately, data indicate that 25% of North American pediatric burn units fail to include emotional aspects of patient care in their discharge planning efforts (Jenkins & Stanwick, 1991).

In summary, even a cursory examination of the issues involved in the prevention and acute and long-term follow-up of the pediatric burn victim clearly reveals the central importance of psychological factors to this population. This overview highlighted the many common points of psychological interface involved in the care of these children. Clinicians and consultants working with this population will be well-served by a solid grounding in developmental theory, developmental psychopathology, behavioral medicine, consultation, and traditional child, adult, and family assessment and treatment skills.

With this overview as a background, we now move to discuss the organization and contents of the subsequent chapters that consider these issues in detail.

BOOK ORGANIZATION AND CONTENTS

The book comprises 11 chapters divided into four sections. As a whole, they provide a detailed review of the medical management, and behavioral functioning and care of victims and their families. The first section consists of the present introductory overview and Chapter 2 authored by Fratianne and Brandt. The latter chapter provides the non-specialist with an overview of the medical treatment of the burned patient from arrival in the emergency room to discharge and extended outpatient follow-up care. The chapter provides details on the classification of burns, standard medical and surgical interventions, and emergent treatment technologies.

The second section concentrates on what is known about the acute and long-term psychosocial sequelae of serious pediatric burn injuries. In Chapter 3, Armstrong, Gay, and Levy describe the common acute psychological reactions of children to burns. An emphasis is placed on distinguishing pathological from nonpathological reactions. Specifically addressed are PTSD and related symptomatology. A developmental framework is elaborated within which adaptive and dysfunctional coping are considered. Chapter 4 extends this discussion with consideration of the long-term psychosocial functioning of pediatric burn victims. Tarnowski and Rasnake present a detailed substantive and methodological overview of the child and adolescent follow-up literature.

The third section focuses on selected topics in the pediatric burn literature. In essence, these are major issues that must be considered by all mental health professionals who provide services to burned children and their families. Chapters are arranged along a logical time sequence that follows the patient from acute inpatient hospitalization to discharge and return to family, school, and community.

In the initial chapter (5) in this section, Brown, Dingle, and Koon-Scott consider consultation and liaison models that have or might be effectively used by pediatric mental health professionals confronted with the challenge of pediatric burn consults. The chapter reviews the available empirical literature on pediatric inpatient consultation while considering the unique circumstances of the burn-injured child and his or her family. Bush and Maron extend this discussion in Chapter 6 with a detailed review of the assessment and treatment of pediatric burn-related pain. There is an emphasis on the management of pain in the context of highly aversive medical procedures that are unique to the burn-injured patient (e.g., debridement). Pharmacological approaches are discussed and the use of cognitive-behavioral interventions to promote coping is highlighted. In Chapter 7, Pruzinsky and Doctor provide readers with a review of the critical role of body image in children's development. The impact of disfigurement on adjustment is emphasized as are assessment and intervention methods that appear to hold promise for this population. In Chapter 8, Kaslow, Koon-Scott, and Dingle integrate some of the material presented in previous chapters by considering the role of family in pediatric illness. Contextual variables associated with child injury are noted.

The chapter draws broadly from the pediatric illness and injury literature and describes how family functioning is affected by burns, and outlines interventions that may be appropriate at different points in the recovery process. Blakeney then considers issues surrounding the transition of the pediatric patient from the hospital or home to the school setting. Chapter 9 reviews the relevant clinical issues and describes methods and programs that may facilitate this transition. The final chapter in the section focuses on the prevention of burn injuries. Indeed, the majority of childhood burns appear to be entirely avoidable. Several novel intervention methods have been developed to reduce the incidence of pediatric burns. Jones and Zaharopoulos review interventions that have been conducted on the individual, small group, and community level. The chapter also considers the emerging literature on individual and group skill-training methods to enhance children's fire safety and related emergency management skills.

In the concluding chapter, Tarnowski and Brown integrate the central issues presented in the previous chapters and place the problems and prospects of burn-injured children and their families in a broad perspective by drawing on the developmental, chronic illness, and rehabilitation literatures. The chapter provides a succinct description of what has been accomplished from a pediatric psychology perspective with these children, identifies salient gaps in the literature, and provides a prospectus for future clinical and research activities.

Overall, the volume emphasizes the unique mental health problems and needs of pediatric burn victims. Although we know a great deal about burns and their medical treatment, we know considerably less about the mental health aspects of children who sustain such injuries and how to best contribute to their recovery. Hopefully, this volume will call increased attention to the plight of these youngsters and their families and will serve as an impetus for further clinical innovation and research.

REFERENCES

American Burn Association. (1984). Guidelines for service standards and severity classifications in the treatment of burn injuries. *Bulletin of the American College of Surgeons, 69,* 24–28.

Artz, C. (1970). Historical aspects of burn management. *Surgical Clinics of North America, 50,* 1193–120.

Artz, C. P., Moncrief, J. A., & Pruitt, B. A. (Eds.). (1979). *Burns: A team approach*. Philadelphia: Saunders.

Baker, M. D., & Chiaviello, C. (1989). Household electrical injuries in children: Epidemiology and identification of avoidable hazards. *American Journal of Diseases of Children, 143,* 59–62.

Barrow, R. E., & Herndon, D. N. (1990). Incidence of mortality in boys and girls after severe thermal burns. *Surgery, Gynecology, and Obstetrics, 170,* 295–298.

Baum, A., Grunberg, N. E., & Singer, J. E. (1982). The use of psychological and neuroendocrinological measurements in the study of stress. *Health Psychology, 1,* 217–236.

Beard, S. A., Herndon, D. N., & Desai, M. (1989). Adaptation of self-image in burn disfigured children. *Journal of Burn Care and Rehabilitation, 10,* 550–554.

Belle, D. (1990). Poverty and women's mental health. *American Psychologist, 45,* 385–389.

Bibace, R., & Walsh, M. E. (1980). Development of children's concepts of illness. *Pediatrics, 66,* 912–917.

Breslau, N. (1985). Psychiatric disorder in children with physical disability. *Journal of the American Academy of Child Psychiatry, 24,* 87–94.

Breslin, P. W. (1975). The psychological reactions of children to burn traumata: A review. *Illinois Medical Journal, 148,* 514–519, 595–597, 602.

Brewster, A. B. (1982). Chronically ill hospitalized children's concepts of their illness. *Pediatrics, 69,* 355–362.

Burbach, D., & Peterson, L. (1986). Children's concepts of physical illness: A review and critique of the cognitive–developmental literature. *Health Psychology, 5,* 307–325.

Burn Injury Reporting System. (1986). *Report from the secretary of state*. Albany: New York State Department of State Office of Fire Prevention and Control.

Caniano, D. A., Beaver, B. L., & Boles, E. T. (1986). Child abuse: An update on surgical management of 256 cases. *Annals of Surgery, 203,* 219–224.

Carvajal, H. F. (1990). Burns in children and adolescents: Initial management as the first steps in successful rehabilitation. *Pediatrician, 17,* 237–243.

Cella, D. F., Perry, S. W., Poag, M. E., Amand, R., & Goodwin, C. (1988). Depression and stress responses in parents of burned children. *Journal of Pediatric Psychology, 13,* 87–99.

Center for Disease Control Division of Injury Epidemiology and Control. (1987). Regional distribution of deaths from residential fires—United States, 1978–1984. *Journal of American Medical Association, 258,* 2355–2356.

Clark, W. R., & Lerner, D. (1978). Regional burn survey: Two years of hospitalized burned patients in New York. *Journal of Trauma, 18,* 524–532.

Cole, M., Herndon, D. N., Desai, M. H., & Abston, S. (1986). Gasoline explosions, gasoline sniffing: An epidemic in young adolescents. *Journal of Burn Care and Rehabilitation, 7,* 532–534.

Constable, J. D. (1983). Some historical aspects of the treatment of burn injuries. In N. R. Bernstein & M. C. Robson (Eds.), *Comprehensive approach to the burned person* (pp. 22–47). New Hyde Park, NY: Medical Examination Publishing Company.

Cromer, B. A., & Tarnowski, K. J. (1989). Noncompliance in adolescents: A review. *Journal of Developmental and Behavioral Pediatrics, 10,* 207–215.

Curreri, P. W., Luterman, A., Braun, D. W., & Shires, G. T. (1980). Burn injury: An analysis of survival and hospitalization time for 937 patients. *Annals of Surgery, 192,* 472–480.

Daniels, D., Moos, R. H., Billings, A. G., & Miller, J. J. (1987). Psychosocial risk and resistance factors among children with chronic illness, healthy siblings, and healthy controls. *Journal of Abnormal Psychology, 15,* 295–308.

Davidson, L. L., Hughes, S. J., & O'Connor, P. A. (1988). Preschool behavior problems and subsequent risk of injury. *Pediatrics, 82,* 644–651.

Davidson, L. L., Taylor, E. A., Sandberg, S. T., & Thorley, G. (1992). Hyperactivity in school-age boys and subsequent risk of injury. *Pediatrics, 90,* 697–702.

Deitch, E. A., & Staats, M. (1982). Child abuse through burning. *Journal of Burn Care and Rehabilitation, 3,* 89–94.

Demling, R. H. (1985). Medical progress: Burns. *New England Journal of Medicine, 313,* 1389–1398.

Demling, R. H. (1987). Fluid replacement in burned patients. *Surgical Clinics of North America, 67,* 15–70.

Dyer, C., & Roberts, D. (1990). Thermal trauma. *Nursing Clinics of North America, 25*, 85–117.

El-Muhtaseb, H., Qaryoute, S., & Ragheb, S. A. (1984). Burn injuries in Jordan: A study of 338 cases. *Burns, 10*, 116–120.

Epstein, L. H. (1992). Role of behavior theory in behavioral medicine. *Journal of Consulting and Clinical Psychology, 60*, 493–498.

Feller, I., Tholen, D., & Cornell, R. G. (1980). Improvements in burn care: 1965–1979. *Journal of American Medical Association, 244*, 2047–2078.

Ferrari, M. (1990). Developmental issues in behavioral pediatrics. In A. M. Gross & R. S. Drabman (Eds.), *Handbook of clinical behavioral pediatrics* (pp. 29–47). New York: Plenum Press.

Frank, H. A., Berry, C., Wachtel, T. L., & Johnson, R. W. (1987). The impact of thermal injury. *Journal of Burn Care and Rehabilitation, 8*, 260–262.

Goodstein, R. K. (1985). Burns: An overview of clinical consequences affecting patient, staff, and family. *Comprehensive Psychiatry, 26*, 43–57.

Green, A. (1984). Epidemiology of burns in childhood. *Burns Including Thermal Injuries, 10*, 368–371.

Gross, A. M., & Drabman, R. S. (Eds.). (1990). *Handbook of clinical behavioral pediatrics*. New York: Plenum Press.

Guyer, B., & Gallagher, S. S. (1985). An approach to the epidemiology of childhood injuries. *Pediatric Clinics of North America, 32*, 5–15.

Hammond, J. S., Ward, C. G., & Pereira, E. (1988). Self-inflicted burns. *Journal of Burn Care and Rehabilitation, 9*, 178–179.

Herbert, T. B., & Cohen, S. (1993). Depression and immunity: A meta-analytic review. *Psychological Bulletin, 113*, 472–486.

Hibbard, R. A., & Blevins, R. (1988). Palatal burn due to bottle warming in a microwave oven. *Pediatrics, 82*, 382–383.

Hobbs, N., & Perrin, J. M. (Eds.). (1985). *Issues in the care of children with chronic illnesses*. San Francisco: Jossey–Bass.

Hurt, F. J., & Tarnowski, K. J. (1990). Behavioral consultation in the management of pediatric burns. *Medical Psychotherapy, 3*, 117–124.

Jay, K. M., Bartlett, R. H., Danet, R., & Allyn, P. A. (1977). Burn epidemiology: A basis for burn prevention. *Journal of Trauma, 17*, 943–947.

Jenkins, H. M. L., & Stanwick, R. S. (1991). A survey of pediatric discharge educational programs in the North American burn units. *Journal of Burn Care and Rehabilitation, 12*, 243–248.

Kaplan, R. M. (1990). Behavior as the central outcome in health care. *American Psychologist, 45*, 1211–1220.

Karoly, P. (Ed.). (1988). *Handbook of child health assessment*. New York: Wiley.

Kavanaugh, C. (1983). Psychological intervention with the severely burned child: Report of an experimental comparison of two approaches and their effects on psychological sequelae. *Journal of the American Academy of Child and Adolescent Psychiatry, 22*, 145–156.

Kazak, A. E. (1989). Families of chronically ill children: A systems and ecological model of adaptation and challenge. *Journal of Consulting and Clinical Psychology, 57*, 25–30.

Klein, R. M., & Charlton, J. E. (1980). Behavioral observation and analysis of pain behavior in critically burned patients. *Pain, 9*, 27–40.

Knudson-Cooper, M. S., & Leuchtag, A. K. (1982). The stress of a family move as a precipitating factor in children's burn accidents. *Journal of Human Stress, 8*, 32–38.

Krasnegor, N. A., Arasteh, J. D., & Cataldo, M. F. (Eds.). (1986). *Child health behavior: A behavioral pediatrics perspective*. New York: Wiley.

Levine, M. D., Carey, W. B., Crocker, A. C., & Gross, R. T. (Eds.). (1983). *Developmental–behavioral pediatrics*. Philadelphia: Saunders.

Libber, S. M., & Stayton, D. J. (1984). Childhood burns reconsidered: The child, the family and the burn injury. *Journal of Trauma, 24,* 245–252.
Linscheid, T. R., Rasnake, L. K., Tarnowski, K. J., & Mulick, J. A. (1989). Behavioral assessment. In J. K. Luiselli (Ed.), *Behavioral medicine and developmental disabilities* (pp. 21–44). Berlin: Springer-Verlag.
Long, R. T., & Cope, O. (1961). Emotional problems of burned children. *New England Journal of Medicine, 264,* 1121–1127.
Lund, C. C., & Browder, J. R. (1944). An estimation of areas of burns. *Surgery, Gynecology, and Obstetrics, 79,* 224–252.
Luther, S. L., & Price, J. H. (1981). Burns and their psychological effects on children. *Journal of School Health, 51,* 419–422.
McCauley, R. L., Stenberg, B. A., Rutan, R. L., Robson, M. C., Heggers, J. P., & Herndon, D. N. (1991). Class C firework injuries in a pediatric population. *Journal of Trauma, 31,* 389–391.
MacKay, A. M., & Rothman, K. J. (1982). The incidence and severity of burn injuries following Project Burn Prevention. *American Journal of Public Health, 72,* 248–252.
McLoughlin, E., Clarke, N., Stahly, K., & Crawford, J. D. (1977). One pediatric burn unit's experience with sleepwear-related injuries. *Pediatrics, 60,* 405–409.
McLoughlin, E., & Crawford, J. D. (1985). Types of burn injuries. *Pediatric Clinics of North America, 32,* 61–75.
McLoughlin, E., & McGuire, A. (1990). The causes, cost, and prevention of childhood burn injuries. *American Journal of Diseases of Children, 144,* 677–683.
McLoughlin, E., Joseph, M. P., & Crawford, J. D. (1976). Epidemiology of high tension injuries in children. *Journal of Pediatrics, 89,* 62–65.
Maddux, J. E., Roberts, M. C., Sledden, E. A., & Wright, L. (1986). Developmental issues in child health psychology. *American Psychologist, 41,* 25–34.
Mahaney, N. B. (1990). Restoration of play in a severely burned three-year-old child. *Journal of Burn Care and Rehabilitation, 11,* 57–63.
Manheimer, D. I., & Mellinger, G. D. (1967). Personality characteristics of the child accident repeater. *Child Development, 38,* 519–533.
Melamed, B. G., & Bush, J. P. (1985). Family factors in children with acute illness. In D. C. Turk & R. D. Kerns (Eds.), *Health, illness, and families: A life span perspective* (pp. 183–219). New York: Wiley.
Miller, M. D., Elliott, C. H., Funk, M., & Pruitt, S. D. (1988). Implications of children's burn injuries. In D. K. Routh (Ed.), *Handbook of pediatric psychology* (pp. 426–447). New York: Guilford Press.
National Safety Council. (1979). *Accident safety facts.* Chicago: Author.
Neugebauer, D. D., Dohrenwend, B. P., & Dohrenwend, B. S. (1980). The formulation of hypotheses about the true prevalence of functional psychiatric disorders among adults in the United States. In B. P. Dohrenwend, B. S. Dohrenwend, S. Gould, B. Link, R. Neugebauer, & R. Wunsch-Hitzig (Eds.), *Mental illness in the United States* (pp. 45–94). New York: Praeger.
Newachek, P. W., & Taylor, W. R. (1992). Childhood chronic illness: Prevalence, severity, and impact. *American Journal of Public Health, 82,* 364–371.
Newachek, P. W., Stoddard, J. J., & McManus, M. (1993). Ethnocultural variations in the prevalence and impact of childhood chronic conditions. *Pediatrics, 91,* 1031–1039.
O'Neil, J. A. (1979). Burns in children. In C. P. Artz, J. A. Moncrief, & B. A. Pruitt (Eds.), *Burns: A team approach* (pp. 138–167). Philadelphia: Saunders.
Patterson, D. R. (1987). Psychological management of the burn patient. *Topics in Acute Care and Trauma Rehabilitation, 1,* 25–39.
Patterson, D. R., Everett, J. J., Bombardier, C. H., Questad, K. A., Lee, V. K., & Marvin, J. A. (1993). Psychological effects of severe burn injuries. *Psychological Bulletin, 113,* 362–378.

Peterson, L., & Mori, L. (1985). Prevention of child injury: An overview of targets, methods, and tactics for psychologists. *Journal of Consulting and Clinical Psychology, 53,* 586–595.

Piaget, J., & Inhelder, B. (1969). *The psychology of the child.* New York: Basic Books.

Pless, I. B., & Douglas, I. W. B. (1972). Chronic illness in childhood. I. Epidemiological and clinical characteristics. *Pediatrics, 47* 405–414.

Powers, P. S., Maher, M., Helm, M. D., Cruise, M., & Luria, W. (1986). Impact of a disaster on a burn unit. *Psychosomatics, 27,* 553–561.

Prescott, P. R. (1990). Hair dryer burns in children. *Pediatrics, 86,* 692–697.

Purdue, G. F., Hunt, J. L., & Prescott, P. R. (1988). Child burning by abuse—An index of suspicion. *Journal of Trauma, 28,* 221–224.

Rape, R. N., Bush, J. P., & Slavin, L. A. (1992). Toward a conceptualization of the family's adaptation to a member's head injury: A critique of developmental stage models. *Rehabilitation Psychology, 37,* 3–21.

Remensnyder, J. P., & Gryska, P. V. R. (1981). Hazards of wood-burning stoves to children. *New England Journal of Medicine, 304,* 915–916.

Roberts, M. C., & Wright, L. (1982). The role of the pediatric psychologist as consultant to pediatricians. In J. Tuma (Ed.), *Handbook for the practice of pediatric psychology* (pp. 251–289). New York: Wiley.

Roberts, R. N., & Gordon, S. B. (1979). Reducing childhood nightmares subsequent to a burn trauma. *Child Behavior Therapy, 1,* 373–381.

Rosen, B. N., & Peterson, L. (1990). Gender differences in children's outdoor play injuries: A review and integration. *Clinical Psychology Review, 10,* 187–205.

Routh, D. K. (Ed.). (1988). *Handbook of pediatric psychology.* New York: Guilford Press.

Rubin, W. D., Mani, M. M., & Hiebert, J. M. (1986). Fluid resuscitation of the thermally injured patient. *Clinics in Plastic Surgery, 13,* 9–20.

Russo, D. C., & Tarbell, S. E. (1984). Child health psychology: Emerging responsibilities of the pediatric health psychologist. *Clinical Psychology Review, 4,* 495–502.

Russo, D. C., & Varni, J. W. (Eds.). (1982). *Behavioral pediatrics: Research and practice.* New York: Plenum Press.

Russo, D. C., Bird, B. L., & Masek, B. J. (1980). Assessment issues in behavioral medicine. *Behavioral Assessment, 2,* 1–10.

Sampson, L. J. (1990). The development of a discharge planning index for use in a pediatric burn unit. *Journal of Burn Care and Rehabilitation, 11,* 365–371.

Showers, J., & Garrison, K. M. (1988). Burn abuse: A four-year study. *Journal of Trauma, 28,* 1581–1583.

Shuck, J. M. (1979). Biologic dressings. In C. P. Artz, J. A. Moncrief, & B. A. Pruitt (Eds.), *Burns: A team approach* (pp. 129–185). Philadelphia: Saunders.

Silverstein P., & Lack, B. O. (1987). Epidemiology and prevention. In J. A. Boswick (Ed.), *The art and science of burn care* (pp. 11–17). Rockville: MD.

Spirito, A., DeLawyer, D. D., & Stark, L. J. (1991). Peer relations and social adjustment of chronically ill children and adolescents. *Clinical Psychology Review, 11,* 539–564.

St. Lawrence, J. S., & Drabman, R. S. (1983). Interruption of self-excoriation in a pediatric burn victim. *Journal of Pediatric Psychology, 8,* 155–159.

Stoddard, F. J., Norman, D. K., & Murphy, M. (1989). A diagnostic outcome study of children and adolescents with severe burns. *Journal of Trauma, 29,* 471–477.

Stoddard, F. J., Norman, D. K., Murphy, M., & Beardslee, W. R. (1989). Psychiatric outcome of burned children and adolescents. *Journal of the American Academy of Child and Adolescent Psychiatry, 28,* 589–595.

Stone, N. H., Rinaldo, L., Humphrey, C. R., & Brown, R. H. (970). Child abuse by burning. *Surgical Clinics of North America, 50,* 1419–1424.

Tarnowski, K. J. (1991). Disadvantaged children and families in pediatric primary care settings. I. Broadening the scope of integrated mental health services. *Journal of Clinical Child Psychology, 20,* 351–359.

Tarnowski, K. J., & Brown, R. T. (in press). Psychological aspects of pediatric disorders. In M. Hersen & R. T. Ammerman (Eds.), *Advanced abnormal child psychology*. Hillsdale, NJ: Lawrence Erlbaum, Inc.

Tarnowski, K. J., & Kaufman, K. L. (1988). Behavioral assessment of pediatric pain. In R. J. Prinz (Ed.), *Advances in behavior assessment of children and families* (Vol. 4, pp. 119–158). Greenwich, CN: JAI Press.

Tarnowski, K. J., Rasnake, L.K., & Drabman, R. S. (1987). Behavioral assessment and treatment of pediatric burns: A review. *Behavior Therapy, 18,* 417–441.

Tarnowski, K. J., Rasnake, L. K., Linscheid, T. R., & Mulick, J. A. (1989a). Ecobehavioral characteristics of a pediatric burn injury unit. *Journal of Applied Behavior Analysis, 22,* 101–109.

Tarnowski, K. J., Rasnake, L. K., Linscheid, T. R., & Mulick, J. A. (1989b). Behavioral adjustment of pediatric burn victims. *Journal of Pediatric Psychology, 14,* 607–615.

Tarnowski, K. J., King, D. R., Green, L., & Pease, M. G. (1991). Congenital gastrointestinal anomalies: Psychosocial functioning of children with imperforate anus, gastroschisis, and omphalocele. *Journal of Consulting and Clinical Psychology, 59,* 587–590.

Tarnowski, K. J., Rasnake, L. K., Gavaghan-Jones, M. P., & Smith, L. (1991). Psychosocial sequelae of pediatric burn injuries: A review. *Clinical Psychology Review, 11,* 371–398.

Tempereau, C. E., Grossman, A. R., & Brones, M. F. (1989). Loss of will to live in patients with burns. *Journal of Burn Care and Rehabilitation, 10,* 464–468.

Thompson, R. H., & Vernon, D. T. A. (1993). Research on children's behavior after hospitalization: A review and synthesis. *Journal of Developmental and Behavioral Pediatrics, 14,* 28–35.

U.S. Fire Administration. (1978). *First in the United States*. Washington, DC: U.S. Department of Commerce, National Fire Data Center.

Varni, J. W. (1983). *Clinical behavioral pediatrics: An interdisciplinary biobehavioral approach*. New York: Pergamon Press.

Varni, J. W., & Dietrich, S. L. (1981). Behavioral pediatrics: Towards a reconceptualization. *Behavioral Medicine Update, 3,* 5–7

Wallander, J. L., Varni, J. W., Babani, L., Banis, H. T., & Wilcox, K. T. (1989). Family resources as resistance factors for psychological maladjustment in chronically ill and handicapped children. *Journal of Pediatric Psychology, 14,* 157–173.

Warden, G. D., Kravitz, M., & Schnebly, A. (1981). The outpatient management of moderate and major thermal injuries. *Journal of Burn Care, 2,* 159–167.

Watson, E. J., & Johnson, A. M. (1958). The emotional significance of acquired physical disfigurement in children. *American Journal of Orthopsychiatry, 28,* 85–97.

Wernick, R. L. (1983). Stress inoculation in the management of clinical pain: Application to burn pain. In D. Meichenbaum & M. E. Jaremko (Eds.), *Stress reduction and prevention* (pp. 191–217). New York: Plenum Press.

Wilson, G. R., Buckland, R., & Sully, L. (1988). Childhood illness as an aetiological factor in burns. *Burns, 14,* 237–238.

Woodward, J. (1959). Emotional disturbances of burned children. *British Medical Journal, 1,* 1009–1113.

Woodward, J., & Jackson, D. M. (1961). Emotional reactions in burned children and their mothers. *British Journal of Plastic Surgery, 13,* 316–324.

2

Medical Management

RICHARD B. FRATIANNE
and CHRISTOPHER P. BRANDT

INTRODUCTION

Burns are among the most serious of injuries occurring in the pediatric population, often resulting in significant short- and long-term disability. Fire and/or burn injuries are the second most common cause of death of young children in the United States, following only motor vehicle accidents. It was estimated that in 1985, over 400,000 children were treated for burns, with 24,000 requiring hospitalization, resulting in almost 1500 deaths (Feller & Jones, 1987). Most deaths are related to major flame burns and/or smoke inhalation as a result of house fires.

ETIOLOGY AND INCIDENCE

The sources of thermal injury include scalds from hot liquids, contact burns from touching hot objects, flame burns, electrical injury, chemical burns, and flash or radiation burns. The incidence and etiology of burns in children vary according to the age, sex, race, and socioeconomic status of the patient (Chatterjee *et al.*, 1986; Feck & Baptiste, 1979). The most common circumstances surrounding a burn also differ as the child pro-

---

RICHARD B. FRATIANNE and CHRISTOPHER P. BRANDT • Department of Surgery, Case Western Reserve University School of Medicine, MetroHealth Medical Center, Cleveland, Ohio 44109.

Behavioral Aspects of Pediatric Burns, edited by Kenneth J. Tarnowski. Plenum Press, New York, 1994.

ceeds through normal developmental stages. In infants and toddlers, age 0–4 years, approximately 85% of all thermal injuries are caused by exposure to scalding liquids (Feldman *et al.*, 1978). The majority of these burns occur in the kitchen or bathroom as a result of a spill of hot liquids related to food preparation or consumption, or from hot tap water used for bathing (see Figure 1). Many children are scalded by tipping over containers of hot liquids from tables and countertops particularly when electric deep fryers and other appliances are left with the cords overhanging the countertop surface. As children become more mobile they are at greater risk for household electrical burns caused by inserting objects into unprotected electrical outlets, and contact burns from exposure to hot surfaces such as irons, stoves, grills, and heaters. For children older than 6 years, flame burns become more likely and often result from children playing with matches or lighters or while playing with or standing near an open fire.

A study conducted by the National Burn Information Exchange in a review of 41,326 patients created in burn centers between 1964 and 1977 revealed that children under the age of 4 sustain burn injuries more

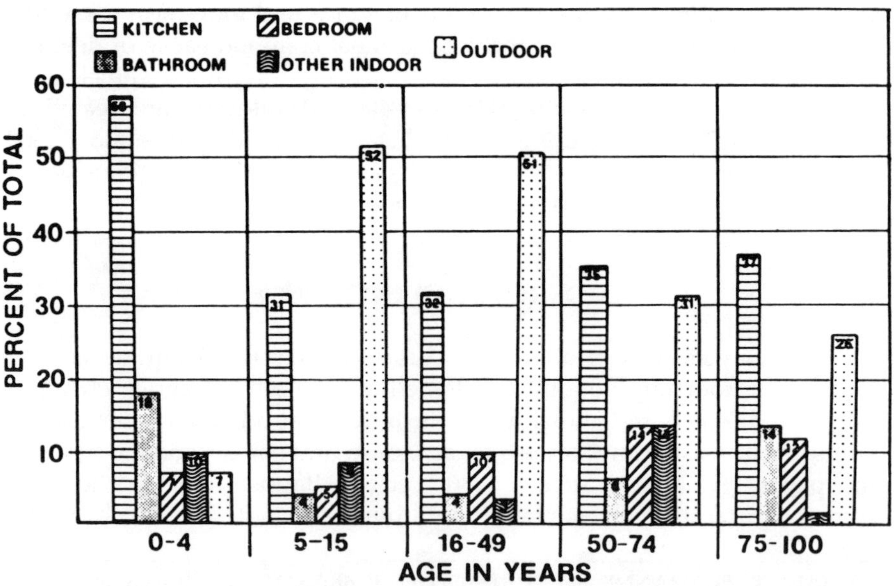

Figure 1. Locations of burn accidents. The most frequent indoor accidents occur in the kitchen, bedroom, and bathroom. [Reprinted with permission of W. B. Saunders Co. Feller, I., & Jones, C. A. (1987). The National Burn Information Exchange. In J. A. Boswick (Ed.), *Surgical Clinics of North America, Burns, 67:2*, 187.]

commonly than any other age group. A comparison of these data with those from 38,674 patients treated in burn centers between 1978 and 1986 revealed an almost identical distribution of patients with the highest incidence occurring in patients in their second year of life (Feller & Jones, 1987) (see Figure 2). The study also reported that in 19,698 patients reviewed, the overwhelming majority of injuries experienced by children up to age 4 occur in the kitchen, with the bathroom being the second most common site. Between ages 5 and 15, the most common site was outdoors, followed by burns sustained in the kitchen. This study also revealed that for children ages 1 and 2, which accounted for 1967 cases, the most common source of scald injury was bathing, second was pulling over pots, pans, and skillets from the stove, followed by pulling over containers of hot liquids, for example, cups filled with hot coffee (see Figure 3). Thus, it is quite clear that children are at greatest risk whenever hot liquids are present. The obvious implication of these data is that increased levels of care and supervision are required for children when they are in the kitchen or bathroom. In adolescent populations, injuries may result from the careless use of gasoline or other flammable substances. Playing with fireworks may result in very serious injuries leading to amputation of body parts or loss of eyes.

The incidence of burns is higher in males than females in all age groups, particularly adolescents. Several studies have also noted a higher incidence in nonwhite than white children (Libber & Stayton, 1984), which is undoubtedly multifactorial in origin and related to various economic, environmental, and social factors. For example, the homes of inner-city families often are heated by space heaters. In older homes that are poorly insulated, fires beginning as a result of faulty appliances may spread with dramatic rapidity and are frequently associated with overwhelming injuries and death in children. Scalds likewise are more common in poor families. For example, in households where gas service has been shut off, hot plates are used to heat water for washing dishes, bathing, and washing clothes. These electric hot plates are frequently positioned on the floor or within reach of children, who may seriously scald themselves when the containers are tipped over.

BURNS RESULTING FROM ABUSE OR NEGLECT

Burns are a common manifestation of child abuse and/or neglect (Holter & Friedman, 1968). Neglected children can be burned as a result of inadequate supervision or insufficient awareness on the part of their caregivers, who may not appreciate the danger that children place them-

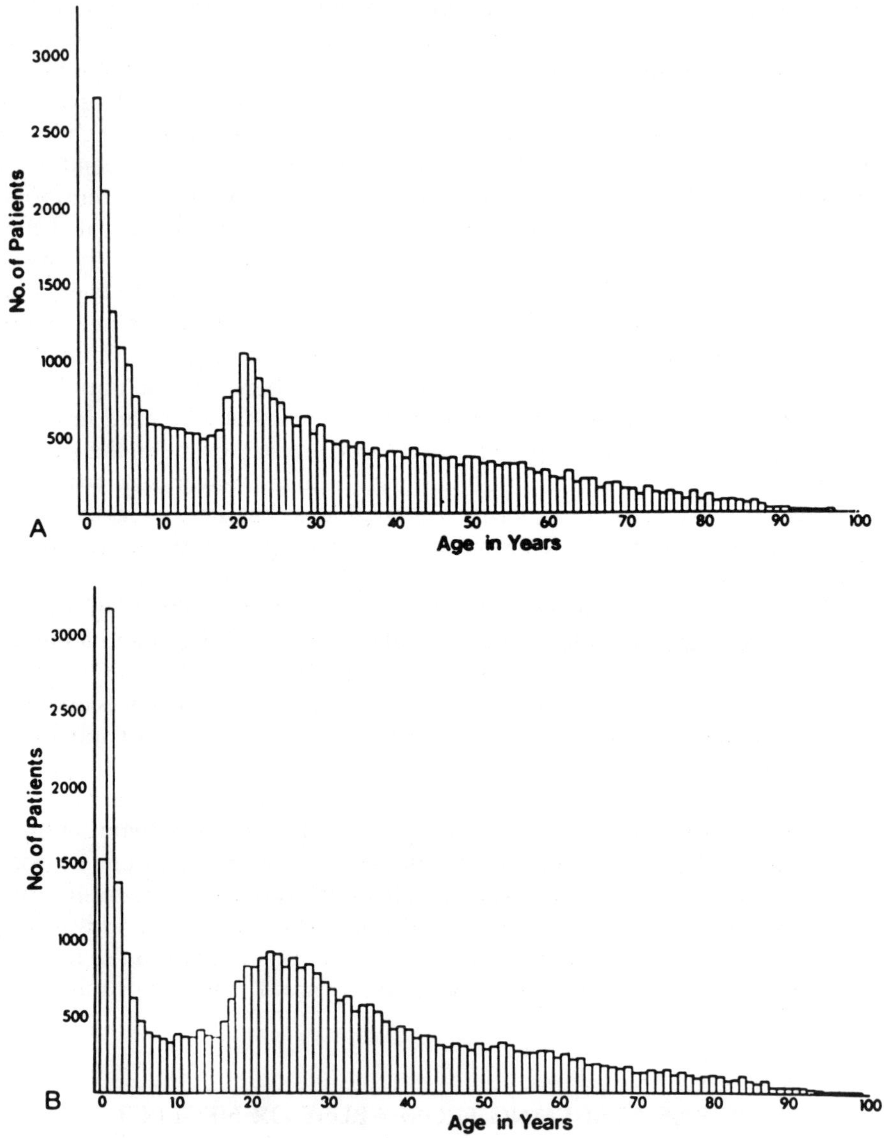

Figure 2. Age distribution of National Burn Information Exchange patients. (A) 1964–1977; (B) 1978–1985. [Reprinted with permission of W. B. Saunders Co. Feller, I., & Jones, C. A. (1987). The National Burn Information Exchange. In J. A. Boswick (Ed.), *Surgical Clinics of North America, Burns, 67:2,* 185.]

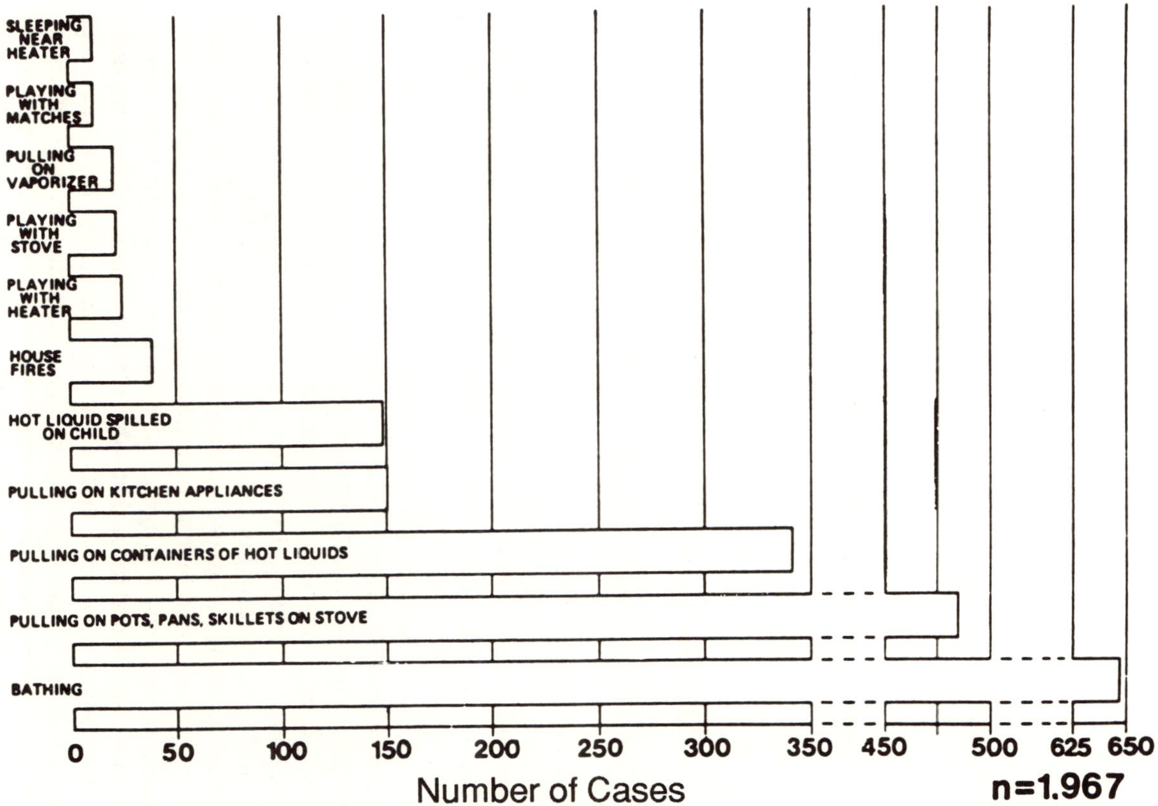

Figure 3. Etiologies of burn accidents involving 1- and 2-year-old children, showing that nearly all accidents are preventable. [Reprinted with permission of W. B. Saunders Co. Feller, I., & Jones, C. A. (1987). The National Burn Information Exchange. In J. A. Boswick (Ed.), *Surgical Clinics of North America, Burns, 67:2*, 187.]

selves in related to sources of heat in the form of hot water or flame. Approximately 25% of children admitted to our Burn Center in Cleveland are reported to the Children's Services of Cuyahoga County as possible cases of abuse/neglect. Abuse burns vary from punishment by burning the child in various parts of the body with lighted cigarettes to deliberately submersing hands in hot water or placing them on hot objects to teach the child not to touch certain things (Hight, Bakalar, & Lloyd, 1979) (see Figure 4). Children who are punished for soiling themselves are frequently placed in hot bath water, often by a caregiver other than the mother, typically the "boyfriend." Since 1970, we have admitted 2455 children. Each year between 12 and 15% of our admissions are determined to be the result of abuse. Investigation into the background of the caregivers reveals that an overwhelming majority of the abusive adults were abused as children and frequently invoke severe punishment as a way of disciplining children in a manner similar to the way they were reared (Lenoski & Hunter, 1977).

HISTORICAL ASPECTS OF BURN TREATMENT

The treatment of burns parallels the advances in control of wound infection. Until the last 20 years, burn wound infection had been the leading cause of death in patients sustaining thermal injury of any etiology. The ancient Egyptians wrapped burns in papyrus and linen soaked with beeswax in the manner similar to the way they prepared nobility for burial. Beeswax contains a substance called propolis, which has antibacterial effects. The Egyptians recognized early on that a burn patient would not survive if the burn wound became infected (Bryan, 1974). Similarly, the Romans developed a dressing utilizing olive oil, oil of flax, and linen impregnated with beeswax (Scarborough, 1969; Sigerist, 1951). From that time forward, there has been a progression of topical unguents placed on burn wounds in an attempt to control infection. In the pre-Listerian era, these included tincture of benzoin, dilute calcium hydroxide dressings, linen saturated with molasses, sodium and calcium chloride dressings, and mercuric chloride. In the post-Listerian era, when bacteria were recognized as the causative agents of infection, treatment was directed more toward using substances that were lethal to bacteria. These included phenol, boric acid, picric acid, and tannic acid dressings. These dressings were quite toxic to tissues and no significant reduction in burn mortality was achieved. The premodern era of burn therapy revealed the first use of occlusive dressings and 0.9% sodium chloride subcutaneously. A report from Sneve (1905) in the United States described using zinc acetate powder and 0.9% sodium chloride intravenously. The dressing used in World War I

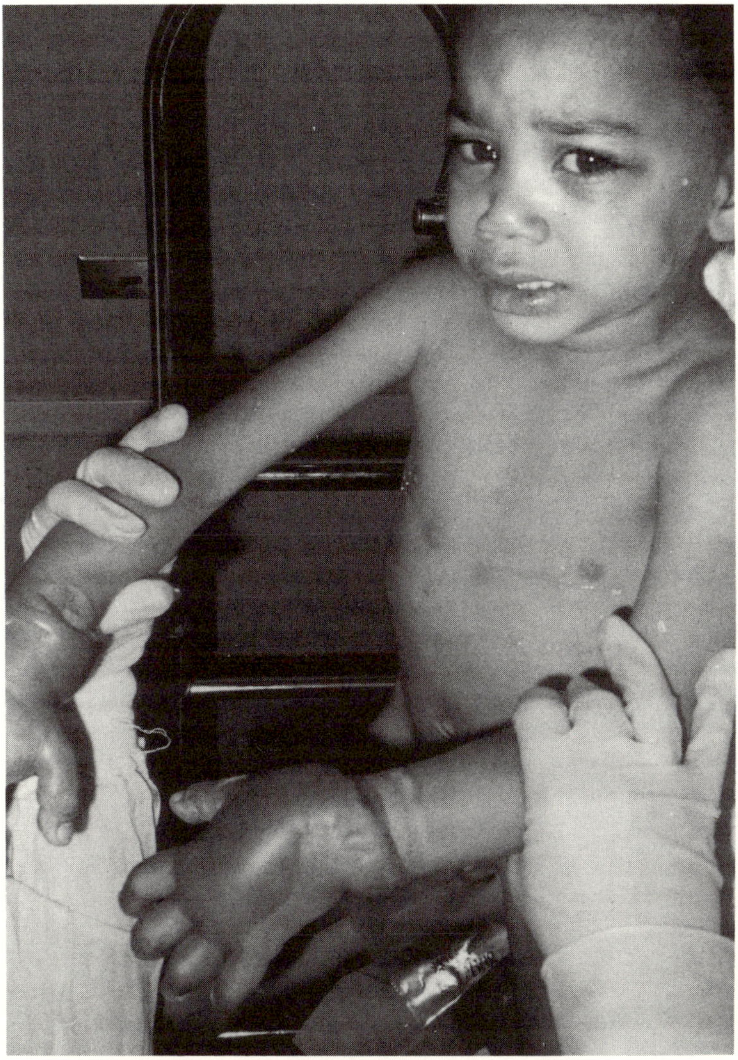

Figure 4. Glove distribution of burns of both hands. Note hemorrhagic blisters of hands and multiple bruises on face and trunk.

was paraffin with sodium chloride intravenously; and in 1926, Carran oil with subcutaneous sodium chloride and the first use of blood transfusions was described. In 1951, the first modern formula for resuscitating burns was developed by Evans (1952), followed in 1954 by the Brooke Army Formula and in 1970 by the Parkland Formula (Table 1).

Silver nitrate, 0.5% solution, was the preferred burn dressing beginning in the early 1930s. Following World War II, mafenide acetate cream was introduced at the Surgical Research Unit at Ft. Sam Houston in San Antonio, Texas, and in 1968, silver sulfadiazine cream was introduced as a topical agent. The latter two agents had antimicrobial effects and the ability to penetrate effectively into devitalized skin (eschar) to bring the antimicrobial action to the deeper layers of the burn wound and prevent deep burn wound sepsis.

When penicillin first became available in 1938, the organism normally colonizing the skin of most individuals was *Streptococcus*. Penicillin was found to effectively eradicate these organisms, and physicians erroneously believed that the problem of early burn wound infection (*Streptococcus* erysipelas) would be solved (Cockshott, 1956). Subsequently, gram-negative infections became more prominent and despite the use of sulfa drugs and streptomycin, which became available in the 1950s and early 1960s, resistant organisms emerged, chiefly *Pseudomonas aeruginosa*. With the development of antibiotics able to control *Pseudomonas* infection, the problem of burn wound sepsis was again thought to be solved. Many saprophytic gram-negative organisms found in the human colon became infective agents in patients who are severely immunosuppressed, as are burn patients at the extremes of age or with burns greater than 40% total body surface area (TBSA). It became apparent that despite broad-spectrum antibiotics, good topical antimicrobial agents, and a much better understanding of the physiology of resuscitation for major burn injuries,

Table 1. Comparison of Resuscitation Formulas

	ml/kg per % burn		
	Evans	Brooke	Parkland
Colloid	1.0	0.5	0
N/saline	1.0	0	0
Ringer's	0	1.5	4.0
D5/W	Maintenance	Maintenance	0

mortality in patients with greater than 50% TBSA burns continued to be high.

In the mid-1970s, a radical change occurred in the care of burns. It was recognized that early tangential excision of partial-thickness wounds led to more rapid reepithelialization of the burn (Janzekovic, 1975). This observation led to a change toward early excision of burns, and later, immediate autograft closure of the wound. With very large burns, intermediate use of allograft (cadaver) skin grafts was also advocated. Coincident with this change in burn therapy from trying to control burn wound infection by application of topical agents to excision and early grafting to close the burn wound, there has been a dramatic increase in survival in patients with very large burns (see Figure 5).

ASSESSMENT OF BURN DEPTH

The severity of a burn injury is related to the depth of burn and to the extent of TBSA involved. Flame injuries, particularly involving combustion of clothing, cause temperatures to reach thousands of degrees and almost uniformly result in full-thickness burns. Although the severity of a scald injury also depends on the TBSA scalded, the depth of the injury will depend on the temperature of the scalding liquid and the length of time the skin is in contact with the offending agent (see Table 2).

Burns are categorized as being first, second, or third degree, depending on the layers of the skin that are involved. A first-degree burn is superficial, and involves only the epidermis or outermost layer of the skin. The typical appearance of a first-degree burn is a pink or light red coloration, with dryness, lack of blistering, and pain on touch. Healing occurs within 3 to 7 days and does not result in scar formation. Treatment for first-degree burns generally includes application of moisturizing agents which help reduce pain and promote healing.

Second-degree burns involve injury to the dermis of the skin. The dermis is the thick, tough layer of skin which gives the skin substance and resistance to abrasion and penetration. Animal dermis forms the "hide" used in making leather products. Second-degree burns can further be described as either superficial partial-thickness involving the upper one-third,or deep dermal burns involving the lower two-thirds of the dermis (see Figure 6). The former will typically appear as bright pink, moist, occasionally blistered, and extremely painful to touch. Such a burn, when pressed by a gloved finger, will blanch and immediately return to its pink coloration signifying that the capillary circulation to the dermis is intact. These superficial second-degree burns will generally heal in 2 to 3 weeks

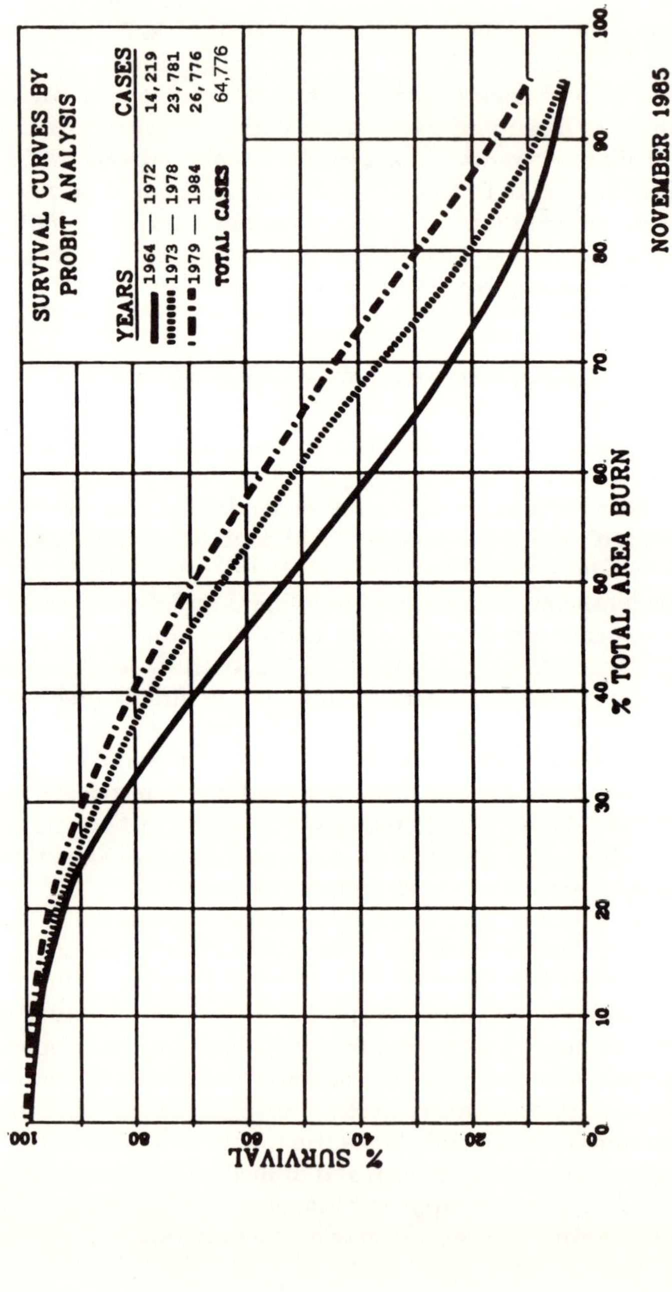

Figure 5. Probit survival curves showing improved survival rates during the period 1964–1984. [Reprinted with permission of W. B. Saunders Co. Feller, I., & Jones, C. A. (1987). The National Burn Information Exchange. In J. A. Boswick (Ed.), *Surgical Clinics of North America, Burns, 67:2*, 179.]

Table 2. Scald Burns in Children: Time of Exposure versus Temperature to Cause Serious Burns

Water temp. (°F)	Time (sec)
120	>300
125	>120
130	30
135	10
140	5
145	3
150	1.5
155	1.0

without skin grafting or significant scarring as long as infection is avoided. Burns of this nature should be covered with barrier-type dressings which include petrolatum-impregnated gauzes (Xeroform), or Op-Cite, a non-adherent dressing that promotes healing (Gerding, Imbembo, & Fratianne, 1988; Gerding *et al.*, 1990).

Deeper second-degree burns will vary in appearance but often are a deep red and the surface is dry with a granular whitish surface. Spontaneous healing of burns of this depth takes greater than 3 weeks and commonly results in hypertrophic scar formation. When hypertrophic scar formation occurs in cosmetic areas or near joints, motion may be restricted and cosmetics are often altered leading to significant functional, psychological, and emotional problems as children grow. At the present time, the preferred treatment for deep second-degree burns, particularly in cosmetic areas or around joints, is early excision and split thickness skin grafting which almost always results in improved cosmesis and better joint function.

Third-degree burns involve the entire thickness of all layers of the skin. These frequently present as white or charred surfaces that are waxy and leathery in appearance. The skin in these lesions loses its pliability and elasticity and thrombosed superficial blood vessels may be visible in the wound. Pain sensation is absent because of the destruction of the nerve endings in the dermis. Wounds of this depth require skin grafting. Extensive full-thickness (third-degree) burns pose significant threat to the life of a child and should be treated in centers specializing in the management of severe burns.

The extent of a burn is measured in terms of percentage of TBSA affected by second- or third-degree injury. Burn diagrams have been developed which outline the surface area percentages for the extremities

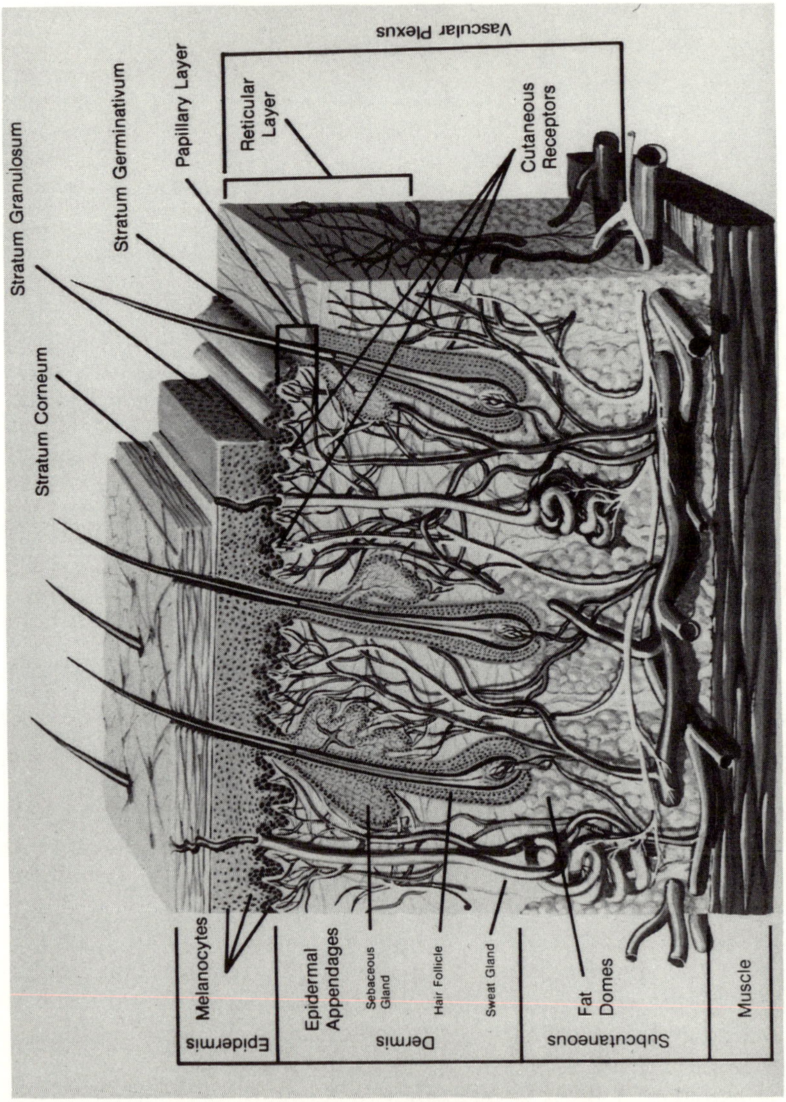

Figure 6. Structure of skin and dermal appendages.

and other portions of the child's body (Wachtel, Kahn, & Frank, 1983) (see Figure 7). This allows for precise calculation of the TBSA burn percentage, which is of critical importance in determining the type of treatment required by the child. The American Burn Association recommends that second-degree burns, either superficial or deep, of greater than 10% TBSA should be admitted to burn centers. It also recommends that third-degree burns of greater than 5% TBSA or any burn that involves the face, neck, hands, feet, or perineum, and all electrical or chemical burns be admitted to a burn center.

FIRST AID FOR MINOR BURNS

There are several principles which govern first aid for burn injuries (Fratianne, 1979). The first principle is to remove the source of heat or offending agent. For scald injuries, this involves removing clothes saturated with hot liquid and then cooling the burn with cool water until the surface of the burn is cool to the touch. For flame injuries, the first order of priority is to extinguish the flames, particularly if clothing is on fire. The burned and hot smoldering clothing should then be rapidly removed and the surface cooled with cool water. In the case of electrical injuries, the first order of priority is to ensure that the source of electric current is no longer in contact with the patient. At that point, if clothing is on fire, the first aid is similar to that for flame injuries. For burns caused by toxic chemicals, rapid flushing with water is essential and removal of clothing saturated with the offending chemical agent should be accomplished as rapidly as possible. Chemical burns should be copiously flooded with water and particular attention must be paid to chemical injuries involving the eye which require irrigation and prompt evaluation in an emergency room facility.

The second general principle is that wounds that are blistered—or if the blister is broken and the wound is pink, painful, and blanches when touched—are most likely partial-thickness burns and will heal if they are kept clean and covered. However, any burn greater than the size of a half-dollar should be evaluated by a medical professional, particularly if the burn involves the face, hands, feet, or perineum. There are a number of "home remedies" that are inappropriate in the modern approach to burn first aid. Applying such things as butter, soap, antiseptics, or harsh cleansing agents is inappropriate. Painful burns feel better when they are covered with agents that block the air from contacting the burn surface. The most appropriate topicals are over-the-counter antibiotic ointments (Neosporin, Bacitracin), aloe-containing gels, or unguents specifically designed for burns. Larger burns and burns that are white and painless

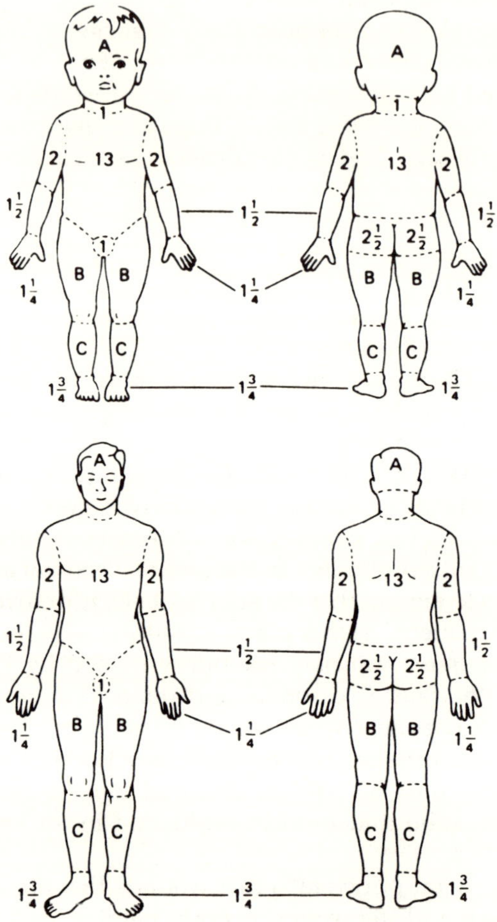

	0 Age	1 year	5 years	10 years	15 years	Adult
A = ½ of head	9½%	8½%	6½%	5½%	4½%	3½%
B = ½ of thigh	2¾%	3¼%	4%	4¼%	4½%	4¾%
C = ½ of leg	2½%	2½%	2¾%	3%	3¼%	3½%

Figure 7. Percent burns by body region. Note difference in proportion of head and thigh areas in children versus adults.

without blanching when touched should have nothing applied but a clean covering and the patient brought promptly to a medical facility for evaluation and treatment. Pain medication for simple, small, and superficial burns may include over-the-counter strengths of ibuprofen or acetaminophen. Whenever there is doubt concerning the size of the burn or the depth, medical attention should be sought promptly.

PHYSIOLOGY OF MAJOR THERMAL INJURY

Burns of greater than 30% TBSA threaten the life of the child. Extensive burns result in severe and prolonged physiologic alterations in the function of the major organ systems (Carvajal, 1980). When one considers the principal functions of the skin, the impact of a major burn injury can be better understood.

Control of Evaporative Water Loss from the Body

When large areas of skin are burned, the water vapor barrier provided by the stratum corneum of the epidermis is lost, allowing for loss of body fluids (extracellular fluid) through the skin. In addition, the physiologic response to the burn injury results in an alteration of capillary endothelium which leads to significant translocation of fluid from the vascular space into the extracellular space. This "capillary leak syndrome" permits loss of water, electrolytes, and albumin which leads to edema formation and hypoalbuminemia. Any child with burns greater than 15% TBSA will require intravenous resuscitation (Graves *et al.*, 1988). The goals of resuscitation are to maintain vital signs within the normal range depending on the age of the child and a urine output of between 1 and 2 ml/kg per hr. The magnitude of the translocation and fluid losses in burns can be appreciated when one considers that with a burn of 50% TBSA, the patient requires the intravenous infusion of crystalloid equal to the total of extracellular fluid volume normally present in the patient, which is approximately 20% of body weight in kilograms.

Control of Body Temperature

Thermal regulation is accomplished by either contracting or expanding the circulation to the skin. Body temperature is carefully controlled by the thalamus via regulation of the dermal circulation in response to adrenergic stimuli. With large surface area burns, heat is rapidly lost from the body. This results in the thalamus resetting the internal temperature thermostat, thus facilitating a dramatic increase in metabolic rate. Metabolism may be accelerated to two and one-half times normal. This results in a tremendous increase in cardiac output and oxygen consumption. There is concomitant stress placed on the hepatic, renal, and pulmonary systems. These changes in metabolism continue until the burn wound is closed.

Protection against Infection

This is accomplished in part by the desquamation of the surface epithelium (squames) that normally occurs with good hygiene. Removing these dead cells gives us the fresh feeling we experience when we towel ourselves after a bath or shower. Sebaceous glands found in the dermis lubricate hair shafts and also have an antibacterial effect. When large areas of skin are burned, not only are these functions lost, but the devitalized tissue offers an excellent culture medium for bacteria that reside on the surface of the skin and in the hair follicles and sebaceous glands. For large burns, current therapy demands excision of the devitalized tissue and should proceed before infection occurs so that early grafting can close the wound more promptly and facilitate return of metabolic rate toward normal (Herndon *et al.*, 1987).

Definition of Body Image

Perhaps the least appreciated but critical function of the skin is that it defines the body image. In children, as well as adults, alterations in body image inevitably affect self-perception. The psychological problems that must be overcome when children become aware of their altered body image are not only profound, but require early intervention by health care professionals including child life specialists, social workers, psychologists, and rehabilitation experts to help children, particularly adolescents, make the necessary adjustments to be able to accept themselves and regain a sense of dignity and self-worth (Bezzeg *et al.*, 1972). The psychologic rehabilitation of burned children begins on the day of admission and often lasts for many years. Special needs for these children include reintegration into society, returning to school, being accepted by their peers, and overcoming the stigma of being "different" in a society which generally makes people who are different feel inadequate.

INITIAL MANAGEMENT OF MAJOR BURNS

The management of a victim with major burns must be performed in a systematic manner that follows the ABCs of major trauma evaluation

(Trunkey, 1978). The principal initial threat to the airway of a burn victim occurs with swelling secondary to burns of the face, neck, or intraoral cavity. Edema formation occurs rapidly when intravenous resuscitation is begun, which may result in compromise of the airway within minutes to hours. Patients presenting with burns in this distribution are frequently intubated prophylactically because delay may make subsequent intubation quite difficult and may require use of a flexible bronchoscope to place the tube through the edematous tissues of the hypopharynx. Evaluation of breathing is done by an assessment of the patient's capacity to ventilate adequately to ensure proper oxygen and carbon dioxide transfer. The principal initial threat to ventilation in burn victims occurs with burns extending from the midaxillary line anteriorly to the opposite midaxillary line. As edema forms beneath the burn tissue, chest wall compliance is decreased, which can rapidly cause reduction in tidal volume and minute ventilation. When this sequence occurs, an escharotomy to relieve the thoracic restriction is required at once. Escharotomies are performed through full-thickness burns and must be carried down through the dermal fascia so that the skin is able to separate freely and restore normal pulmonary dynamics.

Evaluation of the circulation is performed. Circumferential full-thickness burns on an extremity frequently lead to decreased circulation in the distal tissues. Edema formation under the eschar causes progressive compression of the underlying tissue that decreases venous flow from the extremity. If not relieved, this leads to progressive arterial insufficiency. Escharotomies are performed to relieve this constriction and must be carried distally to the furthest point of circumferential burn to restore normal circulatory dynamics to the extremity. The second portion of the evaluation involves the assessment of tissue perfusion and oxygenation. This evaluation is guided by vital signs, capillary refill on burned extremities, acid-base studies on blood gases, urine output, and the patient's sensorium.

FLUID RESUSCITATION

In thermal injury, burn tissue is coagulated and capillary blood flow is not present because the capillaries are thrombosed. Adjacent to this area of destruction, tissues are injured but the capillaries remain open. This adjacent area, referred to as the zone of stasis, is characterized by the presence of vasoactive mediators, principally prostaglandins, thromboxanes, and bradykinin, that results in the "capillary-leak syndrome" leading to the rapid loss of water, electrolytes, and albumin from the vascular space into the interstitial tissues. Burns of greater than 15 to 20% TBSA release such large quantities of these vasoactive substances that there is a generalized edema throughout the body and all tissue is involved. This edema formation secondary to the capillary-leak syndrome principally involves the subcutaneous fat, the intestinal tract, and the central nervous system, although all tissues are involved with edema formation. It is because of this systemic edema formation that patients with larger burns require nasogastric intubation. Because these patients might develop an ileus of the intestinal tract, gastric retention and the threat of emesis and aspiration must be considered. The rapid accumulation of edema fluid in the subcutaneous tissue leads to the problem previously discussed which requires escharotomy. The capillary-leak syndrome is most intense in the first 8 to 12 hr following major thermal injury. During this period, rapid infusion of crystalloids is required to maintain plasma volume and cardiac output. Addition of colloids to the resuscitation fluid during the first 8 to 12 hr generally has a deleterious effect by increasing interstitial oncotic pressure that results in changes in fluid dynamics leading to increased interstitial edema formation. As the capillary-leak syndrome abates, colloids in the form of albumin, plasmanate, or fresh frozen plasma, are added to the resuscitation fluid. Children, especially infants, demand careful attention not only to the restoration of plasma volume and maintenance of cardiac output, but also to maintenance of adequate serum albumin concentrations. In addition, glycogen stores are limited in infants and very young children, and glucose must be administered to guard against the deleterious effects of hypoglycemia in these patients.

A child with a major thermal injury often requires intubation with paralysis, multiple escharotomies with the wound subsequently treated with topical antimicrobial creams, two secure intravenous routes for the rapid administration of large volumes of fluid, an arterial line to monitor blood gases, and *very attentive* nurses and physicians to respond to the moment-to-moment and hour-to-hour changes in the patient's physiologic status (Finkelstein *et al.*, 1992).

INHALATION INJURY

Inhalation injury poses a significant threat to the life of a patient and usually results from fires that occur in a closed space when the victim is forced to breathe the products of combustion for more than a few seconds (DiVicenti, Pruitt, & Reckler, 1971). For those trapped in a fire in which smoke is present, the safest and best place to be is as close to the floor as possible, because heat and smoke and the products of combustion rise, and whatever fresh air is available will be closest to the floor. Similarly, the temperatures can vary significantly in a closed-space fire. Temperatures 6 feet from the floor may reach 200 to 300°F whereas the temperature progressively falls until it may be no more than 100°F at the floor level.

There are three components to inhalation injury and each must be understood correctly for appropriate care to be rendered to the patient (Venus *et al.*, 1981). The first is thermal energy. Breathing heated air, in general, does not cause burns to the lower respiratory tract, inasmuch as the cooling capacity for air passing through the nose and mouth is quite effective. The rich circulation to the mucosa of the nose, mouth, and hypopharynx is able to carry away heat effectively except with temperatures above 150°F. Thermal injury, however, is not uncommon when patients are exposed to breathing superheated steam. This might occur with rapid decompression of a pressure cooker or other similar device. The microscopic water droplets maintain high temperature as the moist air is drawn into the lower respiratory tract. When this occurs, thermal injury to the lower respiratory tract is not uncommon and almost invariably leads to massive pulmonary edema and obstruction of bronchi and alveoli.

The second component of inhalation injury is carbon monoxide. Hemoglobin has an affinity for carbon monoxide that is between 200 and 250 times its affinity for oxygen. By binding avidly to the hemoglobin, carbon monoxide displaces oxygen, lowers oxygen saturation, and decreases oxygen delivery to vital tissues. Carbon monoxide bound to hemoglobin molecules cannot be displaced unless the patient breathes high concentrations of oxygen, preferably 100% delivered by endotracheal tube. Hyperbaric oxygen may also be useful.

Most of the deaths that occur in house fires or fire in closed spaces are secondary to carbon monoxide intoxication rather than burns even though patients may be incinerated after they are dead. Carbon monoxide levels above 55% are almost invariably fatal. Concentrations between 35 and 55% render patients unconscious or stuporous. Carboxyhemoglobin levels of 25 to 35% are frequently associated with agitation and delirium; however, when injuries of this nature are treated promptly with high flow oxygen, recovery is likely unless the patient has been severely hypoxic for more than 5 min. Breathing cigarette smoke on a regular basis can result in 10% carboxyhemoglobin levels in the blood and must be considered when children breathe secondhand smoke.

Carbon monoxide also affects the cytochrome oxidase enzyme system. As a result, oxidative metabolism is impaired. When this function is impaired, hydrogen ion concentration increases in the blood, reflected by metabolic acidosis. Increased fractional inspired oxygen concentrations or hyperbaric oxygen should be maintained until aerobic metabolism is restored as evidenced by a rise in the serum bicarbonate level of the normal range.

The third component of inhalation injury is best described as a chemical pneumonitis that has multiple physiologic derangements associated with it. Acids, aldehydes, and other chemicals formed in the combustion of the material being burned, when dissolved in the secretions of the tracheobronchial tree, become quite destructive to the mucosa and deeper layers. These physiologic derangements result in rapid loss of the ciliary action of the tracheobronchial epithelium, rapid loss of surfactant levels secondary to inhibition of type II pneumonocytes, mucosal edema with airway obstruction at the bronchial and alveolar levels, and chemical irritation of the substance of the lung resulting in a rapid accumulation of interstitial edema that effectively increases the space between capillaries and alveoli resulting in decreased gas exchange characterized by increased pulmonary shunt fractions.

The diagnosis of inhalation injury is made either by bronchoscopy or by ventilation perfusion scans. Bronchoscopic findings may range from mucosal edema to punctate hemorrhages to frank hemorrhages to ulceration of the tracheobronchial mucosa, and survival is inversely related to the severity of these bronchoscopic findings (Trunkey, 1978).

Therapy for inhalation injury is multifaceted; however, one of the most important aspects of therapy remains good bronchopulmonary toilet. Patients with significant inhalation injury should be intubated, which facilitates adequate suction, clapping, turning, and aerosol therapy. Because ciliary action is reduced, clearing of mucus is depressed and, along with the loss of surfactant, causes collapse of the terminal bronchi and alveoli. Atelectasis is common and increases the pulmonary shunt fraction. These physiologic derangements lead to infection and when pneumonia develops there is a significant decrease in the chance of recovery from the inhalation injury. Positive end expiratory pressure (PEEP) should be rapidly instituted to aid in preventing atelectasis as well as improving gas exchange. Children sustaining inhalation injury frequently require endotracheal intubation for 5 to 10 days or longer. These children often require chemical paralysis to tolerate the ventilator. This can be a significant stressor for both patient and parents. Special care must be given to ensure the safety of the child, and parents need ongoing information and consideration during this extremely stressful period.

SURGICAL MANAGEMENT OF LARGE FULL-THICKNESS BURNS

Extensive full-thickness burns are treated initially with topical antimicrobial creams; however, autologous skin grafting will eventually be required for these patients (Herndon *et al.*, 1987). Grafting autologous skin involves removing sheets of skin from unburned areas of the patient using a dermatome, which can be set precisely to obtain grafts from 0.008 to 0.0012 inch in thickness. Grafts of this depth involve the epidermis and the upper layers of dermal tissue. The donor site thus created is equivalent to a fresh partial-thickness burn in many respects. Both donor sites and partial-thickness burns heal by the proliferation of epithelial cells which make up the hair follicles and sebaceous glands in the remaining viable dermis. This process normally takes 7 to 14 days unless infection or vascular compromise or desiccation occur.

The burn to be grafted must be prepared surgically. Burn tissue may be excised tangentially using a variety of instruments to "shave" the burn tissue deeply enough to encounter viable tissue. For very large burns, removal may involve excision of the burned skin and subcutaneous tissue down to the underlying muscle fascia. Fascial excision is done because it involves less blood loss during surgery. Furthermore, autografts have a higher rate of "take" when placed on fascia than on subcutaneous fat. In very large burns, the percent take is of extreme importance because of the paucity of available donor sites.

When there is insufficient autograft to cover the burn wound that has been excised, it may be covered with freshly obtained or frozen human allograft skin, fresh or frozen xenograft (porcine) skin, or a variety of artificial skin "equivalents" that act to protect the freshly excised healthy and viable exposed tissue until suitable autograft sites are available for harvest or reharvest.

The process required to treat a child with greater than 50% full-thickness burns requires multiple surgeries to excise the burn wound and to progressively close the burn wound with skin grafts obtained from the limited donor sites available (Alexander *et al.*, 1981). Face and hands are never used as donor sites; however, all other areas of the body are used as donor sites including scalp and feet. During this time the children are at great risk for infection. They are undergoing rigorous dressing changes that require large doses of narcotics and sedatives to help them endure these procedures, and together with the ventilator, intravenous infusions, transfusions, and blood tests, the patients may be in a state of "delirium" for several weeks or longer. Often during this period, survival is unsure, and it becomes a most arduous emotional trial not only for parents but also for the health care professionals caring for the child.

NUTRITIONAL SUPPORT

Nutritional support is a major priority in the care of the burned child (Law, Dudric, & Abdan, 1974). For children with burns less than 25% TBSA, a diet supplemented with vitamins and extra calories is sufficient to promote healing (Hildreth *et al.*, 1989, 1990). A severe burn injury, however, leads to a degree of hypermetabolism unmatched by any other trauma or medical illness (Allick *et al.*, 1979). The resulting neuroendocrine response to the loss of body heat and proteins through the open wounds leads to marked catabolism, muscle breakdown, and large energy requirement. For burns greater than 50% TBSA, the energy expenditure exceeds twice normal resting requirements. Early and aggressive nutritional support is therefore necessary to compensate for these effects, as well as to promote wound healing. Inadequate nutrition may also increase the risk and incidence of sepsis and organ failure in these severely injured patients.

Nutritional assessment and support is begun within 24 to 48 hr of the burn injury (O'Neil, Hutsler, & Hildreth, 1989). Various formulas have been devised to estimate the caloric energy requirements for each patient based on weight and TBSA. This allows for an initial estimation of necessary energy provision; however, ongoing reassessment is necessary and dependent on each individual's response. The adequacy of the nutritional program is assessed by monitoring body weight, visceral protein levels, calorie counts, and nitrogen balance, and is continued throughout the hospital course until the patient is able to maintain adequate nutrition on his/her own. For the critically ill patient, nitrogen balance studies comparing protein intake to calculated protein loss are commonly used as an estimate of net protein synthesis by the patient.

Nutritional support can be provided via an enteral route using the gastrointestinal (GI) tract, or parenterally using intravenous access. The enteral route is preferred because of relative ease of use, lower cost, and potential complications associated with central venous catheters necessary for parenteral nutrition. There is also increasing evidence that early and continuous use of the GI tract for feeding is associated with a lower incidence of sepsis related to prevention of translocation of intestinal bacteria to the systemic system. With larger burns, enteral feeding may require the placement of feeding tubes into the stomach or small intestine. Specialized high-calorie, protein-rich liquid formulas can then be provided. Some children may only require nocturnal tube feedings as supplements to their intake by mouth. This is desirable, when possible, because it encourages improvements in appetite and eating behavior during the day. A percentage of patients will be unable to tolerate enteral feeding because of intestinal ileus secondary to the original injury or as a result of sepsis; or it may be associated with abdominal trauma suffered with the thermal injury or intrinsic bowel disease. In these patients, adequate nutrition can be supplied via an intravenous catheter. Use of this method requires careful monitoring for electrolytes and glucose abnormalities as well as complications related to catheter insertion, particularly infection.

IMMUNOLOGIC CONSEQUENCES OF MAJOR BURNS

Infection is the primary or contributing cause of death in the majority of patients with burn injury, particularly in those who survive the initial resuscitation. This is a direct result of the profound alterations that occur in the immunologic status of a person suffering a major burn. A number of host defense mechanisms are affected by thermal injury. The skin normally provides a direct barrier to bacterial penetration and this first line of defense is obviously disrupted with thermal injury. The injured tissue which forms exudate and eschar also provides an ideal reservoir for growth of microorganisms.

A major burn also leads to a number of adverse changes in both the humoral and cellular immune systems of the burn victim (Waldmann & Broder, 1977). Lymphocytes are the primary cells involved with the immunologic response to infection. Thymus-derived lymphocytes (T cells) are responsible for cell-mediated immunity while bone marrow-derived lymphocytes (B cells) are responsible for humoral or antibody-mediated immunologic responses. When stimulated, T lymphocytes are activated into helper cells that trigger antibody production against antigens previously experienced by the patient and suppressor cells that regulate the level of inflammatory response. Normally, T helper cells predominate over T suppressor cells; however, after major thermal injury the ratio between helper and suppressor cells is reversed and the patients are unable to recognize recall antigens (Miller & Claudy, 1979). The magnitude of this T cell ratio reversal is proportional to the severity of the injury. In very large burns, immunosuppressive reactions can be observed within 24 hr; moreover, this suppressive activity remains until the patient develops anabolic metabolism and the burn wound closes (Ninnemann, 1981).

Humoral immunity, mediated by B lymphocytes, results in the production of specific antibodies against microorganisms or their breakdown products. There are five major immunoglobulins, three of which are known to have functionally significant antibody activity against microorganisms. These are IgG, IgM, and IgA. Major thermal trauma significantly lowers IgG concentrations, while IgA and IgM are lowered to a lesser degree. The immunoglobulins are part of a complex integrated network that includes the complement system which facilitates ingestion of microorganisms by phagocytic cells. The phagocytic cells that require microorganisms to be opsonized to facilitate their ingestion and destruction include neutrophils and monocytes, which freely circulate in the bloodstream. There are fixed phagocytes (macrophages) which are found primarily in the liver and spleen and make up the reticuloendothelial system. The function of fixed tissue macrophages is likewise significantly depressed following major thermal injury (Miller, 1981).

Other aspects of burn care may also compromise the patient's immunologic response. Multiple surgical procedures, transfusion of blood products, and need for frequent general anesthesia all have been shown to adversely affect the patient's response to infection (Moran & Munster, 1987). Certain antibiotics and other pharmacologic agents may have associated immunosuppressive side effects. In summary, the combination of multiple factors leads to a marked susceptibility of the burn patient to local and systemic infection (Gallin, 1975). Sepsis has become the most difficult problem for the burn surgeon to combat. The investigation of potential methods to proactively modulate the immune system to diminish the adverse immunologic response seen in burn injuries is a major area of research. Preliminary efforts suggest that this will be an increasingly important modality in burn care in the future (Hansbrough, Zapata-Sirvent, & Peterson, 1987).

TISSUE-CULTURED SKIN

Keratinocytes grown in tissue culture have become a modality of treatment for very large burns with very limited donor sites (Rheinwald & Green, 1975). The method for their growth was first described by Green, Kehinde, and Thomas (1979). This process involves taking a square inch biopsy of skin, enzymatically separating the epidermis from the dermis, mincing the epidermis, and separating the keratinocytes. These can then be grown in a variety of tissue culture media, resulting in a sheet of pure keratinocytes, six to eight cell layers thick in approximately 10 to 12 days. Microscopic examination of these cells reveals that the cells adjacent to the plastic container begin to differentiate into basal cells. When the keratinocyte cultures reach confluence, they can be transferred to the excised wound using a Vaseline gauze carrier to facilitate transfer of this gossamer-like sheet of keratinocytes so that the basal cell layer is adjacent to the burn wound (see Figure 8). The original thought was that tissue-cultured keratinocytes would provide closure of very large wounds when donor sites were inadequate; however, experience has revealed that the wound closed with cultured keratinocytes is thin and brittle and is easily abraded (Munster, Weiner, & Spence, 1990). Further, the take of the cultured keratinocytes is quite tenuous because bacterial contamination of the recipient site almost invariably causes the cultured graft to be lost. As a result of these observed inadequacies, attention has been turned to producing a skin equivalent using tissue culture techniques in which fibroblasts are seeded onto a variety of collagen preparations utilizing either gels or matrices (Schafer *et al.*, 1989). As the fibroblasts take up residence, they begin to proliferate and produce collagen. At approximately 10 days,

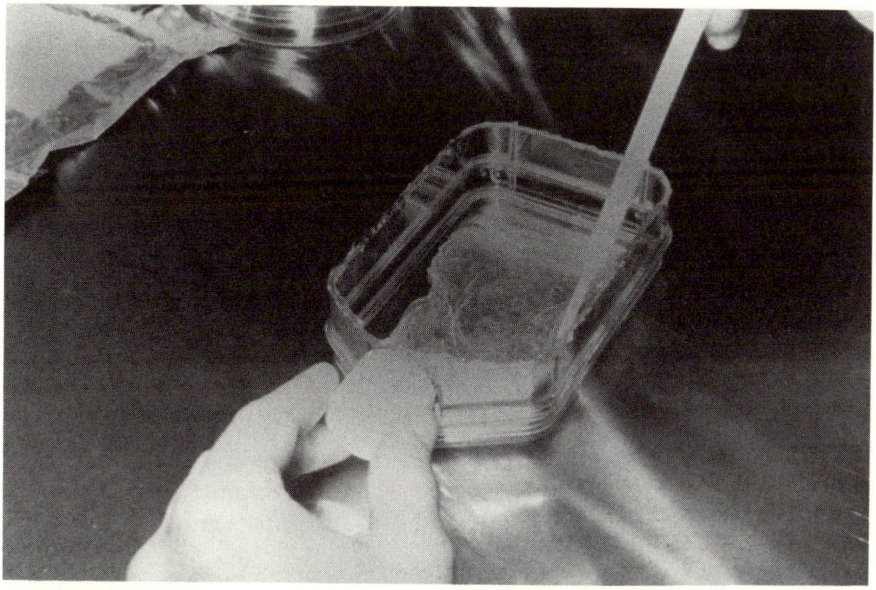

Figure 8. Confluent sheet of keratinocytes enzymatically freed from the culture flask, ready for transfer to the Vaseline gauze carrier.

these cultures can be overseeded with keratinocyte suspensions resulting in an epidermis forming over the previously created dermal equivalent. Although these methods are currently under intense investigation, clinical application remains in a highly experimental phase (Fratianne *et al.*, 1993).

REHABILITATION OF THE BURNED CHILD

Despite the arduous clinical course that children with significant thermal injury are forced to endure, the principal aim of the health care professionals is to restore patients to full function. This requires physical, emotional, and psychosocial rehabilitation, and reintegration into their normal environment. In addition, this process often requires multiple surgical procedures to correct hypertrophic scars, contractures near joints, and cosmesis.

Functional Rehabilitation

Despite the rigorous hospital course that a child with a major burn must undergo, the goals of physical rehabilitation will only be fully achieved if physical and occupational therapy is begun on the day of admission. Initially, this rehabilitation may involve merely the positioning of affected joints in proper anatomic positions to prevent contractures. As children go through the grafting process and the skin grafts become engrafted sufficiently to allow for exercising, joints are manipulated gently through their range of motion. This keeps the healing tissues stretched and pliable to prevent the inevitable contractions that would occur if the child were allowed to assume a position of comfort (e.g., full flexion of affected joints resulting in the fetal position). As the healing process progresses, joints become more painful to move and patients attempt to resist passive exercises that are vital if the joint is to maintain its normal flexibility. This physical and occupational therapy often requires a team approach involving not only occupational and physical therapists, but also the pediatric psychologist, social worker, child life specialists, nurses, and family members. Gaining the cooperation of a child in pain that is magnified by the therapy to be given requires sensitivity, compassion, and skill, but is vital if the child is to be restored to full functioning.

Hypertrophic Scarring

The formation of hypertrophic scars is common when deep partial-thickness burns are allowed to heal spontaneously but require more than 3 weeks to reepithelialize (see Figure 9). These hypertrophic changes also may occur in any grafted area or donor site. Hypertrophic scars are managed by application of skin emollients, massage, and compression dressings utilizing either elastic bandages or custom-made elastic garments (Larson *et al.*, 1971) (see Figure 10). In many cases, healed hypertrophic scars require compression for 6 months to 1 year. The clinical signs of hypertrophic scar involve signs of inflammation in the healing wound, principally edema, vasodilatation, and redness. Contraction of collagen by the formation of fibroblasts differentiating into myofibroblasts is common when deep partial-thickness burns require more than 3 weeks to reepithelialize. It is only when the natural healing process is completed and edema and redness disappear that patients are generally considered for reconstructive surgery if necessary.

Surgical Reconstruction

Skin contractures around joints can be treated with a variety of surgical techniques which include z-plasty, v-y skin advancements, incision with split-thickness graft inlays, excision of the scar with either split-thickness or full-thickness skin grafts, rotation of skin flaps, rotation of

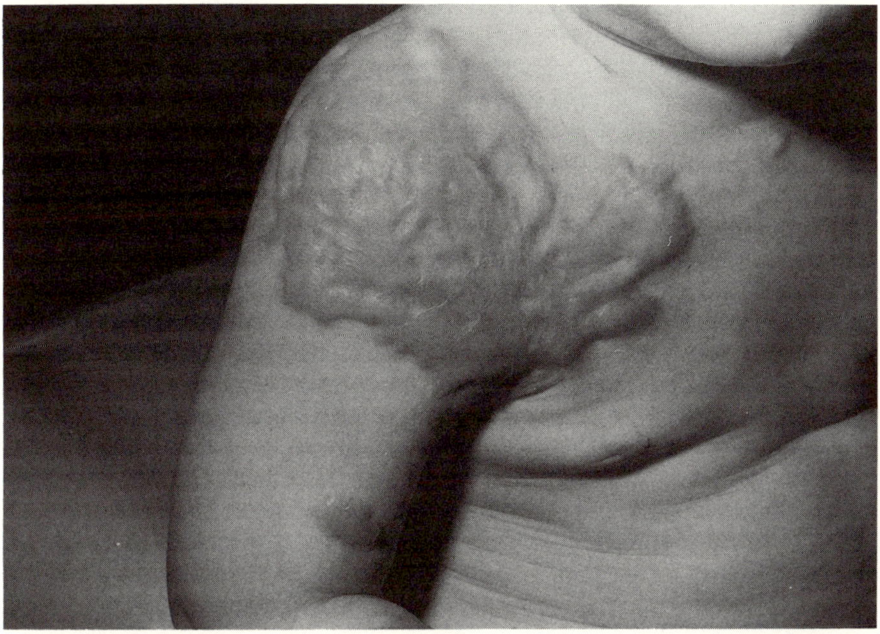

Figure 9. Hypertrophic scar resulting in contracture formation of the anterior axilla.

myocutaneous flaps (rotation of skin with its underlying muscle to preserve blood supply to the skin flap), and free tissue transfers using microvascular anastomosis to reestablish circulation (Earle & Fratianne, 1979). Cosmetic reconstructions often involve all of these modalities plus dermabrasion and dermabrasion with overgrafting with thin split-thickness grafts. Injecting hypertrophic scars with steroids has generally not been effective in ameliorating the hypertrophic changes but may, in some cases, be of some benefit.

It is easy to understand the distress present in both children and parents as they progress through the acute stages of burn care to the rehabilitative phase of their healing only to be told that surgery must be deferred until the wound matures sufficiently. They are then faced with the prospect of multiple plastic surgical procedures, each of which is painful, requires temporary loss of function, and results in a healing scar that may temporarily appear to be uglier than the original scar. The anticipated benefit in function or cosmetics may be delayed for 3 to 4 months while the surgical reconstruction heals. Parental anxiety during the acute phase centers on whether the child will survive. During the recovery phase, it is

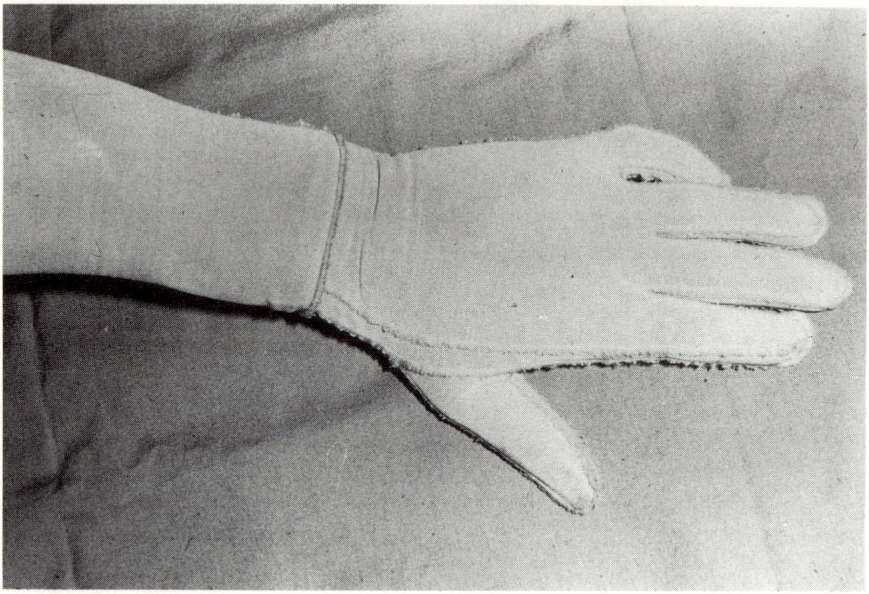

Figure 10. Custom-fitted elastic garments to control hypertrophic scar formation.

centered on how the child can go through the arduous rehabilitative maneuvers necessary to restore joint mobility; and then during the reconstructive phase, it is being faced with the unknown consequences of what is hoped to be restoration of good function and acceptable cosmetics. This entire process, in some cases, requires 2 to 3 years or longer before the ultimate result is achieved. It is, therefore, of great importance to have continuity among the caregivers to help ameliorate, as best possible, the overwhelming emotional stress on both child and parents.

CONCLUSIONS

Although great advances have been made in burn care in the last 20 years with survival reported of children with 80 to 90% TBSA burns, it is quite clear that prevention is the key to safeguarding children who are at great risk of burn injury. Simple measures such as providing smoke detectors on every floor of a dwelling, reducing the thermostat setting on hot water tanks to 125°F, and having a working fire extinguisher in every kitchen would save hundreds of lives and thousands of children from the terror of the burn unit. Parent education is an important factor in burn prevention and requires the cooperation of many segments of the community. For those children suffering major burn injuries, it is important for all health care professionals involved in their care to have an understanding of the magnitude of the sequelae of such a tragedy.

The team consists of health care professionals specializing in burn surgery, plastic surgery, critical care, psychiatry, critical care nursing, psychology, social work, child life, occupational therapy, physical therapy, nutritional support, and pastoral care. On our Unit, "TEAM" means Together Each Accomplishes More. By working together in a compassionate environment where patients, families, and fellow team members are supported and affirmed, the burn team members are able to help patients and families overcome the devastation and scarring which are unavoidable consequences of major burn injuries (Fratianne *et al.*, 1992).

The physical and psychological effects of thermal injury, particularly when they involve large areas of the body surface or cosmetic areas, are profound. The process of recovery from burns is physically arduous involving painful dressing changes, painful exercises of joints that are burned, increased requirements for high-protein and high-calorie nutrients, repeated trips to the operating room, and prolonged periods in an intensive care setting with ventilators, invasive monitoring devices, and high technological supportive measures.

Successful recovery from burn injuries involves far more than just having skin grafts applied. A dedicated team of skilled professional specialists is required to give burned children the best chance of leading happy and fulfilling lives in spite of their physical and emotional scars.

REFERENCES

Alexander, J. W., MacMillan, B. F., Law, E., & Kittur, D. S. (1981). Treatment of burns with widely meshed skin autograft and meshed skin allograft overlay. *Journal of Trauma, 21,* 433–438.

Aulick, L. H., Handler, E. H., Wilmore, D. W., Mason, A. D., Jr., & Pruitt, B. A., Jr. (1979). The relative significance of thermal and metabolic demands of burn hypermetabolism. *Journal of Trauma, 19,* 559–566.

Bezzeg, E. D., Fratianne, R. B., Karnasiewicz, S., & Plank, E. N. (1972). The role of the child care worker in the treatment of severely burned children. *Pediatrics, 50,* 617–624.

Bryan, C. P. (1974). *Ancient Egyptian medicine: The papyrus ebers.* Chicago: Area Press.

Carvajal, H. F. (1980). A physiologic approach to fluid therapy in severely burned children. *Surgery, Gynecology, and Obstetrics, 150,* 379–384.

Chatterjee, B. F., Barancik, J. I., Fratianne, R. B., Waltz, R. C ., & Fife, D. (1986). Burn injury in northeastern Ohio. *Journal of Trauma, 26,* 844–847.

Cockshott, W. P. (1956). The history of the treatment of burns. *Surgery, Gynecology, and Obstetrics, 102*, 116–124.

DiVicenti, F. C., Pruitt, B. A., Jr., & Reckler, J. M. (1971). Inhalation injuries. *Journal of Trauma, 11*, 109–117.

Earle, A. S., & Fratianne, R. B. (1979). Delayed definitive reconstruction of the burned hand: Evolution of a program of care. *Journal of Trauma, 19*, 149–152.

Evans, E. I. (1952). The early management of the severely burned patient. *Surgery, Gynecology, and Obstetrics, 94*, 273–282.

Feck, G., & Baptiste, M. S. (1979). The epidemiology of burn injury in New York. *Public Health Report, 94*, 312–318.

Feldman, K. W., Schaller, R. T., Feldman, J. A., & McMillon, M. (1978). Tap water scald burns in children. *Pediatrics, 62*, 1–7.

Feller, I., & Jones, C. A. (1987). The National Burn Information Exchange. In J. A. Boswick (Ed.), *Surgical Clinics of North America, 67:2* (pp. 167–189). Philadelphia: Saunders.

Finkelstein, J. L., Schwartz, S. B., Madden, M. R., Marano, M. A., & Goodwin, C. W. (1992). Pediatric burns. An overview. *Pediatric Clinics of North America, 39*, 1145–1163.

Fratianne, R. B. (1979). Prehospital and emergency evaluation and treatment of thermal injuries. *Ohio State Medical Journal, 75*, 375–377.

Fratianne, R. B., Yurko, L., Coffee, T., & Brandt, C. (1992). When is enough enough? Ethical dilemmas on the burn unit. *Journal of Burn Care and Rehabilitation, 13*, 600–603.

Fratianne, R. B., Papay, F., Housini, I., Lang, C., & Schafer, I. A. (1993). Keratinocyte allografts accelerate healing of donor graft sites: Possible applications for improved treatment of burns. *Journal of Burn Care and Rehabilitation, 14*, 148–154.

Gallin, J. E. (1975). Abnormal chemotaxis: Cellular and humoral components. In J. A. Bellanti & D. H. Dayton (Eds.), *The phagocytic cell in host resistance* (pp. 227–248). New York: Raven Press.

Gerding, R. L., Imbembo, A. L., & Fratianne, R. B. (1988). Biosynthetic skin substitute vs. 1% silver sulfadiazine for treatment of inpatient partial thickness thermal burns. *Journal of Trauma, 28*, 1265–1269.

Gerding, R. L., Emerman, C., Effron, D., Lukens, T., Imbembo, A. L., & Fratianne, R. B. (1990). Outpatient management of partial thickness burns—Biobrane vs. 1% silver sulfadiazine. *Annals of Emergency Medicine, 19*, 121–124.

Graves, T. A., Cioffi, W. G., McManus, W. F., Mason, A. D., & Pruitt, B. A., Jr. (1988). Resuscitation of infants and children with massive thermal injury. *Journal of Trauma, 28*, 1656–1659.

Green, H., Kehinde, O., & Thomas, J. (1979). Growth of cultured human epidermal cells into multiple epithelia suitable for grafting. *Proceedings of the National Academy of Sciences U.S.A., 76*, 5665–5668.

Hansbrough, J. F., Zapata-Sirvent, R. L., & Peterson, V. M. (1987). Immunomodulation following burn injury. In J. A. Boswick (Ed.), *Surgical Clinics of North America, 67:2* (pp. 69–75). Philadelphia: Saunders.

Herndon, D. N., Gore, D., Cole, M., Desai, M. H., Linares, H., Abston, S., Rutan, T., Van Osten, T., & Barrow, R. (1987). Determinants of mortality in pediatric patients with greater than 70% full-thickness total body surface area thermal injury treated by early total excision and grafting. *Journal of Trauma, 27*, 208–212.

Hight, D. W., Bakalar, H. R., & Lloyd, J. R. (1979). Inflicted burns in children. *Journal of American Medical Association, 242*, 517–520.

Hildreth, M. A., Herndon, D. N., Desai, M. H., & Duke, M. A. (1989). Caloric needs of adolescent patients with burns. *Journal of Burn Care and Rehabilitation, 10*, 523–526.

Hildreth, M. A., Herndon, D. N., Desai, M. H., & Broemeling, L. D. (1990). Current treatment reduces calories required to maintain weight in pediatric patients with burns. *Journal of Burn Care and Rehabilitation, 11,* 405–409.

Holter, J. C., & Friedman, S. B. (1968). Child abuse: Early case findings in the emergency department. *Pediatrics, 42,* 128–138.

Janzekovic, Z. (1975). The burn wound from the surgical point of view. *Journal of Trauma, 15,* 42–62.

Larson, D. L., Abston, S., Evans, E. B., Dobrokovsky, M., & Linares, A. H. (1971). Techniques for decreasing scar formation in the burned patient. *Journal of Trauma, 11,* 807–823.

Law, D. K., Dudrick, S. J., & Abdau, N. I. (1974). The effects of protein caloric malnutrition on immune competence of the surgical patient. *Surgery, Gynecology, and Obstetrics, 139,* 257–262.

Lenoski, E. F., & Hunter, K. A. (1977). Specific patterns of inflicted burn injuries. *Journal of Trauma, 17,* 842–846.

Libber, S. M., & Stayton, D. J. (1984). Childhood burns reconsidered: The family and the burn injury. *Journal of Trauma, 24,* 245–252.

Miller, C. L. (1981). Alteration in macrophage function following thermal injury. In J. L. Ninnemann (Ed.), *The immune consequences of thermal injury* (pp. 49–65). Baltimore: Williams & Wilkins.

Miller, C. L., & Claudy, B. J. (1979). Suppressor T cell activity induced as a result of thermal injury. *Cellular Immunology, 44,* 201–208.

Moran, K., & Munster, A. M. (1987). Alterations of the host defense mechanism in burned patients. In J. A. Boswick (Ed.), *Surgical Clinics of North America, 67:2* (pp. 47–55). Philadelphia: Saunders.

Munster, A. M., Weiner, S. H., & Spence, R. J. (1990). Cultured epidermis for the coverage of massive burn wounds. *Annals of Surgery, 211,* 676–680.

Ninnemann, J. L. (1981).Suppression of lymphocyte response following thermal injury. In J. L. Ninnemann (Ed.), *The immune consequences of thermal injury* (pp. 66–89). Baltimore: Williams & Wilkins.

O'Neil, C. E., Hutsler, D., & Hildreth, M. A. (1989). Basic nutritional guidelines for pediatric burn patients. *Journal of Burn Care and Rehabilitation, 10,* 278–284.

Rheinwald, J. G., & Green, H. (1975). Serial cultivation of strains of human epidermal keratinocytes: The formation of keratinizing colonies from single cells. *Cell, 6,* 331–344.

Scarborough, J. (1969). *Roman medicine*. Ithaca: Cornell University Press.

Schafer, I. A., Shapiro, A., Kovach, M., Lang, C., & Fratianne, R. B. (1989). The interaction of human papillary and reticular fibroblasts and human keratinocytes in the contraction of three-dimensional floating collagen lattices. *Experimental Cell Research, 183,* 112–125.

Sigerist, H. E. (1951). *A history of medicine: Primitive and archaic medicine*. London: Oxford University Press.

Sneve, H. (1905). The treatment of burns and skin grafting. *Journal of American Medical Association, 45,* 1–8.

Trunkey, D. D. (1978). Inhalation injury. *Surgical Clinics of North America, 58,* 1133–1140.

Venus, B., Matsuda, T., Copiozo, J. B., & Mathru, M. (1981). Prophylactic intubation and continuous positive airway pressure in the management of inhalation injury in burn victims. *Critical Care Medicine, 9,* 519–523.

Wachtel, T. L., Kahn, V., & Frank, H. A. (1983). *Current topics in burn care*. Rockville, MD: Aspen Systems Corporation.

Waldmann, T. A., & Broder, S. (1977). Suppressor cells in the regulation of the immune response. In R. S. Swartz (Ed.), *Progress in clinical immunology* (Vol. 13). New York: Grune & Stratton.

3

Acute Reactions

F. DANIEL ARMSTRONG, CARYL L. GAY, and JACQUELINE D. LEVY

INTRODUCTION

Conventional wisdom has long suggested that a number of acute psychological problems may be encountered by burn-injured youth (Noyes, Andreasen, & Hartford, 1971), but the research in this area has been limited by small and sometimes biased samples, infrequent inclusion of comparison samples, and a wide range of dependent measures that vary in reliability and validity (Tarnowski, Rasnake, Gavaghan-Jones, & Smith, 1991). Simply describing the problems observed may be insufficient for fully understanding the phenomenon, particularly when this understanding is needed to develop an appropriate intervention. A given behavior problem may result from a variety of different factors, and failure to adequately assess the context, beyond the immediate burn experience, may lead to the selection of an ineffective treatment. Therefore, we will identify factors that may influence our understanding and assessment of children's acute reactions to burns and burn therapy, reviewing the available literature on the occurrence of acute problems and treatment alternatives. We will then describe a strategy for developing prevention interventions with this population. For purposes of this chapter, we will focus on burns occurring in children and adolescents that require hospitalization.

F. DANIEL ARMSTRONG, CARYL L. GAY, and JACQUELINE D. LEVY • Department of Pediatrics, University of Miami School of Medicine, Miami, Florida 33101.

Behavioral Aspects of Pediatric Burns, edited by Kenneth J. Tarnowski. Plenum Press, New York, 1994.

METHODOLOGICAL CONSIDERATIONS

Reviews of the literature focusing on psychosocial assessment and treatment of children and adolescents with burns have consistently referred to an empirical data base characterized by multiple methodological limitations (Miller, Elliott, Funk, & Pruitt, 1988; Tarnowski, Rasnake, & Drabman, 1987; Tarnowski *et al.*, 1991). Unfortunately, there have been few improvements in the methodological rigor applied to research on pediatric burns, so several aspects of this chapter are based on descriptive or anecdotal observations. There are, however, a number of reasons for the limitations that exist. The state of published research directly reflects the clinical difficulty involved in developing psychosocial treatments for children who are burned. There are many factors that may independently, concurrently, or interactively influence the problems experienced by children and adolescents in a burn unit. Given the complexity of the potential interactions between these factors, it is very difficult to develop a treatment research design that can adequately control for all of them. This is particularly true when the number of children and adolescents hospitalized for burns, while substantial, represents such a wide variety of experiences dispersed across multiple treatment centers throughout the United States. Thus, although it is appropriate to critically evaluate the methodology of-studies in this area, such evaluation must carry with it a realistic appraisal of the practical limitations of research at this time.

Treatment research on the psychosocial aspects of pediatric burns has been predominantly characterized by case reports with no experimental control, single subject reversal and multiple baseline designs, or group comparisons with limited small samples (Miller *et al.*, 1988; Patterson *et al.*, 1993; Tarnowski *et al.*, 1991) where statistical power and appropriateness of control groups are of substantial concern. These issues must be considered before one is able to make valid inferences or come to any generalizable conclusions based on the research findings. Because there are often limited numbers of patients available for study, subject characteristics such as premorbid psychopathology (Tarnowski *et al.*, 1991), age (Tarnowski *et al.*, 1991), and socioeconomic status (Molinaro, 1978) are often not considered. Much of the experimental work done in this area has relied on single subject methodology (Tarnowski *et al.*, 1987), a legitimate form of scientific inquiry in situations where a few similar individuals are used to study the effectiveness of a specific intervention (Kazdin, 1982). Unfortunately, this type of design may have limited generalizability to the broader population, and studies that utilize group design strategies seldom include appropriate comparison or control groups (Tarnowski *et al.*, 1991). Assessment methodology has also been limited by lack of consistency in measurement of adjustment, with some studies relying on unstructured interviews (e.g., Knudson-Cooper, 1981; Miller, Gardner, & Mlott, 1976; Molinaro, 1978), and incidental report of functioning (Tarnowski *et al.*, 1991) that have no demonstrated validity with the population. Others have used measures with demonstrated reliability, validity, and standardization (e.g., Blakeney, Herndon, Desai, Beard, & Wales-Seale, 1988; Herndon *et al.*, 1986; Knudson-Cooper, 1981; Love, Byrne, Roberts, Browne, & Brown, 1987; Stoddard, Norman, & Murphy, 1989; Tarnowski, Rasnake, Linscheid, & Mulick, 1989a), but there has been no consistent use of a given measure across studies, so generalization of findings has been limited. Finally, some findings are based on case studies (e.g., Seligman, Carroll, & Macmillan, 1972; Stoddard, 1982; Stoddard & O'Connell, 1983) that may represent a biased sample of burned children because cases are often selected to illustrate specific clinical processes (Tarnowski *et al.*, 1991).

CONTEXT OF ACUTE REACTIONS TO BURNS

There are at least six major categories of factors that may influence the child's reaction to a burn, including: (1) biologic aspects of the burn; (2) characteristics of the patient and burn episode; (3) developmental variables; (4) social support and resources; (5) treatment setting factors; and (6) availability and effectiveness of intervention services. Although it is possible that any one of these factors may exert primary influence, it is most likely that a unique combination of factors will determine the level of behavioral adaptation (or maladaptation) experienced by a particular child. Understanding the role of these factors may be critical in understanding the behavior observed, eventually resulting in an effective and acceptable form of intervention.

Biologic Considerations

There are numerous variations in the biologic response to a burn in children (Fratianne & Brandt, this volume), often making comparisons of adaptive functioning across children quite difficult. Among those factors considered important are burn degree and extent, burn location, and degree of functional impairment (Stoddard *et al.*, 1989; Tarnowski *et al.*, 1991). Other factors that are less frequently identified include those related to the unique biologic makeup of the patient, including pain tolerance, recovery of associated organ systems, and the biologic response to pharmacologic intervention (McGrath, 1990). Some of these factors may have a logical and direct link to functional impairment (e.g., the child with limited response to narcotic analgesia may experience higher levels of pain and anxiety behavior). Others may be less established (e.g., degree of depression resulting from severe burns to the face and hands of an adolescent). Research in this area suggests that a number of these factors may play an important role in pediatric adjustment (McGrath, 1991; Stoddard *et al.*, 1989; Tarnowski *et al.*, 1991), but there are numerous relationships that have not been examined yet.

Historical Considerations

Several historical (preburn) factors may be associated with the child's functioning following a burn, with one-third to one-half of children treated for burns having preburn behavioral difficulties (Miller *et al.*, 1988). Unfortunately, most of the studies reporting this relationship are limited by retrospective designs that include no comparison samples. Tarnowski *et al.* (1991) suggest that the presence of preburn behavioral or developmental difficulties, temperament, activity level, school performance, peer interactions, and coping strategies may influence both the likelihood of being burned as well as the quality of a patient's recovery from such injuries.

Preburn adjustment is sometimes confounded, however, by the nature of the setting in which the burn occurs. Children with developmental delays, psychiatric disorders, and behavioral problems (Libber & Stayton, 1984) or even preburn illnesses (Wilson, Buckland, & Sully, 1988) may have a preburn pattern of behavior that places them in a situation that is more likely to result in injury than for other same-age peers without these problems (Miller *et al.*, 1988). Alternatively, a child who is burned as a result of direct child abuse (e.g., submerged in a tub of scalding water) may have already been in an environment where other abusive acts likely occurred. As a consequence, this child may have been already at risk for behavioral or psychological problems before the burn event occurred (Hammond, Nebel-Gould, & Brooks, 1989; Purdue, Hunt, & Prescott, 1988). In contrast, a child in a well-functioning family who suffers a burn as a result of an environmental hazard (e.g., a house fire caused by faulty electrical wiring) is not as likely to have premorbid adjustment difficulties. Predicting the adjustment of children based on their premorbid functioning may require more than a topographical description of that level of adjustment pre- and postburn. The temporal pattern and situational specificity of behavior may differ substantially across children. Likewise, the type and intensity of intervention necessary for each child postburn may differ as well.

Other psychological factors may play an important role in postburn adjustment. Studies of children at risk because of health-threatening events or diseases suggest that the coping strategies utilized by the child may affect coping with the disease. Although the direction of the relationship has not been established, children (or parents of children) with sickle-cell disease who utilize and model active coping strategies accompanied by high levels of social support have been found to have fewer disease symptoms and reduced health care utilization (Armstrong, Lemanek, Pegelow, Gonzalez, & Martinez, 1993; Gil, Williams, Thompson, & Kinney, 1991). Patterns of coping have not been identified in children with burns; instead, a range of both problem-focused and emotion-focused coping responses have been described in adolescents as they attempt to cope with different aspects of burn sequelae (Sutherland, 1988). It may be that a particular type of coping leads to improved outcome, because the active coping approach may provide a greater repertoire of responses to the demands of treatment than a more passive approach. However, it is equally likely that children with fewer injury-related problems are able to better utilize more active coping strategies. Further, the effectiveness of an individual's coping may depend on the specific demands of a situation, and not on the universal effectiveness of one approach to coping.

Developmental Issues

The developmental level of the child with burns will have a substantial effect on the acute reaction to the injury and its treatment. The age of the child at the time of the burn will affect whether the child is able to understand the event that produced the burn, the need for the burn treatment procedures (e.g., hydrotherapy and/or physical therapy), and the potential outcome following treatment (Bush & Harkins, 1991; Maron & Bush, 1991; Miller *et al.*, 1988). These factors may result in the child labeling the burn event as an unpredictable and nonpreventable event or feeling guilty about causing or failing to prevent the burn. They may also influence the degree to which the child accepts the need for treatment and attempts to comply, or rejects and interferes with treatment. Finally, the child's ability to understand the long-term implications of the burn may lead to either minimal distress or significant concerns about long-term appearance and social acceptance (Maron & Bush, 1991). Each and all of these factors may have an impact on the degree of psychological adjustment observed in the acute care setting.

Second, the frequency and quality of patient distress behavior is likely to differ as a function of age, resulting in behavior patterns in infants and toddlers that are quite different from those found in adolescents. Studies of children's responses to invasive medical procedures used in the treatment of cancer suggest that younger children exhibit higher levels of behavioral distress (e.g., crying, screaming, flailing) than older children

(Jay, Ozolins, Elliott, & Caldwell, 1983; Katz, Kellerman, & Siegel, 1980). However, while the observed level of distress behavior may differ by age, the subjective experience may not (Jay, 1988). Although no studies have reported age differences in the behavior of children treated for burns, this may be more related to limited research in this area than to the absence of differences.

Third, comparability of detected psychological problems in children of different ages may be quite difficult. Children across ages, and even within age ranges, may differ widely in their ability to self-report their current level of psychological functioning (McGrath, 1990). Concordance between self-reported adjustment and ratings by significant others in children of varying ages has not always been demonstrated (Karoly, 1991). Reliance on predefined occurrence of emotional behaviors may also be limited by age. For instance, social withdrawal, depressed affect, increased sleep, and overall reduced activity level may be an appropriate characterization of depression in an adolescent, but some of these behaviors may represent adaptive psychological coping with intense pain in a younger child or infant (Craig & Grunau, 1991).

Children's ability to understand the need for procedures, and their ability to learn what is necessary to comply with medical staff requests, may be substantially affected by their level of cognitive development (Bush & Harkins, 1991; Miller *et al.*, 1988). Failure to consider a child's capacity for understanding may lead to behavior that is inappropriately attributed to poor motivation rather than lack of understanding. Further, differential interpretation of similar events by children at different levels of cognitive development may occur (McGrath, 1990). For instance, a child functioning at a concrete level of development may view hydrotherapy only in terms of its aversive and painful qualities, and thus a procedure to be avoided. However, a child functioning at a more abstract reasoning level may view the same event in terms of later healing and appearance, resulting in greater adherence with the procedure and interventions designed to lessen the aversive intensity associated with the procedure. Thus, not only can the child's developmental level of understanding affect the behavior observed, but it may also affect the degree to which intervention is effective.

Social Support and Available Resources

Social support from family, friends, and medical staff may be associated with improved adaptive functioning and less psychological difficulty in children with burns (Benians, 1988a; Blakeney, Portman, & Rutan, 1990; Cella, Perry, Kulchycky, & Goodwin, 1988; Kaslow, Koon-Scott, & Dingle, this volume). Although there has been substantial research examining the role of social support in adult adjustment with chronic illness, the construct of social support is not as well defined with children. In several studies examining the role of parental presence during invasive medical procedures (one suggested form of social support), researchers have suggested that while children state an overwhelming preference for parent presence, most children exhibit lower levels of behavioral distress when their parents are absent than when present (Gonzalez *et al.*, 1989; Shaw & Routh, 1982).

There are a number of factors that must be considered when examining the role of social support with children. The behavior of adults in the medical setting may have a number of different functions (Blount *et al.*, 1989; Zabin & Melamed, 1980). Some adult behaviors may be perceived by the child as supportive and reassuring, serving to reinforce adaptive coping and emotional regulation by the child. Touching, stroking, and talking calmly are examples of this kind of social support. However, other adult behaviors may serve as stimulus cues for the onset of invasive or painful procedures, thus serving to increase pediatric distress (Blount, Davis, Powers, & Roberts, 1991; Gonzalez *et al.*, 1989; Zabin & Melamed, 1980). In fact, several researchers have suggested that behaviors that could readily be labeled forms of social support (e.g., statements of reassurance) are the behaviors that most commonly precede and follow instances of child distress behavior (Blount *et al.*, 1989; Jacobsen, Manne, Gorfinkle, & Schorr, 1990). Other researchers have suggested that some adult behavior may be less related to the distress of the child than to that of the adult observing the child, functioning to alleviate uncomfortable levels of arousal experienced by the adult (Armstrong, 1992). Thus, although social support theoretically may be associated with children's acute adjustment, emerging data suggest that it is important to examine the functional outcome of these support behaviors to determine the role they actually play.

Treatment Setting Factors

Children's behavior occurs within an environmental context, and the stimulus characteristics of the setting may play a critical role in determining the child's adjustment to the burn and treatment. Russo and Varni (1982) discussed the "normal person, abnormal situation" that often occurs when otherwise healthy children and families are confronted with a life-threatening illness or injury. In these situations, the stimulus characteristics of the setting may produce "abnormal" behavior that is attributed, sometimes erroneously, to some characteristic of the child. Armstrong (1992) has further used an aversive conditioning model to describe the behavior of children treated for cancer. With this model, the cues for aversive events are constantly present, making high levels of vigilance and anxiety more the norm than the exception. Further, each of the components of treatment is likely to result in immediate discomfort or pain, and will usually be perceived as aversive. Under these stimulus conditions, the initial behavior to be expected will be agitation and overt distress leading to attempts to escape the situation. If the aversive nature of the situation cannot be changed, then a learned helplessness (Seligman *et al.*, 1972) response may lead to withdrawal and apathy. Cataldo and his colleagues also presented a similar model for understanding children's adjustment to intensive care unit (ICU) settings (Cataldo, Jacobs, & Rogers, 1982).

Burn treatment of children closely follows these models. Following the burn episode the child is confronted with a series of experiences involving pain and discomfort that often equal or exceed that experienced during the original injury episode. Caregivers and medical staff are often only marginally able to reduce or eliminate pain and associated uncomfortable sensations. Further, many of the procedures necessary for treating the burn (e.g., dressing changes, debridement, hydrotherapy, physical therapy) involve increased, rather than decreased, discomfort for the child. Given the aversive nature of these procedures, the child's response is often protest, heightened vigilance for future invasive procedures, and extreme behavioral protest when the procedure is performed. Because escape from the situation is limited or prevented and the procedures are performed repeatedly, the child's distress behavior may eventually habituate somewhat, leading to learned helplessness. However, in contrast to other diseases involving pain and repeated invasive procedures, the level of habituation obtained by many children with burns is considered minimal without consistent intervention and the presence of a supportive coach (Elliott & Olson, 1983).

Research conducted in other intensive care settings (e.g., pediatric ICUs, bone marrow transplantation units) has identified a number of setting factors that may contribute to high levels of acute distress. Classical conditioning may play an important role in associating health care providers (and their attire) with increased rates of distress behavior. Children in ICU settings are sometimes hypervigilant of their surroundings because there are often few cues provided that signal the absence of impending aversive procedures. This hypervigilance may interfere with other necessary components of healing, specifically eating and sleeping. Another consequence of the ICU setting is the necessity of 24-hr monitoring. In the ICU, children often lose track of day/night cycles because the lights and monitors are always on. When sleep occurs, it is likely to be interrupted by necessary monitoring (e.g., checking vital signs). The disruption of normal eating and sleeping cycles, combined with the side effects of many drugs used in the ICU, may lead to decreases in both food intake and hours of sleep. In extreme cases, children with no previous psychiatric history have displayed psychotic behavior termed "ICU psychosis," a usually temporary but disturbing condition for the child and family (Cataldo *et al.*, 1982; Miller *et al.*, 1988).

Although conceptual models are useful in guiding research endeavors, it is important to develop empirical support for the model. Sometimes, the data that emerge conflict significantly with the model. This was demonstrated in an observational study of 40 children treated in a pediatric burn unit (Tarnowski, Rasnake, Linscheid, & Mulick, 1989b). Conventional wisdom suggests that the environment of the burn unit typically produces high levels of negative behavior, and low levels of positive behavior and activity. In fact, Tarnowski and his colleagues found that one-fourth of children's observed verbalizations and vocalizations were positive, and negative vocalization, verbalization, and motor responses occurred less than 15% of the time. Nearly 60% of children's behavior was classified as neutral and occurred during a variety of activities. Positive behavior occurred most often in the presence of other people and when the child was engaged in some unit activity, often with unit child life staff. Thus, although this study represents the experience of children on one specialized burn unit, it challenges the belief that the burn experience is universally and continuously aversive to children.

Providing care to a child in a burn unit may be aversive for the health care staff as well, leading to a pattern of behavior that may unintentionally interfere with the child's adjustment. When repeatedly confronted with a child whose behavior is characterized by pain complaints, the first reaction for a health care provider is to provide assistance in alleviating discomfort. However, when such assistance is in ineffective, and the child's distress behavior continues, escape from the situation is a normal behavioral response. When escape is prevented, then emotional responses similar to those of the child (e.g., agitation, anger, depression) may occur for the health care provider as well. Under these circumstances, the health care worker may then attribute negative characteristics to the child rather than the situation. With such attributions, unintended changes in care behaviors, including reduced pain medication administration, may occur (Armstrong, Pegelow, Gonzalez, & Martinez, 1992).

Intervention Accessibility and Quality

One of the potential contributing factors to the level of adjustment is the degree to which intervention services are available during the acute phase of treatment. The burn experience is likely to produce some form of acute distress and psychological difficulty for almost every child treated. However, the intensity and duration of this difficulty may be affected by whether psychosocial services are unavailable, available on consultation, or available within the framework of a prevention-focused multidisciplinary model (Brown, Dingle, & Koon-Scott, this volume). For example, one pattern of adjustment can be anticipated if a child is appropriately medicated for pain, has nonintrusive medical monitoring to allow extended and regular periods of sleep, and is provided relaxation training and supportive counseling. However, a different, and potentially more intense and disruptive pattern of behavior may occur if services are provided only when the child's behavior interferes with treatment or physical functioning. The type and quality of psychosocial services provided to the child's family may also significantly affect adjustment (Kaslow *et al.*, this volume).

COMMON ACUTE BEHAVIORAL/PSYCHOLOGICAL PROBLEMS

In the expanding body of literature on the psychosocial adaptation and functioning of those who have sustained acute burn injuries, particular attention has been focused on a number of common psychological and psychiatric symptoms that have been documented among burn patients. These reactions include the development of diagnosable psychiatric disorders, emotional responses to the traumatic event and the recovery process, social withdrawal, and various behavior problems. To better understand the current methods of treatment, it is necessary to outline and define the most common acute problems encountered by staff that care for children who have endured the devastating effects of severe burn injury.

Anxiety and Depression

Anxiety and depression are two frequently reported psychological responses following burn injuries (Patterson *et al.*, 1993). Stoddard *et al.* (1989) found a somewhat elevated rate of depression for children and adolescents on long-term follow-up as compared with other groups. Other research indicates that although it appears that children and adolescents are more at risk for an anxiety or depressive disorder in response to burns, most appear to have the resources for eventual and comparatively normal coping (Bowden, Feller, Tholen, Davidson, & James, 1980; Byrne *et al.*, 1986; Knudson-Cooper & Thomas, 1988). Anxiety disorders in burned children are thought to be secondary to the trauma of the burn, to the medical procedures, and to the social rejection resulting from scars. These anxieties are mitigated by successfully coping with the feared stimuli (Stoddard *et al.*, 1989).

Posttraumatic Stress Disorder (PTSD)

PTSD has been described as the "development of characteristic symptoms following a psychologically traumatic event that is generally outside the range of human experience" (American Psychiatric Association, 1980). Some events may induce symptoms in some people, yet not in others, as is the case with major burns. Symptoms include anxiety and the reexperiencing of the event, such as in the form of intrusive recollections, nightmares, or associations with environmental stimuli. Also characteristic of the disorder are disturbances in mental and social function, such as diminished alertness or memory, low mood, sleep disorders, and phobic behavior. PTSD seems to occur more frequently in adult and pediatric burn patients than in comparable nonburn samples (Patterson *et al.*, 1993; Stoddard *et al.*, 1989). In a review of the literature on psychological reactions during hospitalization, Patterson *et al.* (1993) noted that PTSD appears to be a common, but generally transient, complication that resolves without specific intervention other than standard hospital care. However, another study of posttraumatic adaptation and distress among adult burn survivors by Roca, Spence, and Munster (1992) found a delayed emergence of symptoms approximately 4 months following discharge from the hospital. This indicates that the symptoms may not resolve in the absence of therapeutic intervention and there may exist the need for longitudinal observation of *all* burn survivors so that assessment and appropriate treatment of the disorder may be provided for them. Whether or not these results are generalizable to the pediatric burn population remains to be seen. Although symptoms consistent with a diagnosis of PTSD may be detected in burned children at follow-up (Saigh, 1989), there is a need for further research investigating the epidemiology, developmental response patterns, and intervention methods that are applicable specifically to pediatric burn-related PTSD (Tarnowski *et al.*, 1991).

Social Adjustment and Withdrawal

For burned children and adolescents, research on the role of social factors in children's adjustment has provided mixed results. Problems with the resumption of relationships with peers and other issues involving social adjustment, including withdrawal, depression, delinquency, and aggressiveness have been reported (Molinaro, 1978). However, several studies failed to identify a significant relationship between burn severity and the psychosocial adjustment of burned children (Blakeney *et al.*, 1988; Love *et al.*, 1987; Molinaro, 1978). Although some research supports the notion that the severity of disfigurement is associated with poorer social adjustment (Stoddard *et al.*, 1989), there is evidence to the contrary, that injury visibility does not play a significant role in adjustment (Bowden *et al.*, 1980; Molinaro, 1978; Tarnowski *et al.*, 1989a).

Dietary Noncompliance

Another issue that can confound the acute treatment of postburn pediatric patients involves dietary noncompliance. There are several factors that affect this issue that should be considered when faced with a child who is unwilling to eat and on whom a lecture on the value of adequate nutrition is wasted. According to White and Kamples (1990), the reasons for dietary noncompliance can be categorized into (1) normal psychosocial factors and (2) hospital/injury factors. The former include: the separation anxiety that the child and parents experience when the role of caregiver is transferred from the parent to the hospital; the guilt that parents feel in not being able to ameliorate their child's distress and the resulting discord that the child senses and to which he or she may react by not eating; the premorbid personality and behavioral traits of the child, who has a history of exercising control over adults. The hospital/injury factors include: the child's physiologic state, which can be disturbed by anything from nausea to exhaustion to pain; the unfamiliar food the child is given to eat; the atypical burn unit schedules; the multiple "strangers" (medical staff) who are subjecting the child to painful procedures; the well-meaning visitors who provide unauthorized snacks to the children, disrupting their feeding schedules. All of these factors can have a negative effect on the pediatric burn patient's willingness to adhere to a nutritional program.

Emotional Responses

Several studies have examined clusters of emotional responses of pediatric burn survivors and their families. Watson and Johnson (1958) reported that children who suffered from burns that resulted in the loss of a body part "frequently anticipated rejection, expressed anger, guilt, and wished that others experienced mutilation." Stoddard (1982) looked at the emotional response of children to burns at different developmental levels: before the age of 18 months, the children incorporated the burn into their own body image; at school age, the children recognized the change and grieved the loss; and adolescents responded with anger, guilt, and anxiety.

Distressed emotional responding is not limited to those suffering from the actual injury and may occur in members of the patient's family, particularly mothers (Vigliano, Hart, & Singer, 1964; Wright & Fulwiler, 1974).

Factors associated with the extent of the emotional response of the burn victim appear to be the amount of time since the injury, burn severity, maternal adjustment to the situation, and other family variables, such as infrequent visitation at the hospital (Browne *et al.*, 1985; Byrne *et al.*, 1986; Knudson-Cooper, 1981).

Adaptive Coping

Although it is sometimes assumed that children who have suffered burn injuries will exhibit severe long-term adjustment problems, a review of the literature suggests that only a minority of children with burns are at risk for later psychological difficulties (Tarnowski *et al.*, 1991). While this minority has been the focus of the research in pediatric burns, little attention has been given to the majority of burned children who have been found to exhibit no severe psychopathology either acutely or at extended follow-up. Patterson *et al.* (1993) suggest that it is not the case that severely burned individuals experience long-term permanent deterioration of psychological functioning. They reported that for the majority of hospitalized burn patients, the injury was a "temporary, albeit painful, disruption from life's routine; one after which they will eventually resume their normal preinjury functioning" (p. 371). Tarnowski *et al.* (1991) have proposed that attention be focused on the identification of the variables related to stress-resiliency in children; adaptive resources, and the protective factors in high-risk, stress-resilient children and families. This information could lead to more effective treatment approaches.

TREATMENT OF ACUTE PROBLEMS

Fifteen years ago, clinical and research interest in the psychological treatment and behavioral management of severely burned children was quite limited. Most of the literature focused on adult burn victims and did not give specific attention to pediatric burn patients. With the higher survival rates documented in recent years (Feller, Tholen, & Cornell, 1980), however, considerably more attention and research has been directed toward identifying the psychological impact of burn treatment and developing effective intervention approaches for severely burned children and their families (Kavanaugh, 1983; Stoddard *et al.*, 1989; Tarnowski *et al.*, 1987). Psychological and behavioral interventions have the dual function of facilitating the administration of necessary medical procedures and improving quality of life for the pediatric burn victims and their families.

For clinicians confronted with developing treatment plans for children with burns, the task is no less daunting than for the researcher. There is no clear evidence that any single type of intervention is universally effective with all children in all situations. In fact, treatment may necessarily involve a carefully designed multiple-component plan that systematically targets the critical and often idiosyncratic factors affecting adjustment. There are some components that seem essential to any intervention program. First, attention to the acute aspects of burn care should include a structured environment where the child receives clear information about what procedures and tasks are necessary, and when these are likely to occur. Second, appropriate pharmacological pain management should be in place for all children, with the principal goal being to have the child pain free within the limits of safety (Konigova, 1992). Although there are differing opinions about the pediatric pain experience, children who are pain free, and who are not anticipating that there will be a new onset of pain in the immediate future, are less likely to develop hypervigilance and high levels of anxious behavior. In addition, these children are more likely to be receptive to other psychosocial interventions. Third, social support during the burn unit stay, characterized by parent/family presence and age-appropriate opportunities for play with peers, may be a nonspecific but essential component in aiding acute and long-term adjustment (Benians, 1988a; Mahaney, 1990).

Beyond these basic intervention components, specific interventions targeting specific problems need to be developed. Treatment of distress associated with debridement, social withdrawal following abuse, or depression following facial burn may each require specific yet different strategies. In some cases, only one of these problems may be present. In others, multiple problems may coexist that require a coordinated intervention plan. In the following sections, we review some general intervention strategies and components that have demonstrated promise in the psychosocial treatment of pediatric burn victims.

Treatment Approaches

Psychological intervention and behavioral management may be necessary at any stage of treatment and recovery, and therefore would be most efficiently utilized as an integral part of a multidisciplinary team approach (Gillman & Mullins, 1991). In a review of the effectiveness of experimental interventions for hospitalized children, Vernon and Thompson (1993) concluded that children receiving such intervention experience less psychological upset than children who do not. Furthermore, timely and efficient management of treatment-related behavior problems can decrease the distress experienced by the burned child and the staff providing burn treatment as well as facilitate optimal recovery with minimal complications.

General Treatment Issues

Unpredictability and lack of control over aversive stimuli have been associated with negative outcomes among pediatric burn patients. Lack of control over dressing changes may result in learned helplessness on the part of the patient, characterized by withdrawal, reduced food intake, and depressed behavior (Kavanaugh *et al.*, 1991). However, allowing children and adolescents to participate in dressing changes and related procedures can dramatically reduce the distress associated with the procedure (Lasoff & McEttrick, 1986). Consequently, intervention plans for pediatric burn patients should be designed to maximize predictability and the child's sense of control over the treatment.

A second issue relevant to all intervention programs is the need for parental involvement. Benians (1988b) studied the influence of parental visiting on the survival and recovery of severely burned children and found that daily parental visits resulted in significantly better outcomes. However, as noted earlier, parental presence may not be sufficient, depending on the behavior that is problematic (Brantley, Stabler, & Whitt, 1981; Gonzalez *et al.*, 1989). It seems critical to examine the quality of the parents' support, perhaps focusing the intervention on supporting parents' attempts to more effectively aid in their children's coping. It is often difficult for parents to respond so as to facilitate children's engagement in an aversive situation, when in reality the parents' primary role, up to the point of the illness or injury, is to help their children avoid situations that cause distress. In fact, the parents' own negative affect resulting from observing the child in pain may interfere with their ability to provide social support (Armstrong, 1992). Interventions may need to provide parents with a way to (1) manage their own psychological and physiological arousal and (2) engage in parenting behaviors that facilitate adaptive coping in the child and result in increased parental competence with a situation that has not been previously encountered.

In cases where the burn event is a result of parent neglect or abuse, intervention is typically needed at multiple levels. Child protective services may be involved and there may be legal restraints on the parent's ability to be present. In this case, interventions to target potential separation anxiety and social withdrawal need to be considered. If the parent is present and will retain custody, there may be a heightened level of child distress related to the parent's association with the burn episode. Intervention may need to focus on gradually reducing distress within the parent–child relationship and possibly initiating family treatment as well (Blakeney *et al.*, 1988). Further, parent training and supervision to prevent further abuse/neglect may need to be part of the program (Knudson-Cooper & Thomas, 1988).

Analgesic Pain Management

Behavioral approaches are often used in conjunction with pharmacologic interventions for the management of burn-related pain (Maron & Bush, 1991). Providing a schedule of pain medication that results in continuous, rather than intermittent, pain relief often results in substantial reductions in associated pain behaviors (Patterson, 1992). Several factors may account for this pattern. First, when pain is adequately and consistently controlled, anxiety related to the anticipated onset of pain is reduced. Second, when pain is controlled, pain behaviors (e.g., complaints of pain, crying, requests for medication) are less likely to occur, and therefore are less likely to be reinforced by the removal of pain following medication administration. Finally, when children are pain free, there is greater likelihood that they will engage in other developmentally appropriate activities, eat, sleep, and comply with other aspects of therapy. In turn, these activities may result in lower levels of anxiety, depression, and social withdrawal. Thus, one of the first behavioral interventions that needs to be considered on the burn unit is a behavioral assessment of the effectiveness of the analgesic pain control strategy. These strategies are discussed in greater detail by Bush and Maron (this volume).

Self-Regulation Techniques

Relaxation Training

Both self-mediated arousal reducing strategies (e.g., progressive muscle relaxation and visual imagery) and operant approaches have been shown to be effective in reducing behavioral distress in children with burns (Elliott & Olson, 1983). However, relaxation training has been found to be of limited effectiveness during the acute phase of burn treatment (Patterson, 1992). Often, patients are too exhausted or disoriented to focus or maintain the concentration required by most relaxation techniques. Further, the fast pace of the burn unit may not be conducive to the intensive training required to master these techniques. When relaxation strategies are used, simple techniques, such as focusing on the breathing process, appear to work best (Patterson, 1992).

Cognitive Interventions

Cognitive interventions can generally be divided into two types: avoidance strategies and reappraisal techniques (Patterson, 1992). Avoidance or distraction techniques involve the patient in mental imagery or self-talk. Reappraisal techniques involve the patient in thinking about the sensory experience in a less anxiety-provoking way.

Distraction techniques have been used to help young children cope with the pain associated with hydrotherapy, debridement, and application of topical medications. Cartoon watching during the hydrotherapy and debridement procedures has been combined with rewarding children with stars to reduce behavioral distress (Kelly, Jarvie, Middlebrook, McNeer, & Drabman, 1984). For the two children in the study, behavioral distress decreased 43 and 31% from baseline levels. Reappraisal techniques can help the patients to think of the painful procedures in a way that promotes a sense of healing, not further tissue damage (Patterson, 1992), but the development of age-appropriate strategies is critical in optimizing treatment effectiveness.

Behavioral Approaches

Behavioral approaches have been effectively used in the management of pediatric burn patients, primarily with regard to pain, noncompliance, food refusal, nightmares, and self-excoriation. Given the aversive nature of burn treatment, many of the behavioral strategies have focused on reducing behavioral distress associated with painful procedures or reducing/eliminating behaviors that reduce burn treatment effectiveness or cause physical harm (e.g., self-excoriation). Other strategies have focused on increasing behaviors necessary for healing, including eating or participating in physical therapy. Finally, behavioral strategies focusing on nonspecific aspects of the burn experience (e.g., PTSD symptoms, generalized anxiety, social withdrawal) have also been employed.

A number of operant procedures have demonstrated success in alleviating distress and pain behavior, particularly when used in combination with analgesic therapy. Positive reinforcement (e.g., praise, providing stickers and other concrete rewards) for compliance with debridement and hydrotherapy (Elliott & Olson, 1983), dietary regimens (White & Kamples, 1990), and physical therapy (Adriaenssens, Eggermont, & Pyck, 1988) often result in clinically significant improvement. Most of the studies in this area focus on a specific problem in one or two children, and have been reviewed in detail elsewhere (Miller *et al.*, 1988; Tarnowski *et al.*, 1987).

Positive reinforcement techniques are sometimes difficult to implement, because the distress behavior of the child may be so frequent and intense that other adaptive behaviors do not occur frequently enough to have the reinforcing consequence applied on a clinically effective schedule. In these cases, extinction or negative reinforcement strategies may be necessary to reduce the distress behavior so that alternative behaviors can be reinforced.

As noted earlier, there are other specific behaviors besides pain and behavioral distress that may produce problems for the child with burns and the burn unit staff. Because these behaviors are common and may significantly impede the administration of appropriate medical care, strategies that have proven effective in reported cases are specifically described below.

Compliance with Occupational and Physical Therapy

Occupational and physical therapy are often a necessary part of burn treatment to prevent contracture and restricted range of motion. The scar tissue needs to be stretched through positioning, splinting, and exercises that often cause extreme pain. Because of the painful nature of these therapies, it is often difficult to obtain children's cooperation, particularly when they do not comprehend the rationale for treatment. Because pain behaviors often interfere with the administration of necessary therapies, management of pain behaviors can be an important component in burn recovery. Reinforcement procedures for reducing pain behavior have been found to be effective for decreasing resistance and increasing compliance with standard medical procedures (Varni, Bessman, Russo, & Cataldo, 1980).

Food Refusal

Severe burns result in a dramatic increase in the body's need for replacement fluids and supplemental calories. Furthermore, significant weight loss (>10%) after a burn injury has been associated with slow rates of healing and depressed immune function. Severe weight loss (>20%) has been associated with sepsis. Weight loss greater than 30–40% of previous weight usually results in death. In extreme cases, oral intake can be supplemented by tube feedings and parenteral feedings, though such measures are not preferred because they may result in complications such as sepsis, diarrhea, and withdrawal (Curreri, Luterman, Braun, & Shires, 1980).

Reducing children's energy expenditure can reduce children's caloric needs and increase the likelihood that their nutritional needs can be met through oral intake. Even with such measures, encouraging oral intake is often met with behavioral resistance. Behavioral contracting and contingency management has been found to be quite effective in motivating burned children to eat more (Zide & Pardoe, 1976). Although the expectations for the child's oral intake must be clear and firm, the child should be given as much control as possible over their eating. However, if the child does not eat enough to meet his or her nutritional needs, nasogastric (NG) feedings may need to be initiated. In this situation, it is critical that the NG tube be presented as a step taken to help the child with nutrition. Often tube feeding is initiated following a threat to use it as a punishment for noncompliance with oral intake. Combinations of NG feeding with positive reinforcement schedules for oral intake may optimize success because the child is provided adequate nutrition during a time when a difficult behavior, eating, is gradually shaped using positive approaches. Punitive approaches to eating problems are generally unsuccessful and only produce concurrent increases in negative affect. Consistent, flexible, and supportive approaches seem far more advantageous in treating this problem (White & Kamples, 1990).

Nightmares

PTSD symptoms, such as sleep disturbance and nightmares, are commonly associated with burn trauma (Noyes *et al.*, 1971) and have typically been treated through the use of systematic desensitization and extinction. One case study examined the effectiveness of a multicomponent intervention that combined response prevention techniques with systematic desensitization to reduce nightmares in a 5-year-old girl. The onset of nightmares invariably involved the girl clutching her nightgown. At the first sign of clutching, the girl was awakened, thereby preventing the nightmare. Desensitization with the same subject utilized gradual exposure to a ten-item hierarchy of fire-related pictures. This combined approach was effective in eliminating the nightmares. This case demonstrates the importance of targeting both the arousal elicited by thoughts about the burn event through systematic desensitization, as well as specifically targeting the operant, in this case early behaviors associated with the nightmares. Clearly, more research is needed in the area of treating PTSD-like symptoms among pediatric patients.

Self-Excoriation

Intense itching often accompanies the natural healing process of burned tissue, particularly grafted tissue (Brodland & Andreasen, 1974). A response-interruption device was used to prevent scratching in a 10-month-old infant with burns to the lower extremities. The child's scratching was significantly interfering with the healing of the skin graft, and the intensity of the itching sensation and the age of the child precluded effective reinforcement of alternative behaviors. Therefore, a device consisting of a divider worn about the waist that precluded the infant from reaching her legs and feet was used. This prevented self-excoriation without unduly restricting appropriate movement.

Treatment of Associated Problems

Burn Psychosis

Burn psychosis has been described as a syndrome of delirium, clouded consciousness, disorientation, memory disturbances, impaired intellect and judgment, labile affect, and hallucinations or delusions (West & Shuck, 1978). Disturbances generally appear during the first few days of hospitalization and often remit spontaneously. Management of burn psychosis usually involves a multimodal approach. Initially, the possibility of a physiological basis should be evaluated. Patients need to be placed under close supervision to ensure that they do not harm themselves or others. In addition, patients and their families need to be assured that such episodes are not unusual after a severe burn injury and do not reflect chronic mental illness. In handling the psychotic episodes, the patient needs to be reoriented frequently with orienting statements, clocks, calendars, and access to radio or television (West & Shuck, 1978). Consistency and predictability among medical staff and family visits may also help the patient remain oriented.

Disfigurement and Body Image

The disfigurement of burn patients often results in increased body image concerns and acute social readjustment difficulties. Even burned children who appear to have adjusted to their altered body image may experience painful self-consciousness during adolescence and young adulthood. Although these concerns have been reported (Beard, Herndon, & Desai, 1989; Jessee, Strickland, Leeper, & Wales, 1992) there are currently no studies on treatment approaches to this problem. However, strategies including a desensitization component (rehearsal), a competence component, and an exposure/reinforcement component may prove effective, and are often included as components of reentry programs for children (discussed by Blakeney, this volume).

Although general behavioral strategies are promising, the reports describing their use highlight the difficulty of developing a standardized intervention for these problems. Case reports utilize different behavioral treatment components (or set of components) targeted specifically to the problems presented by the child. Until studies are available that demonstrate the generalizability of a specific intervention to a number of children with similar characteristics, clinicians will be forced to use variants of these general intervention strategies in the absence of unequivocal support documenting either the validity or effectiveness of these methods.

For each of the problems described above, a creative approach to assessing, conceptualizing, and intervening seems critical. It is incumbent on psychosocial professionals to develop conceptual models that can be used to test the effectiveness of interventions, either in single cases or with groups of children with similar problems and background characteristics. This requires attention to the multiple factors associated with the acute adjustment of children with burns, an understanding of the relationship between these factors and the behaviors observed, and an application of intervention techniques that are empirically supported for other similar behaviors.

Some strategies may be effective with some problems in some children, but these may need to be adapted as new situations arise. Reliance on the existing empirical literature, supportive and competent colleagues, and collaboration with parents and medical staff are critical features of effective intervention for acute psychological and behavioral problems in children treated for burns.

ACKNOWLEDGMENTS. We are grateful to Charles Elliott, Ph.D., Jay Caulk, R.N., and the staff of the Pediatric Burn Unit at Oklahoma Children's Memorial Hospital in Oklahoma City, Oklahoma, for providing the practical foundation that made this chapter possible.

REFERENCES

Adriaenssens, P., Eggermont, E., & Pyck, K. (1988). The video invasion of rehabilitation. *Burns, 14*, 417–419.

American Psychiatric Association. (1980). *Diagnostic and statistical manual of mental disorders* (3rd ed.). Washington, DC: Author.

Armstrong, F. D. (1992). Psychosocial intervention in pediatric cancer: A strategy for prevention of long-term problems. In T. Field, N. Schneiderman, & P. McCabe (Eds.), *Stress and coping in infancy and childhood* (pp.197–218). Hillsdale, NJ: Lawrence Erlbaum and Associates.

Armstrong, F. D., Pegelow, C. H., Gonzalez, J. C., & Martinez, A. (1992). Impact of children's sickle cell history on nurse and physician ratings of pain and medication decisions. *Journal of Pediatric Psychology, 17*, 651–664.

Armstrong, F. D., Lemanek, K. L., Pegelow, C. H., Gonzalez, J. C., & Martinez, A. (1993). Impact of lifestyle disruption on parent and child coping, knowledge, and parental discipline in children with sickle cell anemia. *Children's Health Care, 22*, 189–203.

Beard, S. A., Herndon, D. N., & Desai, M. (1989). Adaptation of self-image in burn-disfigured children. *Journal of Burn Care and Rehabilitation, 10*, 550–554.

Benians, R. C. (1988a). The influence of parental visiting on survival and recovery of extensively burned children. *Journal of Burn Care and Rehabilitation, 14*, 31–34.

Benians, R. C. (1988b). The influence of parental visiting on survival and recovery of extensively burned children. *Burns, 14*, 31–34.

Blakeney, P., Herndon, D., Desai, M., Beard, S., & Wales-Seale, M. (1988). Long-term psychosocial adjustment following burn injury. *Journal of Burn Care and Rehabilitation, 9*, 661–665.

Blakeney, P., Portman, S., & Rutan, R. (1990). Familial values as factors influencing long-term psychological adjustment of children after severe burn injury. *Journal of Burn Care and Rehabilitation, 11*, 472–475.

Blount R. L., Corbin, S. M., Sturges, J. W., Wolfe, V. V., Prater, J. M., & James, L. D. (1989). The relationship between adult's behavior and child coping and distress during BMA/LP procedures: A sequential analysis. *Behavior Therapy, 20*, 585–601.

Blount, R. L., Davis, N., Powers, S. W., & Roberts, M. C. (1991). The influence of environmental factors and coping style on children's coping and distress. *Clinical Psychology Review, 11*, 93–116.

Bowden, M. L., Feller, I., Tholen, D., Davidson, T. N., & James, M. H. (1980). Self-esteem of severely burned patients. *Archives of Physical Medicine and Rehabilitation, 61*, 449–452.

Brantley, H. T., Stabler, B., & Whitt, J. K. (1981). Program considerations in comprehensive care of chronically ill children. *Journal of Pediatric Psychology, 6*, 229–237.

Brodland, G. A., & Andreasen, N. J. C. (1974). Adjustment problems of the family burn patient. *Social Casework, 55*, 13–18.

Browne, G., Byrne, C., Brown, B., Pennock, M., Streiner, D., Roberts, R., Eyles, P., Truscott, D., & Dabbs, R. (1985). Psychological adjustment of burn survivors. *Burns, 12*, 28–35.

Bush, J. P., & Harkins, S. W. (1991). Conceptual foundations: Pain and child development. In J. P. Bush & S. W. Harkins (Eds.), *Children in pain: Clinical and research issues from a developmental perspective* (pp. 1–30). Berlin: Springer-Verlag.

Byrne, C., Love, B., Browne, G., Brown, B., Roberts, R., & Streiner, D. (1986). The social competence of children following burn injury: A study of resilience. *Journal of Burn Care, 7*, 247–252.

Cataldo, M. F., Jacobs, H. E., & Rogers, M. C. (1982). Behavioral/environmental considerations in pediatric inpatient care. In D. C. Russo & J. W. Varni (Eds.), *Behavioral pediatrics: Research and practice* (pp. 271–298). New York: Plenum Press.

Cella, D. F., Perry, S. W., Kulchycky, S., & Goodwin, C. (1988). Stress and coping in relatives of burn patients: A longitudinal study. *Hospital and Community Psychiatry, 39*, 159–166.

Craig, K. D., & Grunau, R. V. E. (1991). Developmental issues: Infants and toddlers. In J. P. Bush & S. W. Harkins (Eds.), *Children in pain: Clinical and research issues from a developmental perspective* (pp. 171–193). Berlin: Springer-Verlag.

Curreri, P. W., Luterman, A., Braun, D. W., & Shires, G. T. (1980). Burn injury: Analysis of survival and hospitalization time for 937 patients. *Annals of Surgery, 192*, 472–480.

Elliott, C. H., & Olson, R. A. (1983). The management of children's distress in response to painful medical treatment for burn injuries. *Behaviour Research and Therapy, 21*, 675–683.

Feller, I., Tholen, D., & Cornell, R. G. (1980). Improvements in burn care: 1965–1979. *Journal of the American Medical Association, 244*, 2074–2078.

Gil, K. M., Williams, D. A., Thompson, R. J., & Kinney, T. R. (1991). Sickle cell disease in children and adolescents: The relation of child and parent pain coping strategies to adjust. *Journal of Pediatric Psychology, 16*, 643–663.

Gillman, J. B., & Mullins, L. L. (1991). Pediatric pain management: Professional and pragmatic issues. In J. P. Bush & S. W. Harkins (Eds.), *Children in pain: Clinical and research issues from a developmental perspective* (pp. 117–148). Berlin: Springer-Verlag.

Gonzalez, J. C., Routh, D. K., Saab, P. G., Armstrong, F. D., Shifman, L., Guerra, E., & Fawcett, N. (1989). Effects of parent presence on children's reactions to injections: Behavioral, physiological, and subjective aspects. *Journal of Pediatric Psychology, 14*, 449–462.

Hammond, J., Nebel-Gould, A., & Brooks, J. (1989). The value of speech-language assessment in the diagnosis of child abuse. *Journal of Trauma, 29*, 1258–1260.

Herndon, D. N., LeMaster, J., Beard, S., Bernstein, N., Lewis, S. R., & Rutan, T. C. (1986). The quality of life after a major thermal injury in children: An analysis of 12 survivors with greater than or equal to 80% total body, 70% third degree burns. *Journal of Trauma, 26*, 609–619.

Jacobsen, P. B., Manne, S. L., Gorfinkle, K., & Schorr, O. (1990). Analysis of child and parent behavior during painful medical procedures. *Health Psychology, 9*, 559–576.

Jay, S. M. (1988). Invasive medical procedures: Psychological intervention and assessment. In D. K. Routh (Ed.), *Handbook of pediatric psychology* (pp. 401–425). New York: Guilford Press.

Jay, S. M., Ozolins, M., Elliott, C. H., & Caldwell, S. (1983). Assessment of children's distress during painful medical procedures. *Health Psychology, 2*, 133–147.

Jessee, P. O. Strickland, M. P., Leeper, J. D., & Wales, P. (1992). Perception of body image in children with burns, five years after burn injury. *Journal of Burn Care and Rehabilitation, 13*, 33–38.

Karoly, P. (1991). Assessment of pediatric pain. In J. P. Bush & S. W. Harkins (Eds.), *Children in pain: Clinical and research issues from a developmental perspective* (pp. 59–82). Berlin: Springer-Verlag.

Katz, E. R., Kellerman, J., & Siegel, S. E. (1980). Behavioral distress in children with cancer undergoing medical procedures: Developmental considerations. *Journal of Consulting and Clinical Psychology, 48*, 356–365.

Kavanaugh, C. (1983). Psychological intervention with the severely burned child: Report of an experimental comparison of two approaches and their effects on psychological sequelae. *Journal of the American Academy of Child Psychiatry, 22*, 145–156.

Kavanaugh, C. K., Lasoff, E., Eide, Y., Freeman, R., McEttrick, M., Dar, R., Helgerson, R., Remensynder, J., & Kalin, N. (1991). Learned helplessness and the pediatric burn patient: Dressing change behavior and serum cortisol and beta-endorphin. *Advances in Pediatrics, 38*, 335–363.

Kazdin, A. E. (1982). *Single-case research designs: Methods for clinical and applied settings*. London: Oxford University Press.

Kelly, M. L., Jarvie, G. J., Middlebrook, J. L., McNeer, M. F., & Drabman, R. S. (1984). Decreasing burned children's pain behavior: Impacting the trauma of hydrotherapy. *Journal of Applied Behavior Analysis, 17*, 147–158.

Knudson-Cooper, M. S. (1981). Adjustment to the visible stigma: The case of the severely burned child. *Social Science in Medicine, 15*, 31–44.

Knudson-Cooper, M. S., & Thomas, C. M. (1988). Psychosocial care of the severely burned. In H. F. Carvajal & D. H. Parks (Eds.), *Burns in children* (pp. 345–362). Chicago: YearBook Medical Publishers.

Konigova, R. (1992). The psychological problems of burned patients. The Rudy Hermans Lecture 1991. *Burns, 18*, 189–199.

Lasoff, E., & McEttrick, M. A. (1986). Participation versus diversion during dressing change: Can nurses' attitudes change? *Issues in Comprehensive Pediatric Nursing, 9*, 391–398.

Libber, S. M., & Stayton, D. J. (1984). Childhood burns reconsidered: The child, the family, and the burn injury. *Journal of Trauma, 24*, 245–252.

Love, B., Byrne, C., Roberts, J., Browne, G., & Brown, B. (1987). Adult psychosocial adjustment following childhood injury: The effect of disfigurement. *Journal of Burn Care and Rehabilitation, 8*, 280–285.

McGrath, P. A. (1990). *Pain in children: Nature, assessment, and treatment*. New York: Guilford Press.

McGrath, P.A. (1991). Intervention and management. In J. P. Bush & S. W. Harkins (Eds.), *Children in pain: Clinical and research issues from a developmental perspective* (pp. 83–115). Berlin: Springer-Verlag.

Mahaney, N. B. (1990). Restoration of play in a severely burned three-year-old child. *Journal of Burn Care and Rehabilitation, 11*, 57–63.

Maron, M., & Bush, J. P. (1991). Burn injury and treatment pain. In J. P. Bush & S. W. Harkins (Eds.), *Children in pain: Clinical and research issues from a developmental perspective* (pp. 275–294). Berlin: Springer-Verlag.

Miller, M. D., Elliott, C. H., Funk, M., & Pruitt, S. D. (1988). Implications of children's burn injuries. In D. K. Routh (Ed.), *Handbook of pediatric psychology* (pp. 426–447). New York: Guilford Press.

Miller, W. C., Gardner, N., & Mlott, S. (1976). Psychosocial support in the treatment of severely burned patients. *Journal of Trauma, 16*, 722–725.

Molinaro, J. R. (1978). The social fate of children disfigured by burns. *American Journal of Psychiatry, 135*, 979–980.

Noyes, R., Andreasen, N. J. C., & Hartford, C. E. (1971). The psychological reaction to severe burns. *Psychosomatics, 12*, 416–422.

Patterson, D. R. (1992). Practical applications of psychological techniques in controlling burn pain. *Journal of Burn Care and Rehabilitation, 13*, 13–18.

Patterson, D. R., Everett, J. J., Bombardier, C. H., Questad, K. A., Lee, V. K., & Marvin, J. A. (1993). Psychological effects of severe burn injuries. *Psychological Bulletin, 113*, 362–378.

Purdue, G. F., Hunt, J. L., & Prescott, P. R. (1988). Child abuse by burning—An index of suspicion. *Journal of Trauma, 28*, 221–224.

Roca, R. P., Spence, R. J., & Munster, A. M. (1992). Posttraumatic adaptation and distress among adult burn survivors. *American Journal of Psychiatry, 149*, 1234–1238.

Russo, D. C., & Varni, J. W. (1982). Behavior pediatrics. In D. C. Russo & J. W. Varni (Eds.), *Behavioral pediatrics: Research and practice* (pp. 3–24). New York: Plenum Press.

Saigh, P. A. (1989). The validity of DSM-III posttraumatic stress disorder classification as applied to children. *Journal of Abnormal Psychology, 98*, 189–192.

Seligman, R., Carroll, S., & Macmillan, B. G. (1972). Emotional responses of burned children in a pediatric intensive care unit. *Psychiatric Medicine, 3*, 59–65.

Shaw, E. G., & Routh, D. K. (1982). Effect of mother presence on children's reaction to aversive procedures. *Journal of Pediatric Psychology, 7*, 33–42.

Simons, R. D., McFadd, A., Frank, H. A., Green, L. C., Malin, R. M., & Morris, J. L. (1978). Behavioral contracting in a burn care facility: A strategy for patient participation. *Journal of Trauma, 18*, 257–260.

Stoddard, F. J. (1982). Body image development in the burned child. *Journal of the American Academy of Child Psychiatry, 21,* 502–507.

Stoddard, F. J., & O'Connell, K. G. (1983). Dysphoria in children with severe burns. *Journal of Children in Contemporary Society, 15,* 41–50.

Stoddard, F. J., Norman, D. K., & Murphy, M. (1989). A diagnostic outcome study of children and adolescents with severe burns. *Journal of Trauma, 29,* 471–477.

Sutherland, S. (1988). Burned adolescents' descriptions of their coping strategies. *Heart and Lung, 17,* 150–157.

Tarnowski, K. J., Rasnake, L. K., & Drabman, R. S. (1987). Behavioral assessment and treatment of pediatric burn injuries: A review. *Behavior Therapy, 18,* 417–441.

Tarnowski, K. J., Rasnake, L. K., Linscheid, T. R., & Mulick, J. A. (1989a). Behavioral adjustment of burn victims. *Journal of Pediatric Psychology, 14,* 607–615.

Tarnowski, K. J., Rasnake, L. K., Linscheid, T. R., & Mulick, J. A. (1989b). Ecobehavioral characteristics of a pediatric burn injury unit. *Journal of Applied Behavior Analysis, 22,* 101–109.

Tarnowski, K. J., Rasnake, L. K., Gavaghan-Jones, M. P., & Smith, L. (1991). Psychosocial sequelae of pediatric burn injuries: A review. *Clinical Psychology Review, 11,* 371–398.

Varni, J. W., Bessman, C. A., Russo, D. C., & Cataldo, M. F. (1980). Behavioral management of chronic pain in children: Case study. *Archives of Physical Medicine and Rehabilitation, 61,* 375–378.

Vernon, D. T. A., & Thompson, R. H. (1993). Research on the effect of experimental interventions on children's behavior after hospitalization: A review and synthesis. *Developmental and Behavioral Pediatrics, 14,* 36–49.

Vigliano, A., Hart, L. W., & Singer, F. (1964). Psychiatric sequelae of old burns in children and their parents. *American Journal of Orthopsychiatry, 34,* 753–761.

Watson, E. J., & Johnson, A. M. (1958). The emotional significance of acquired physical disfigurement in children. *American Journal of Orthopsychiatry, 28,* 85–97.

West, D. P., & Shuck, J. M. (1978). Emotional problems of the severely burned patient. *Surgical Clinics of North America, 58,* 1189–1204.

White, S., & Kamples, G. (1990). Dietary noncompliance in pediatric patients in the burn unit. *Journal of Burn Care and Rehabilitation, 11,* 167–174.

Wilson, G. R., Buckland, R., & Sully, L. (1988). Childhood illness as an aetiological factor in burns. *Burns, 14,* 237–238.

Wright, L., & Fulwiler, R. (1974). Long range emotional sequelae of burns: Effects of children and their mothers. *Pediatric Research, 8,* 931–934.

Zabin, M. A., & Melamed, B. G. (1980). Relationship between parental discipline and children's ability to cope with stress. *Journal of Behavioral Assessment, 2,* 17–38.

Zide, B., & Pardoe, R. (1976). The use of behavior modification therapy in a recalcitrant burned child. *Plastic and Reconstructive Surgery, 57,* 378–382.

4

Long-Term Psychosocial Sequelae

KENNETH J. TARNOWSKI
and L. KAYE RASNAKE

INTRODUCTION

Recent advances in the medical care of burns have resulted in an increased survival rate for pediatric and adult burn victims (see Fratianne & Brandt, this volume). Although technological and surgical innovations have resulted in reduced mortality rates, purportedly there has been a concomitant increase in the physical and psychosocial morbidity associated with the treatment and rehabilitation of pediatric burn patients (e.g., debridement, extended hospitalization) (Tarnowski, McGrath, Calhoun, & Drabman, 1987). Pediatric burn survivors must often live with permanent disfigurement and physical disabilities (Hurt & Tarnowski, 1990; Tarnowski & Brown, in press-a,b; Tarnowski & Rasnake, 1989; Tarnowski, Rasnake, & Drabman, 1987). In addition, the parents and uninjured siblings of pediatric burn survivors are considered to be an at-risk population as they must face the numerous challenges associated with the traumatic injury of a family member.

KENNETH J. TARNOWSKI • Department of Psychology, University of South Florida, Fort Myers, Florida 33919. **L. KAYE RASNAKE** • Department of Psychology, Denison University, Granville, Ohio 43023.

Behavioral Aspects of Pediatric Burns, edited by Kenneth J. Tarnowski. Plenum Press, New York, 1994.

Several studies have examined the postburn psychological adjustment of adult burn victims (see review by Patterson *et al.*, 1993). Andreasen and colleagues reported that 20% of adult survivors exhibit mild adjustment problems while an additional 10% display moderate or more severe psychological difficulties (Andreasen & Norris, 1972; Andreasen, Norris, & Hartford, 1971). Malt (1980) reviewed the literature and concluded that approximately 30% of victims exhibit long-term problems. A more recent comprehensive review of the adult burn literature by Patterson *et al.* (1993) cited evidence to support the notion that the majority of adult burn patients (e.g., 90%) adjust quite well to their injuries. Although many patients demonstrate clinically significant distress following severe burn injury, the majority of such reactions appear to be transient.

Recently, increased attention has been devoted to assessing the multiple problems of pediatric burn victims (Tarnowski, McGrath *et al.*, 1987; Tarnowski & Rasnake, 1989; Tarnowski *et al.*, 1987; Tarnowski, Rasnake, Linscheid, & Mulick, 1989a,b). A recent review of the behavioral assessment and treatment literature by Tarnowski *et al.* (1987) revealed that there exists a small but developing data base concerning clinical interventions for acute problems frequently exhibited by pediatric burn victims (e.g., distress during medical procedures, consummatory behavior, sleep-related problems, and self-excoriation). Unfortunately, little attention has been devoted to increasing our understanding of the long-term psychosocial sequelae associated with pediatric burn injuries. Once concerns about acute survival have been resolved, persistent and predictable questions about long-term sequelae emerge. Although such questions will be directed at a variety of professionals (e.g., surgeons, nurses), mental health professionals will ultimately bear the greatest responsibility for addressing such concerns in an informed manner.

The purpose of the chapter is to provide a substantive and methodological review of the research literature addressing the psychosocial outcome of childhood burn injuries. The chapter is an updated version of the recent review by Tarnowski, Rasnake, Gavaghan-Jones, and Smith (1991).* The first section details the results of studies that have focused on the adjustment of burned children following burn injuries. The second section reports on studies that have focused on parental and/or family adjustment following child injury.

*This chapter is based on an article by Tarnowski, Rasnake, Gavaghan-Jones, and Smith that appeared in *Clinical Psychology Review*, *11*, 371–398. Used with permission of Pergamon Press.

CHILD STUDIES

A variety of approaches have been used to study the psychosocial adjustment of children who have sustained burn injuries. A subset of studies have used school and vocational variables to index long-term outcome. Other studies have examined specific symptomatology such as anxiety, depression, withdrawal, and impaired self-concept. Unfortunately, much of the information on the long-term adjustment of children is derived from uncontrolled case studies. However, these case reports are of importance from both historical and contemporary perspectives, as they have served as the foundation from which much of the existing clinical lore about long-term sequelae has been derived. Discussion of these reports is followed by presentation of larger sample investigations, most of which have improved methodological rigor.

In an early case report, Watson and Johnson (1958) examined the ego responses of children who had sustained traumatic bodily injury. Based on clinical observations and psychiatric interviews, it was reported that the children frequently anticipated rejection, expressed anger and guilt, and wished that others experienced mutilation. They concluded that serious physical threat disrupts personality integration resulting in hostility and anger. More recently, a similar conclusion, at least for adolescent patients, was reached by Stoddard (1982) who examined the impact of severe burns on the body image development of three children of different ages. Using clinical data, Stoddard asserted that children burned before the age of 18 months incorporated the burn into their body image, school-aged children recognized a bodily change and grieved the loss, and adolescents tended to respond to burns with anger, anxiety, and guilt. In another case report, Stoddard and O'Connell (1983) noted that severely burned young children coped remarkably well and failed to exhibit chronic dysphoric symptomatology.

Using a slightly older population, Sutherland (1988) evaluated the postburn adjustment of eight subjects (age 13–20 years, M = 18) with a range of injury of 10–85% total body surface area (TBSA) (M = 42%). The minimum amount of time postburn was 14 months and the maximum was 476 months (M = 28 months). All subjects reported continued "phobic neurosis" related to events associated with the burn injury. Gender differences were identified with women being much less comfortable with public display of scars. Although an uncontrolled study with a limited sample, the authors suggested that the adolescents generally had healthy postburn adjustment as evidenced by report that they had resumed preburn or age-appropriate activities.

Using a semistructured interview, Riss, Andersen, Pederson, and Hall (1992) collected information on the psychosocial status of 25 patients (12–58 years of age) 7 to 21 years postinjury. Three groups were identified based on age at the time of injury. Two groups are appropriate for consideration here: adults burned in childhood and over 16 years of age at the time of the interview ($N = 8$), and the children less than 16 years of age at the time of the interview ($N = 3$). TBSA for these subjects ranged from 30 to 49% and all burns were second and third degree. No behavior disorders were identified in the sample. Two subjects reported that the injury had adversely affected their sibling relationship and six subjects reported peer taunting. Nine of the eleven subjects reported no opposite-sex relationship difficulties; four reported social problems when scars were visible. The authors of this uncontrolled investigation suggest a positive prognosis for individuals who had suffered childhood burn injuries.

Clarke and Martin (1978) examined the adjustment of 56 subjects (ages 13–21 years) who had sustained burn injuries 1 to 16 years prior to the interview. Unfortunately, neither the prevalence of adjustment problems nor the content of the interview were reported. The authors noted several factors believed to be related to positive postburn adjustment. These variables included lack of visible injuries, young age at time of burn, rural community residence, and families with extensive social support networks. At 1-year follow-up, Giljohann (1979) noted other variables thought to be associated with positive outcome: resilient premorbid personalities, completed surgical reconstruction, regular visitation by families, and treatment of the child by family as a normal family member. Facial scarring was judged to be an important obstacle to attainment of adequate adjustment.

A major methodological problem that plagues research in the area concerns the premorbid psychopathology that may be present in pediatric burn victims. Basically, the issue is that if one assesses the adjustment of burn victims following their injury, one cannot be certain that any detected psychopathology is a function of the behavioral and emotional sequelae of the burn injury or reflects maintenance or exacerbation of psychopathological conditions that existed prior to injury. Two case reports have examined the impact of preburn adjustment and family functioning on children's postburn adjustment. Quinby and Bernstein (1971) presented a series of seven case studies, approximately one-half of which came from disorganized or marginally functional families. Outcome assessment was based on projective testing and staff reports. Cases were followed for varying durations and the authors concluded that: (1) dramatic regressive behavior may occur during hospitalization but is not necessarily predictive of later adjustment, (2) a subset of children experience a tragic future following burns, particularly if they live in maladjusted families, and (3) crisis intervention may be needed but is often spurned because of denial of problems by family members. Seligman, Carroll, and MacMillan (1972) evaluated four burned children between the ages of 5 and 13 years. Through clinical observations and review of psychosocial medical histories, the children's early development and preburn personality, emotional responses to the injury and hospitalization, and long-term adjustment to the physical and emotional trauma of burns were assessed. Seligman *et al.* reported that familial and individual emotional problems were evident premorbidly and related to the occurrence of the burn injuries.

In general, case studies suggest that burned children evidence marked psychopathology. However, these conclusions do not appear to be warranted given the serious methodological limitations inherent in these reports. In essence, anecdotal clinical descriptions of a small number of patients are offered as evidence. Nonstandardized assessment methods were generally used, the contents of which were not reported. No control subjects were evaluated, little information was presented concerning patient characteristics, and length of patient follow-up varied widely. The cases presented may represent a biased sample of burned children as they were selected, in some instances, to illustrate specific clinical processes. In summary, the validity and generalizability of findings from these case presentations is severely limited.

Other investigations of the adjustment of burned children have used standardized assessment instruments and enhanced methodological controls. The characteristics of these study samples also vary widely in terms of participant ages, burn severity, and disfigurement.

Using a nonburned comparison group, Jesse, Strickland, Leeper, and Wales (1992) explored the impact of burn injuries on body image. Five years postinjury, the body image scores of 32 pediatric burn patients (ages 5–15 years) were compared with those of an age-matched normal control group. The body image (as assessed through human figure drawings) of the burn-injured children did not differ significantly from those of the controls. This is particularly interesting given that 50% of the children had burns over their entire body and 42% had suffered burns of 51% or greater TBSA. The authors suggest that body image forms the core for the development of self-concept, and these children appear to be at minimal risk for impaired self-concept. However, no multidimensional index of self-concept was used in the investigation and the developmental impact of injuries sustained at different points in the life span was not assessed.

Orr, Reznikoff, and Smith (1989) extended this analysis in a study of patient-rated body image, self-esteem, and depression in a sample of adolescents and young adults who had been burned within 10 years of the study. The mean age at time of burn was 12.7 years (range 4–20), the mean time since burn injury was 5.2 years (range 0–10), the mean TBSA was 27.3% (range 1–90), and 75% of the subjects sustained burns in socially sensitive areas (e.g., face, hands). A participant response rate of 61% was reported. Analyses revealed that perceived social support was associated with a more positive body image, higher levels of self-esteem, and less depression. Significant gender differences were reported (higher body image scores for boys and young men). Of interest was the failure to find a relationship between the assessment variables and burn TBSA or location. In general, the findings underscore the clinical importance of social support for burn-injured adolescents and young adults.

One outcome of interest is the degree to which burned children (and adults) function in educational and occupational realms. Chang and Herzog (1976) compared the pre- and postburn life status of 51 individuals with particular emphasis on school and job adjustment. Subjects were 37 males and 14 females between the ages of 1 and 88 years. The average duration of follow-up was 25.6 months postburn and average TBSA was 31.2%. Fifty-seven percent of the sample had involvement of the hands or face. Interviews were conducted to obtain information concerning the burn injury, preburn status, and postburn status. Results indicated that the average duration of absence from school was 6 months and the majority of children required special tutoring while in the hospital. Of those children in school, 75% reported involvement with preburn peer groups. Depression was commonly associated with burns of the hands and face but began to diminish 1 year postinjury. Academic functioning was also studied by DeWet, Cywes, Davies, and Riet (1979). Their sample included 25 pediatric burn patients (10 males, 15 females) ranging in age from 6 months to 11 years at the time of injury, and 4 to 22 years at follow-up. Extent of burns ranged from 30 to 75% TBSA. An unstructured patient and parent interview was conducted that focused on scholastic achievement and employment history. Based on end-of-year exam grades and employment stability, 12% of the patients were rated as having made good adjustment, 60% reasonable adjustment, and 28% poor adjustment (not attending school or unemployed during the 6 months preceding the interview). Additionally, 40% of the subjects were reported to be aggressive, 28% depressed, and 32% withdrawn. A major weakness of this study is that no standardized ratings or clinical diagnoses of psychopathology were obtained. Although grades and employment data are acceptable functional outcome measures, criteria for establishing "good" versus "poor" adjustment and interrater reliability data were not reported. Based on the results of these studies, it is difficult to discern the risk that burn-injured children may be at for academic impairment.

In an effort to assess problems encountered by burn-injured children on reentry into social settings, Molinaro (1978) evaluated the social behavior of 18 children, ranging in age from 7 to 19 years. Subjects had completed at least one full semester of school following their burn injury and participated in several open-ended interviews designed to determine withdrawal behavior in socially significant areas (e.g., school, play). Children were classified into one of three groups: no, moderate, and severe withdrawal. Results indicated that 8 children showed marked withdrawal and 4 showed moderate withdrawal. No relationship was established between withdrawal and severity of burn, location of scars, sex, or facial/hand disfigurement. Four of the six children in the "no withdrawal" group had experienced previous psychiatric intervention, while only 1 of the 12 other children had received such services. Molinaro concluded that significant problems are encountered by children with regard to social reentry, particularly in the area of peer relationships. It was further suggested that psychiatric intervention is associated with better adjustment. Study limitations include lack of a control group, use of subjective interview data, and selective nature of the sample (only those who were available for interview during a 1-month period). In addition, limited demographic information concerning subject characteristics (e.g., mean age, severity of burn, mean length of time since burn injury, visibility of disfigurement) prevents an evaluation of sample representativeness.

Many of the studies reviewed thus far have attempted to describe the adjustment of pediatric burn victims without benefit of standardized measures of adjustment. Using a well-validated assessment instrument, Tarnowski *et al.* (1989b) examined the relationship of a variety of biopsychosocial variables to maternal ratings of children's psychosocial adjustment in a sample of 68 (41 male, 27 female) burned children. Criteria for study inclusion were: (1) age at the time of the study greater than 2 years and less than 17 years, (2) time lapse since discharge from the burn unit greater than 1 year but less than 5 years, and (3) burn injuries involving at least 10% TBSA. Children were a mean of 8.1 years of age and had a mean TBSA of 18.72%. Mothers rated their children's behavioral adjustment using the Achenbach Child Behavior Checklist (CBCL; Achenbach & Edelbrock, 1983). Regression analyses were conducted to examine the contribution of demographic (sex, age, SES, and family intactness), burn injury (TBSA, percent full-thickness burns, percent partial-thickness burns, days hospitalized, and number of body parts injured), and injury visibility (presence of facial burns, burns on other visible body parts) variables to four CBCL summary scores. Time since the burn injury was additionally controlled for in all analyses. Regardless of which classification criterion was used, the models accounted for little variance and a consistent pattern of nonsignificant findings emerged. Examination of the means for the four CBCL summary scores (T-transformed) revealed that all scores were well within normal limits. However, examination of the frequency distribution of total behavior problem scores revealed that 13% of the sample had T-scores in excess of 70. Results of this study are limited in that no data were available concerning children's premorbid level of psychosocial adjustment and findings were based exclusively on maternal reports of child behavioral adjustment. Finally, the study focused on what might be viewed as intermediate outcome (1–5 years postinjury).

Stoddard, Norman, and Murphy (1989) examined the incidence of psychiatric disorders among pediatric burn victims using a standardized interview schedule and DSM-III criteria (American Psychiatric Association, 1980). Thirty children were studied ranging in age from 7 to 19 years. Time since burns ranged from 6 months to 17 years (M = 8.86 years) and TBSA ranged from 5 to 95% (M = 38.4%). Children and parents were interviewed regarding the child's symptomatology and diagnoses were made for past and present disorders and for the presence of full or partial symptom complex. The reported incidence of phobias (20–30%), overanxious disorders (36.7%), depression (10–50%), posttraumatic stress disorder (53.3%), oppositional disorder (23%), enuresis (30%), and encopresis (10%) were quite high. Factors related to more pronounced psychopathology included larger TBSA, severe disfigurement, low SES, and parental emotional problems. It should be noted that estimates of the incidence of psychopathology included children who: (1) displayed partial symptoms and who did not meet diagnostic criteria for a disorder and (2) exhibited symptoms at any time since injury, not necessarily at the time of follow-up. The percentage of children displaying full syndromes at the time of follow-up was much lower (0–30%). Finally, a high study participation refusal rate (35%) may have resulted in a biased sample and results await replication.

An extension of this investigation was reported by Stoddard, Norman, Murphy, and Beardslee (1989). The burned victims described in Stoddard, Norman, and Murphy (1989) were contrasted with a matched group of noninjured controls using child and parent DICA as dependent variables. The authors reported that 74% of the burned children met the criteria for a DSM-III diagnosis at the time of the interview as compared with 40% of the comparison group; 87% of the burned children met the criteria for a diagnosis in their lifetime as compared with 53% of the controls. Burn-injured children were significantly more likely to currently meet criteria for an anxiety disorder than controls.

Several studies have documented that nondisabled individuals have more negative attitudes toward disabled individuals with physical disfigurement as opposed to those without such deformation (English & Palla, 1971; MacDonald & Hall, 1969). In general, greater social discrimination is associated with visible disabilities (Salfilios-Rothschild, 1970). Studies have examined the relationship between location and severity of burn injuries and postburn adjustment. Several studies have focused on the visibility of injuries particularly facial scarring, and their relationship to adjustment. Goldberg, Bernstein, and Crosby (1975) assessed the relationships among facial disfigurement, career plans, and rehabilitation outlook in 34 adolescents (10 female, 24 male) who had sustained burn injury. Criteria for participation required that the 12- to 18-year-old subjects exhibit some facial scarring and be 1 year or more postinjury at the time of study recruitment. Results indicated that the severity of facial disfigurement correlated with rehabilitation outlook and career plan variables. In general, subjects with more severe disfigurement had vague plans and less optimism about their futures. Goldberg *et al.* (1975) postulated that disfigurement alters children's self-image which, in turn, impacts their view of the future including formulation of career plans. An earlier study by Goldberg (1974) compared two groups of disabled children who differed with respect to the visibility of their disability. Burned children ($N = 22$) ages 11–15 years were assessed at an average of 5.5 years postinjury (range: 2–11 years). All burned children had facial disfigurement. The contrast group consisted of 26 children ages 11–15 who had congenital heart disease (e.g., aortic stenosis). Results indicated that children in the congenital heart disease group scored higher (better adjusted) on the vocational aspirations and origin of interest in vocational aspiration variables. Goldberg (1974) interpreted this finding as evidence that an invisible congenital handicap had a less deleterious effect on vocational maturity in comparison with a visible disability. Although this is an important finding, this study has several methodological weaknesses that reduce confidence in the validity of this interpretation of the data. SES was not controlled for in this investigation and it is likely that the burned subjects were from a lower SES group than were children in the congenital heart group. Subjects may have differed on a variety of other demographic and subjective characteristics in addition to those assessed. A multivariate analysis would have been the preferred analysis. Adjusting the alpha level for the number of comparisons (Bonferroni correction) resulted in no significant group differences.

Other studies have suggested that burned children with visible disfigurement have more adjustment difficulties. Love, Byrne, Roberts, Browne, and Brown (1987) examined psychosocial and biological variables associated with adjustment in 42 adult survivors of childhood burn injury. All subjects scored within the normal range on an index of psychosocial adjustment to illness. Burn severity failed to explain significant variability. Patients were divided into high and low adjustment groups (median split) and analyses indicated that less well adjusted patients were more disfigured and less socially engaged. The majority of patients were preadolescent at the time of injury (*M* = 12.7 years) and, thus, burns occurred at a developmental stage when body image and peer acceptance are of critical import. Although the representativeness of the study was established via comparison with nonparticipants, the number of statistical contrasts in this investigation was high (29), study *N* limited, and multivariate analyses should have been employed.

In a similar study of the status of adolescent and adult survivors burned as children, Blakeney, Herndon, Desai, Beard, and Wales-Seale (1988) examined subjects aged 14–32 years who presented with a mean TBSA of 55.3% and mean third-degree TBSA of 44.7%. Subjects were divided into three groups based on extent of burn. A battery of standardized instruments were used. No test differences emerged in contrast between burned subjects and normative test samples. In addition, no differences were found among the three groups of study patients. Age at time of injury, gender, intelligence, facial disfigurement, attitude toward self/body failed to relate to psychological disturbance. Aspects of family environment (cohesion and independence) were found to be related to disturbance. Subjects with heightened psychopathology viewed their families as less cohesive, independent, assertive, and self-sufficient than less disturbed patients. Generalizability of these findings is limited as no separate comparisons were conducted for adult versus adolescent subjects. Contrasts between patients with and without facial burns were limited because of the small number of subjects (*N* = 4) without facial injuries.

In a follow-up to their 1988 investigation, Blakeney, Portman, and Rutan (1990) attempted to further evaluate the impact of family functioning, burn severity, and time since injury on postburn adjustment. Subjects (*N* = 44) were 12 years or older (*M* = 17 years) and 1 year or more postinjury (*M* = 7 years). All subjects had sustained third-degree burns of at least 40% TBSA (*M* = 60%). Multiple regression analyses revealed that differences in psychological adjustment were accounted for largely by three family variables: cohesion, conflict, and independence. Subjects were divided into good and poor adjustment groups. Poorly adjusted patients described their families as passive dependent, constrictive, and less cohesive. In addition, the poorly adjusted group differed from the well-adjusted subsample in terms of time since injury (6 years versus 10 years, respectively). Findings provide additional support that family functioning appears crucial in mediating adjustment. Findings also suggest that the process of adjustment may be lengthy and that better adjustment may be found as a function of time since burn injury.

Using a prospective longitudinal design, Beard, Herndon, and Desai (1989) reported on six severely burned children (>80% TBSA) who were followed for a 2-year period. Subjects were of primary school age and were 0–16 months postburn at the initial assessment. Although no criteria were specified, the authors found that children exhibited below-average age-related development at the time of initial evaluation, with one-half of the subjects rated average at follow-up (16 months to 3 years postburn), and two additional children rated as average at extended follow-up (3–5 years postburn). Self-esteem and behavior rating data indicated that all but one subject evidenced adequate scores at follow-up. Investigator qualitative ratings of parental assistance suggested that "facilitative" parenting resulted in more rapid clinical improvement. Such nonblinded qualitative global ratings might be considered retrospective and subjective in nature. However, the study does touch on a neglected topic in this literature, namely, parent effects on child psychosocial sequelae.

Knudson-Cooper (1981) examined the relationship between severe childhood burns and three measures of adjustment in young adults: social integration (social involvement and education/career status), emotional adjustment, and self-esteem. Eighty-nine subjects (41 male, 48 female) between the ages of 16 and 28 participated. Time elapsed since the burn ranged from 4 to 23 years and the mean patient TBSA was 27%. One independent variable of interest in this study was the cosmetic impact of the burns, both in terms of severity of disfigurement and location of the scars. These data were obtained using photographs from patients' medical records. In terms of social integration, a rough nonstatistical comparison of percentages for Knudson-Cooper's sample and U.S. census data indicated little difference between the burned responders and the U.S. population in terms of SES, education, marriage, social involvement, and other demographic indices. For self-esteem, the obtained mean was slightly, but not significantly, above the mean reported for the normative standardization sample. Self-esteem was not found to be significantly related to sex, TBSA, age at burn, time since burn, or facial burn involvement. Results suggested that severe burns had little or no adverse impact on social and emotional adjustment.

One specific subgroup of burned children that has received little attention is the massive burn-injured patient. With marked improvements in the medical management of thermal injuries, many of these children now survive extensive injury. Herndon *et al.* (1986) studied the quality of life of 12 children (9 males, 3 females) who had survived such injuries. The children's burns involved 80–95% TBSA (71–89% third-degree burns). Children ranged in age from 0.8 to 12.4 years at the time of injury and were evaluated 0.8 to 2.8 years following discharge. Psychological assessment consisted of a standard child mental status evaluation conducted by two independent psychoanalysts, a parent interview, and parent completion of the Louisville Behavior Checklist (LBC; Miller, 1967). The psychoanalysts rated each child in the areas of body image, self-esteem, anxiety level, fears, interpersonal relationships, and active mastery and adaptation on a 5-point scale. Eleven of the twelve subjects were rated as having moderate to severe problems in all areas. Conversely, data from the LBC suggested a much lower incidence of behavioral problems.

Summary

There is little consensus among the reviewed child studies concerning the adjustment of children following burn injury. There is suggestive evidence of impairment in scholastic and vocational adjustment (Chang & Herzog, 1976). Similarly, Molinaro (1978) reported that children and adolescents had difficulties in social adjustment and resumption of relationships with peers following burn injuries. These investigations also noted significant levels of depression, withdrawal, delinquency, and aggressiveness. Conversely, in a study using a standardized behavioral rating scale, only a minority of burned children and adolescents were found to exhibit problems at follow-up (Tarnowski *et al.*, 1989b). Beard *et al.* (1989) found 83% of subjects to have intact self-esteem. Mixed results also emerged from studies that assessed the impact of burn injury visibility, especially facial burns. Several studies found disfiguring burns to be associated with depression, vague career plans, increased psychopathology, and lower vocational aspirations (Chang & Herzog, 1976, Giljohann, 1979; Goldberg, 1974; Love *et al.*, 1987; Salfilios-Rothschild, 1970; Stoddard, Norman, & Murphy, 1989), while other studies did not find injury visibility to be a significant factor in adjustment (Blakeney *et al.*, 1988; Jesse *et al.*, 1992; Knudson-Cooper, 1981; Molinaro, 1978; Tarnowski *et al.*, 1989b). Six studies failed to identify a significant relationship between burn severity and psychosocial adjustment (Blakeney *et al.*, 1988; Giljohann, 1979; Goldberg, 1974; Goldberg *et al.*, 1975; Love *et al.*, 1987; Molinaro, 1978). Studies have reported data supporting gender differences in self-esteem (Sutherland, 1988) and body image (Orr *et al.*, 1989). In general, demographic variables (e.g., age, sex, SES, family intactness) failed to influence the results of several other studies (Blakeney *et al.*, 1988; Knudson-Cooper, 1981; Molinaro, 1978; Tarnowski *et al.*, 1989b). However, family factors and social support have been found to relate to adjustment (Beard *et al.*, 1989; Blakeney *et al.*, 1990; Orr *et al.*, 1989). Finally, conflicting findings were obtained within one study that examined children with massive burn injuries (Herndon *et al.*, 1986). Psychoanalysts' ratings indicated a high level of psychopathology, whereas results using a standardized rating scale indicated a much lower incidence of psychosocial maladjustment.

The methodological shortcomings of the reviewed studies preclude one from being able to establish generalized and definitive conclusions concerning the psychological sequelae of pediatric burns. In general, sample sizes have been small, participation response rates have been poor, and sample representativeness has been questionable. A major weakness of some studies is that child and adult patients were not considered separately (Chang & Herzog, 1976). In other studies, there is insufficient information concerning sample characteristics and demographics (Goldberg *et al.*, 1975; Molinaro, 1978). Few studies made any attempt to assess children's premorbid level of psychopathology. Only two investigations employed a control group (Goldberg, 1974; Stoddard, Norman, Murphy, & Beardslee, 1989). The control group in the Goldberg (1974) study, however, was not matched with the burned sample on the important variable of SES (Goldberg, 1974). Eight studies compared burned children's scores on standardized measures against the test standardization norms (Beard *et al.*, 1989; Blakeney *et al.*, 1988, 1990; Herndon *et al.*, 1986; Knudson-Cooper, 1981; Love *et al.*, 1987; Orr *et al.*, 1989; Tarnowski *et al.*, 1989b). This strategy was not possible in many instances as nonstandardized assessment measures were employed (Chang & Herzog, 1976; Clarke & Martin, 1978; DeWet *et al.*, 1979; Giljohann, 1979; Herndon *et al.*, 1986; Knudson-Cooper, 1981; Miller *et al.*, 1976; Molinaro, 1978). One study, in fact, stated that no direct questions were asked with respect to psychological symptomatology and that this information was obtained solely through incidental report (DeWet *et al.*, 1979). Six studies used structured or semistructured interviews (Goldberg, 1974; Goldberg *et al.*, 1975; Riss *et al.*, 1992; Stoddard, Norman, & Murphy, 1989; Stoddard, Norman, Murphy, & Beardslee, 1989; Sutherland, 1988), but only three reported interrater reliability data (Goldberg, 1974; Stoddard, Norman, & Murphy, 1989; Stoddard, Norman, Murphy, & Beardslee, 1989). Finally, the multiple statistical comparisons used in some studies capitalized on chance findings (Goldberg, 1974; Love *et al.*, 1987). Subject and study characteristics for these investigations are presented in Table 1.

FAMILY STUDIES

A logical extension of studies that assess children's adjustment involves the assessment of parental responses to children's burn injuries, hospitalization, and extended medical treatment. The focus on maternal adjustment is quite appropriate given evidence suggesting that children's

Table 1. Studies of the Psychosocial Adjustment of Burned Children and Their Families

Study	Subjects	% burns	Time since injury	Assessment procedures	Design	Results
Child studies						
Watson & Johnson (1958)	N = 5 3.5–14 years 2 males	NR[a]	NR	Clinical obs. and interview	Uncontrolled case study	Children's play showed revenge fantasies, anger, anticipation of rejection, disruption of personality integration, desire to see siblings suffer
Quinby & Bernstein (1971)	N = 7 7–13 years 3 males	NR	NR	1. Clinical obs. 2. Projective tests	Uncontrolled case study	Pts had different outcome that appeared to be a function of family functioning and premorbid adjustment
Seligman *et al*. (1972)	N = 4 5–13 years 1 male	% 3rd = 38–53%	Hospital course	Clinical obs. and interview	Uncontrolled case study	Family discord predated injury; numerous psychosomatic complaints during hospitalization but declined at 3–4 months follow-up
Goldberg (1974)	Burned N = 22 11–15 years 15 males Heart dis. N = 26 11–15 years 13 males	NR	2–11 years	Goldberg Scale of Vocational Development	Contrasted groups	Children with heart disease scored higher than burned children on vocational aspiration index

Goldberg *et al.* (1975)	N = 34 12–18 years 24 males	NR	> 1 year	Goldberg Scale of Vocational Development	Within group; correlational	Severity of facial disfigurement related to career plans and rehabilitation outlook
Miller *et al.* (1976)	N = 17 17 months–15 years	>30%	1 year	Unstructured parent interview	Within group; descriptive	Subjects' postburn adjustment judged to be adequate in school and no problems with peer or body image
Clark & Martin (1978)	N = 56 13–21 years 28 males	NR	1–16 years	Unstructured pt and parent interview	Within group; descriptive	Positive outcome associated with earlier age at time of injury, minimal scarring, living in rural community, extended social support network
Molinaro (1978)	N = 18 7–19 years	NR	Had attended ≥1 semester of school	Semistructured interview	Within group; descriptive	No relationship found between burn injury variables and withdrawal, 8 pts markedly, 4 moderately, 6 not withdrawn
DeWet *et al.* (1979)	N = 25 1–22 years 10 males	BSA = 30–75%	2–11 years	Unstructured pt and parent interview	Within group; descriptive	12% of subjects had "good," 60% "reasonable," 28% "poor" adjustment
Chang & Herzog (1976)	N = 51 1–88 years 37 males	BSA M = 31%, 57% with 2nd and 3rd	M = 26 months, SD = 12 months	Structured interview	Within group; correlational	75% of pts continued with preburn peer group; facial and hand burns associated with greater depression; % BSA related to duration of disability; 14% adolescents delinquent

(continued)

Table 1. (*Continued*)

Study	Subjects	% burns	Time since injury	Assessment procedures	Design	Results
Giljohann (1979)	*N* = 18 adolescents	NR	NR	Unstructured pt and parent interview	Within group; descriptive	8 pts rehabilitated in areas of work, home, leisure; 3 pts rehabilitated in two areas, 3 pts in one area, 3 in no areas
Knudson-Cooper (1981)	*N* = 89 16–28 years 41 males	BSA = 2–89%, *M* = 27%	4–23 years	1. Self-report 2. Coopersmith Self-Esteem 3. Medical records	Within group; correlational; contrasted group (test norms, U.S. census data)	Burned pts self-esteem not significantly different from normative sample; rating of cosmetic impact not related to self-esteem; pts did not differ from census data on social integration
Stoddard (1982)	*N* = 3 18 months–15 years 2 males	% 2nd & 3rd = 10–67%	Hospital course	1 Unstructured pt and parent interviews 2. Projective tests 3. Dream analysis	Uncontrolled case study	Pts of various ages incorporate burns into body image in different manner
Stoddard & O'Connell (1983)	*N* = 3 1–6 years 2 males	BSA = 30–95%	NR	Clinical obs.	Uncontrolled case study	Pts did not exhibit chronic dysphoria
Herndon *et al.* (1986)	*N* = 12 8 months–12 years 9 males	BSA = 80–90%, % 3rd = 71–89%	0.8–2.8 years	1. Mental status 2. Parent interview 3. Louisville Checklist	Within group; descriptive	Psychoanalyst rating indicated 11/12 children severe problems; rating scale data showed ⅓ with problems

Love *et al.* (1987)	*N* = 42 adults (>16 years) burned as children	38.1% major (BSA *M* = 14.2%), 61.9% minor/moderate (BSA *M* = 7%)	Major 6.5 years, minor 7.7 years	1. Medical records 2. Billings & Moos Coping Scale 3. Participation in Social and Recreation Activities 4. Social Support Scale 5. Psychosocial Adjustment to Illness Scale	Multiple within groups; correlational	Burn severity failed to explain variability in assessment measures; subanalyses indicated that less well adjusted had more disfigurement and less socially engaged
Blakeney *et al.* (1988)	*N* = 37 14–32 years *M* = 19.6 years 22 males	BSA 5–91%, *M* = 55.3%, 3rd = 44.7%	2–31 years, *M* = 11.8 years	1. Minnesota Multiphasic Personality Inventory 2. Suicide Probability Scale 3. Body Attitude Scale 4. Family Environment Scale	Within group; correlational	No differences emerged between subjects grouped according to severity; most disturbed had poorer family adjustment
Beard *et al.* (1989)	*N* = 6 primary school age	>80%	0–5 years	1. Standard interview 2. Piers-Harris Self Esteem Inventory 3. Self-drawing 4. Incomplete Sentences for Children 5. Louisville Behavior Checklist	Within group; descriptive	By 16 months to 3 years postburn 50% demonstrated average developmental progression and 83% showed high or moderate levels of self-esteem; adjustment related to parental behaviors

(*continued*)

Table 1. (*Continued*)

Study	Subjects	% burns	Time since injury	Assessment procedures	Design	Results
Orr *et al.* (1989)	$N = 121$ 14–27 years	1–90%, M = 27.3%	0–10 years, M = 5.2 years	1. Beck Depression Inventory 2. Rosenberg Self-Esteem Scale 3. Perceived Social Support Inventory for Family and Friends 4. Semantic Differential	Within group; correlational	Perceived social support predictive of body image, self-esteem, depression; males showed more positive body image; relationship between body image and self-esteem, and between body image and depression
Stoddard, Norman, & Murphy (1989)	$N = 30$ 7–19 years $M = 13.3$ years 13 males	BSA = 5–95%, M = 38.4%	6 months to 17 years, M = 8.9 years	Diagnostic Interview Schedule for Children	Within group; correlational	High rates of anxiety and depressive disorders; poorer adjustment related to more extensive burns, greater disfigurement, lower SES, reported parental adjustment problems
Stoddard, Norman, Murphy, & Beardslee (1989)	2 samples: 1. Burned $N = 30$; $M = 13.3$ years 2. Control $N = 30$; $M = 13.3$ years	5–95%	⩾6 months	Standardized interview: Diagnostic Interview for Children and Adolescents—Child Version and Parent Version	Contrasted groups	Burned children significantly higher rate of anxiety disorders compared with matched controls

Tarnowski *et al.* (1989b)	*N* = 68 2–16 years *M* = 8.1 years 41 males	>10%, *M* = 18.7%	>1 year but <5 years, *M* = 3.9 years	1. Medical records 2. Child Behavior Checklist	Within group; correlational	Mean adjustment ratings did not differ from nonburned children; 13% of pts clinically deviant scores; little variance accounted for on basis of variety of biopsychosocial predictor variables
Blakeney *et al.* (1990)	*N* = 44 *M* = 17 years	>40%, *M* = 60%	>1 year, *M* = 7 years	1. Interview 2. Family Environment Scale 3. Suicide Probability Scale	Within group; descriptive	50% of subjects were well adjusted; family functioning variables and time since burn injury differentiated well from poorly adjusted children
Jessee *et al.* (1992)	2 samples: 1. Burn pts *N* = 32; 5–15 years 2. Nonburned controls *N* = 32; 5–15 years	1–100%	5 years	Human Figure Drawings	Contrasted groups	No difference in body image between burned and control children
Riss *et al.* (1992)	*N* = 11 12–32 years	30–49%	7–21 years	Semistandardized interview	Within group; descriptive	Optimistic prognosis; no significant psychological impairment; high divorce rate in parents

(continued)

Table 1. *(Continued)*

Study	Subjects	% burns	Time since injury	Assessment procedures	Design	Results
Child and family studies						
Woodward (1959)	3 samples: 1. Burn pts $N = 198$; <15 years at injury 2. Sibs of pts $N = 608$ 3. Nonburned controls $N = 50$	>10%	2–6 years	1. Medical records 2. Structured parent interview 3. Teacher questionnaire	Multiple within groups; correlational	81% of mothers rated burned children disturbed; 26% rated severity of maladjustment as in need of professional intervention; disturbance not related to burn characteristics; pts siblings described as less disturbed than random controls; mothers of burned pts more disturbed than control mothers
Woodward & Jackson (1961)	2 samples: 1. Tx group $N = 71$ 2. Sample described in Woodward (1959)	>10%	>1 year	Unstructured parent interview	Contrasted groups	Emotional adjustment (global maternal judgment) of children who received social worker supportive treatment better than that of untreated burn group after 1 year
Long & Cope (1961)	$N = 19$ 9 months–17 years 17 males	NR	Hospital course	1. Psychiatric interview 2. Clinical obs.	Within group; descriptive	High incidence of family disturbance noted that predated burns. Pts often found to evidence premorbid psychopathology; regression, aggression common responses

Vigliano *et al.* (1964)	$N = 10$ 6–16 years	BSA > 15%, $M = 20\%$	>1 year	1. Medical records 2. Unstructured interview 3. Projective tests 4. Parent questionnaire	Within group; descriptive	Children reluctant to discuss disfigurement; immature drawings with weak and inadequate bodies; anxiety symptoms; mothers often depressed with marital discord; psychological disturbance in 9 pts and 8 mothers
Martin (1970)	$N = 50$ 7 months–14 years	NR	Up to 12 months	1. Unstructured interview 2. Clinical obs.	Within group; descriptive	37% younger children experiencing 1 of Bowlby's 3 stages of separation/loss; children <2 years reacted strongly to separation; fathers isolated; mothers depressed
Wright & Fulwiler (1974)	2 samples: 1. Burned $N = 12$; 8–13 years 2. Matched nonburned controls $N = 12$	BSA = 5–50%	1.5–5 years	1. PPVT 2. Bradley Self-Concept 3. Rosenweig Picture Frustration Test 4. Children's Manifest Anxiety Scale	Contrasted groups	No difference between burned pts and controls on PPVT, Rorschach, Rosenweig, or CMAS; some nonsignificant group differences on projective drawings; mothers of burned pts evidenced more psychopathology than control mothers
Sawyer *et al.* (1983)	$N = 37$ 8–16 years 19 males	BSA > 5%	>3 years	1. Semistructured pt and parent interviews 2. Child Behavior Checklist 3. Teacher Rutter Scale	Within group; correlational	Facial and hand burns associated with behavior problems among adolescents; % BSA not related to adjustment; maternal emotional disturbance and frequent geographic moves associated with adolescent psychopathology

(continued)

Table 1. (*Continued*)

Study	Subjects	% burns	Time since injury	Assessment procedures	Design	Results
Browne *et al.* (1985)	3 samples: 1. Adult: $N = 340$; >16 years; burned as adults 2. Adult: $N = 42$; >16 years; burned as children 3. Child: $N = 145$; <16 years	NR	NR	All samples: 1. Medical records 2. Billings & Moos Coping Scale 3. Participation in Social and Recreation Activities 4. Social Support Scale 5. Psychosocial Adjustment to Illness Scale Mothers, sample 3: 6. Family Environment Scale 7. Child Behavior Checklist	Multiple within groups; correlational	15.7% of child pts maladjusted; adjustment not function of burn severity; poorly adjusted from families with less religious and moral emphasis, mothers with poor adjustment and avoidance methods of coping
Byrne *et al.* (1986)	$N = 145$ Major $M =$ 8.6 years; minor $M =$ 7.9 years	Major $N = 67$, BSA $M =$ 16.1%, SD = 3.02	Major $M = 4.9$ years, minor $M = 4.8$ years	1. Child Behavior Checklist 2. Psychosocial Adjustment to Illness Scale 3. Family Environment Scale	Within group; correlational	More severe burns, longer time since burn, and higher SES associated with better adjustment

[a]NR, not reported.

responses to hospitalization and medical care are directly influenced by parental emotional states (Tarnowski & Brown, in press-b). In addition, it is clear that catastrophic illness and injury significantly impact family functioning. This section reviews those studies that have examined the adjustment of family members in addition to that of the burned child.

One of the earliest reports assessing both pediatric burn injury patients and their mothers was published by Woodward (1959). Woodward was interested in comparing the emotional adjustment of burned children with their siblings and a random control group. One hundred and ninety-eight children who had suffered burns of 10% TBSA or greater when they were less than 15 years of age participated in the study. Controls included 608 siblings and 50 random control subjects, matched for age, sex, and neighborhood distribution (SES approximation). Mothers were interviewed using a structured interview. Variables assessed included the child's current emotional adjustment and the status of children's preburn emotional adjustment based on maternal opinion and recollection of the child's prior functioning. For those children attending school, teachers were sent questionnaires developed by the authors to assess teacher perceptions of emotional and behavioral adjustment, absenteeism, school performance, and attitude. Evidence of emotional disturbance was noted for 81% of the burned children. Emotional adjustment was reportedly not correlated with age, gender, TBSA, percentage of whole skin loss, or length of hospital stay. Adjustment did correlate with frequency of parental visitation during hospitalization and maternal self-reports of emotional adjustment. Mothers of burned children reported more emotional disturbance than mothers of control children and their families were larger and poorer. In general, teacher responses were consistent with parental report of children's adjustment.

In a follow-up study, Woodward and Jackson (1961) assessed the impact of providing psychosocial support to parents (mothers) of burned children during and after the child's hospitalization. Details of their methodology were not provided. Psychosocial support was provided by social workers through an unspecified number of home visits after the burned child was discharged. Using a global subjective judgment of emotional disturbance (maternal judgment, social worker opinion), 90% of the burned children were considered to be disturbed at the time of their return home with 20% still "unsettled" at the end of 1 year. The authors concluded that this outcome compared favorably with data from the previous study by Woodward in which 81% of untreated children continued to evidence problems at 1 year postdischarge (using the same criteria to determine maladjustment). While the authors concluded that the emotional sequelae of pediatric burns can be favorably impacted, the methodological limitations of this study are considerable. The most serious problems are lack of clearly specified criteria for defining emotional disturbance, no description of the components of treatment, and exclusive reliance on global maternal impressions of child disturbance as an outcome measure. No data are provided on the number of dropouts from treatment, preburn adjustment, and important subject characteristics (e.g., SES). Thus, it is difficult to determine how representative the study sample was of the burn population.

Other studies have provided support for Woodward's (1959) findings on maternal disturbance. Both Vigliano, Hart, and Singer (1964) and Wright and Fulwiler (1974) reported high rates of maternal disturbance following pediatric burn injuries. Rate and extent of disturbance among child victims is less clear. Ten burn victims (ages 6–16 years) and their mothers were the subjects of study for Vigliano *et al.* (1964). Children had recovered from the acute phase of the burn injury (at least 15% TBSA) no less than 1 year prior to the assessment. Unstructured psychiatric interview and psychological assessment methods were used to evaluate child and maternal functioning. Psychological disturbance was reported in 90% of the children and 80% of mothers. Children were described as evidencing body image disturbance and fear of injury and harm. Mothers were described as depressed, guilty, and fearful.

Results of the Wright and Fulwiler (1974) study of the long-term consequences of burn injury for children and mothers suggested that child burn injury has a more psychologically deleterious effect on mothers than on children. Twelve burned children and their mothers were compared with a control group of subjects matched according to age, sex, SES, race, and hospitalization experience. Children and mothers were assessed with a variety of psychological measures. Assessment protocols were scored by experienced clinicians blind to subject group membership. Only 2 of the 31 child variables distinguished groups while differences emerged on 10 of the 28 maternal variables. The authors concluded that mothers of burned children experienced more emotional disturbance than did their children and that the pattern of findings may be related to premorbid parental disturbance and/or greater child resiliency.

Martin (1970) extended the investigation of child and maternal adjustment reactions to include paternal adjustment. Martin studied the relationship of parents' and children's reactions to hospitalization. Interviews were conducted with parents at the time of the injury, during hospitalization, and at 3, 6, and 12 months postinjury. Children were observed during hospitalization. Fifteen children were identified as "emotionally disturbed" premorbidly and were not included in the analysis of consequent adjustment difficulties. Consistent with Woodward (1959) and Vigliano *et al.* (1964), follow-up data suggested that 40 of the 48 children who survived

(83%) demonstrated behavioral disturbance (e.g., sleep disturbance, increased dependency, aggression) at 3 months postinjury, and 23 (48%) continued to evidence disturbance at 12 months. Martin (1970) noted that many of the fathers isolated themselves, while mothers' reactions generally paralleled those of their children. Mothers often blamed themselves for the injury, but more frequently projected blame. Martin concluded that the behavioral disturbances of burned children are related to disturbances in maternal behavior that result from the experience of the burn injury and hospitalization (e.g., loss of physical contact) and the mother's attribution of responsibility for the injury. Martin's assertion that age, stage of development, and relationship with the primary caregiver influence reactions to burn injuries and hospitalization is consistent with research in the area of children's responses to hospitalization (Katz, Kellerman, & Siegel, 1980; Maddux, Roberts, Sledden, & Wright, 1986). However, the methodological limitations of this investigation render equivocal conclusions with respect to the reactions of children to burn injuries. The anecdotal nature of this study coupled with lack of blind raters and absence of a control group limits the validity of the findings. The suggestion of such a high rate of behavioral disturbance in burned children is particularly suspect.

Rather than focusing on specific child responses to injury, other studies have attempted to assess the impact of overall family functioning on the general adjustment of the child burn victim. Sawyer, Minde, and Zuker (1983) attempted to identify variables that define the child who is at risk for burn-related adjustment problems. Children (8–11 years) and adolescents (12–16 years) ($N = 37$) were assessed using standardized parent and teacher ratings. Semistructured interviews were conducted with children and mothers. Subjects in the adolescent group were found to differ (more deviant) from the younger children on several parameters (internalizing, activity, and social scales). Twenty-two percent of the children in the younger group scored in the deviant range compared with 40% of the older patients. No significant differences were found on rating scales for children burned at different ages or who were injured at various lengths of time prior to the investigation. Parent emotional distress was defined as maternal self-report that a visit was made to a health-care provider for "bad nerves." Although the relative frequency of emotional distress in mothers was not reported, subanalyses suggested that patients with emotionally distressed mothers were more likely to obtain deviant ratings. In addition, pediatric patients with visible burn injuries, and those subjected to multiple home moves appeared to be an at-risk group. These findings do not support the notions that burn victims demonstrate improvement in their adjustment as a function of time since the injury and that age at the time of injury is a critical determinant of later adjustment.

Limitations of the study include a relatively small sample size, no data on children's premorbid adjustment, reliance on maternal reports of children's behavioral adjustment, and reliance on subjective and arbitrary criteria to define maternal emotional disturbance (report by mother that she had seen her physician because of "bad nerves").

Using similar assessment methods, findings for 145 children selected from a sample of 1385 patients admitted to a regional burn unit were presented in two reports (Browne *et al.*, 1985; Byrne *et al.*, 1986). Sixty-seven children in the sample had sustained major burn injuries (TBSA $M = 16.1\%$). This group had a mean age of 8.6 years and mean time since injury was 4.9 years. Seventy-eight children sustained minor burns (TBSA $M = 8.4\%$). These children were a mean of 7.9 years of age and time since injury was 4.8 years. Parents completed standardized psychological measurements. The prevalence of poor child behavior adjustment was estimated to be 15.7% of the sample. Children's behavioral adjustment did not vary as a function of burn severity. However, considering scores on family variables, poorly adjusted children came from families with less moral and religious emphasis and tended to have mothers with inadequate psychosocial adjustment who engaged in avoidance methods of coping, emotional distancing, and few recreational activities. Byrne *et al.* divided children into high- and low-competency groups based on the maternal rating scale data. A discriminant function analysis was used to identify the combination of biological and psychosocial variables that best distinguished the more from less competent children. An unexpected finding was that the more socially competent children had more severe burns. Byrne *et al.* speculated that these children may have received more social support from health professionals and others. Additional factors associated with greater social competence were: (1) longer time since burn, (2) mothers who viewed their child's adjustment more positively, (3) families of higher SES, (4) larger families, and (5) families with high intellectual/cultural emphasis and high participation in social/recreational activities. Collectively, these variables correctly classified 75.2% of the children. Mother's adjustment did not distinguish high and low socially competent children.

Summary

The status of children's postburn adjustment remains unclear. Time since injury has been noted to influence the extent of disturbance. As time since injury increases, some studies found that fewer subjects exhibited maladjustment (Blakeney *et al.*, 1990; Goldberg *et al.*, 1975; Martin, 1970;

Woodward, 1959). However, at least one study found evidence to the contrary (Sawyer *et al.*, 1983). The relationship between burn severity and emotional adjustment is also unclear. The unexpected finding reported by Byrne *et al.* (1986) that increased burn severity was associated with better adjustment deserves further consideration. This finding is consistent with data from other studies that have demonstrated a positive relationship between adjustment and severity/visibility of handicap (Bruhn, Hampton, & Chandler, 1971; Goldberg, 1974; Heisler & Friedman, 1981).

Additionally, family maladjustment has emerged as an important factor in the adjustment of burned children. Studies have reported high rates of guilt, depression, anxiety, and hostility in mothers of pediatric burn victims (Woodward, 1959; Wright & Fulwiler, 1974). The relationship between maternal adjustment and child adjustment is not clear. Some studies have not identified a relationship between maternal adjustment and child functioning (Byrne *et al.*, 1986; Knudson-Cooper, 1981), while others have reported evidence that poor maternal adjustment is related to child dysfunction (Skipper & Leonard, 1968; Vadaro, 1973). Other family variables such as infrequent visitation during hospitalization have been associated with poor child adjustment (Browne *et al.*, 1985). Family variables including large family size of higher SES and high social involvement have been shown to be related to good child adjustment. Again, of critical importance is the issue of premorbid child/family psychopathology (Long & Cope, 1961; Martin, 1970).

Any conclusions made about child and family responses to burn injuries based on the current literature must be tentative. Many of the studies reviewed in this section had small sample sizes or samples that may not be representative of the population. In the Browne *et al.* (1985) study, significant differences emerged between interviewed and noninterviewed subjects with respect to type of burn discharge status and years since burn injury. The authors noted that these differences "were not viewed as clinically important" (p. 33). This would appear to be rather arbitrary since time of injury has appeared as a variable of importance in other investigations. Often important subject characteristics were not reported such as SES, hand and facial involvement, and estimates of premorbid functioning (Vigliano *et al.*, 1964; Woodward, 1959). Lack of control groups (Martin, 1970; Vigliano *et al.*, 1964), or control groups not matched on important variables (e.g., SES) (Woodward, 1959), limit confidence in the reported findings. Perhaps the most pervasive criticism of this literature is that judgments of adjustment are often based on subjective maternal reports, clinical judgment, ratings by nonblinded raters, or use of idiosyncratic and nonstandardized assessment instruments.

CONCLUDING COMMENTS

It is a commonly held belief that the *majority* of burned children evidence serious adjustment problems at follow-up. This belief appears to have emerged, in part, from the results of early reports that suggested rates of psychopathology for burned children in the range of 70–80%. However, early studies consisted largely of uncontrolled case reports, and conclusions concerning psychopathology were based on anecdotal reports and subjective clinical impression. In the present chapter, we have detailed the numerous methodological problems present in the follow-up studies of burned children and their families that constrain the validity and generalization of the findings. In many cases, studies had such serious methodological problems as to render the data uninterpretable. However, several of the more recent investigations were more methodologically rigorous, and we believe that some general conclusions can be derived from the collective literature.

First, more recent studies that employed standardized assessment methods found lower rates of psychopathology than studies relying on nonstandardized assessment approaches or clinical judgment. On the basis of several studies, rates of child psychopathology on the order of 15–20% have been noted. This conclusion is globally consistent with recent estimates of psychopathology for adult burned patients (Malt, 1980; Patterson *et al.*, 1993). However, it should be noted that higher rates of psychopathology (≤ 30%) were reported in the study sample that was assessed with a structured diagnostic interview (Stoddard, Norman, & Murphy, 1989). In discussing the methodological limitations of this investigation earlier in the chapter we noted that although a relatively high percentage displayed partial symptoms, fewer children actually exhibited full syndromes. Patterson *et al.* (1993) have noted that there may be a pervasive tendency to overattribute dysfunction to burn patients. This may be largely attributable to the fact that burns are devastating injuries and that observation of patient symptoms (e.g., depressive symptoms, anxiety, marginal coping) during the acute phase (i.e., inpatient hospitalization) may lead one to erroneously predict extended psychosocial turmoil. Finally, it is important to note that, at least for adults, the incidence of severe psychological distress for burned patients appears consistent with that observed for other types of hospitalized patients (Rodin & Voshart, 1986).

To date, most investigations have considered psychopathology in either a very general (e.g., disturbed versus nondisturbed) or specific manner (e.g., presence of specific anxieties). Clearly, the use of specific psychiatric diagnostic criteria could provide a reference point for future research. However, one cautionary note should be sounded. Independent child and parent interviews often yield different findings, with parents endorsing more externalizing behavioral symptoms and children reporting more subjective symptoms (Herjanic & Reich, 1982) or parents reporting significantly fewer symptoms than children (Earls, Smith, Reich, & Jung, 1988). Earls *et al.* described a summary diagnostic procedure that helps to resolve discrepancies between informants through systematic stepwise consideration of information. For more detailed information on the use of structured diagnostic interviews, the reader is referred to Costello, Edelbrock, and Costello (1985), Gutterman, O'Brien, and Young (1987), and Welner *et al.* (1987).

Second, as previously noted, a problem that continues to plague research in this area concerns the difficulty in adequately assessing the premorbid psychopathological status of children and families. Of course, this is not only an issue for this line of research but is also of critical importance to other areas of psychopathology research. Specific to burn injuries, several adult studies have revealed that a significant proportion of patients presented with preexisting psychiatric disorders. The incidence of previous reported psychiatric history range from 28% (Brezel, Kassenbrock, & Stein, 1988) to 75% (Davidson & Brown, 1985). Although not without difficulties, the assessment of preexisting psychopathology in burned adults is facilitated by the existence of previous medical and psychological treatment histories. In addition, unstructured or structured interviews can be conducted directly with the patient to establish lifetime history of psychiatric morbidity/treatment. The child analogue of this sort of premorbid estimation is often difficult to accomplish because many burned children are toddlers without school history. In addition, although no study has attempted to obtain standardized retrospective ratings from school personnel concerning children's premorbid psychosocial functioning, this approach also has problems in that teachers may be biased in their ratings of children who are currently hospitalized for severe burn injury (e.g., may provide more positive ratings). Grades and attendance records may be used to index limited aspects of premorbid competence. With these younger populations, one is largely restricted to reliance on parents as the source of data concerning premorbid adjustment. There exist several examples in the child literature describing the use of such a strategy. For example, Rutter and colleagues (Brown, Chadwick, Shaffer, Rutter, & Traub, 1981; Rutter, Chadwick, Shaffer, & Brown, 1980) assessed children's premorbid functioning in an investigation of the psychiatric sequelae of head injuries. It was noted that even for children with very serious injuries, the appearance of "new" psychiatric disorder was, in part, a function of preexisting behavioral disturbance (Brown *et al.*, 1981). Children in this investigation were aged 5–14 years. It is possible that this interviewing strategy might be effectively adapted for application to younger children. It should also be noted that similar problems arise when one is interested in obtaining a valid index of premorbid family functioning. Finally, it is important to understand that the assessment of premorbid functioning is not just critical to the study of burn injury sequelae, but has major implications for those interested in accident prevention. For example, we now have preliminary evidence that certain premorbid child characteristics (e.g., conduct problems, high levels of motor activity) are related to increased occurrence of accidental injury (Langley, McGee, Silva, & Williams, 1983). Thus, assessing preexisting behavioral competencies and deficits in burn injury victims will: (1) assist in differentiating sequelae that are unique to the injury versus those that are a continuation/ exacerbation of preexisting conditions and (2) contribute to much needed injury prevention research efforts. Parenthetically, we would like to note that many of the study foci and methodological controls utilized in the child studies described herein have been derived from strategies previously employed in the context of studies of adult burn victims. However, although the adult burn psychological assessment and treatment literature is more fully developed than the child literature, specific methodological advances (e.g., estimation of premorbid psychological functioning) in the former area may have limited applicability to the study of pediatric victims. At this point, the field awaits the development of novel methodological controls and/or the effective adaptation of existing strategies used in adult research. Concerning the adult burn literature, the interested reader is referred to several excellent substantive and methodological reviews (Eyles *et al.*, 1984; Malt, 1980; Patterson *et al.*, 1993).

Third, data suggest that outcome is domain-specific. That is, burn trauma may affect functioning in one psychosocial domain (e.g., social) but have little to no impact on other areas (e.g., academic). Use of narrow-band assessment instruments may provide a distorted picture of these children. If one only examines the construct of anxiety and burned children do not evidence problems on a measure at follow-up, it cannot be concluded that children are not experiencing burn-related psychological sequelae. Obviously, children may be experiencing problems in other psychological domains that were not assessed. Patterson *et al.* (1993) have noted that in many instances it may be more prudent to focus on general constructs such as distress and suffering as opposed to invoking psychopathology-based models.

The studies reviewed here have attempted to address a series of related questions including: (1) what are the child and family psychosocial sequelae associated with serious burn injury, (2) how many pediatric victims exhibit poor outcome, and (3) what specific injury, treatment, and patient demographic variables are associated with poor psychosocial prognosis. Based on the literature, it is apparent that these questions can only be answered with extensive qualification. Given the methodological problems that characterize studies in this area, we conclude that definitive answers await further inquiry. However, we believe that the series of studies reviewed here to provide suggestive evidence concerning the relative importance of several demographic, biologic, and injury-related variables. In many instances, the influence of such variables have been investigated in isolation. Nonetheless, some general trends can be discerned: (1) although counterintuitive, several studies have failed to find a relationship between burn severity and psychological outcome, (2) data are mixed concerning the impact of injury visibility on outcome, (3) there is evidence that maladjustment is mitigated as a function of time since injury, (4) data suggest that age at time of injury can impact outcome; however, findings are mixed with some studies reporting poorer outcome in younger children (preadolescent) while others note heightened difficulties for those burned during adolescence, (5) gender may be important with a tendency for boys to exhibit more externalizing and girls more internalizing problems, (6) career adjustment appears to be negatively affected, (7) poor maternal and family adjustment is associated with poor child adjustment, (8) length of hospitalization has not been found to be a critical determinant of outcome, (9) there are few empirical data concerning body image, and social and peer interactions, (10) several studies suggest few problems with self-esteem, and (11) a subset of parents evidence compromised psychological functioning when assessed subsequent to their child's burn injury.

In this review, we encountered many studies that examined a similar set of variables with mixed results. In attempting to reconcile these interstudy differences, it becomes apparent that the most poignant question may not be "Do burned children evidence negative psychosocial outcome?" As noted above, the evidence to date suggests that a minority of burned pediatric patients constitute an at-risk population for later psychosocial impairment. However, knowing this does little to further our understanding of these patients, their families, and mediating processes. This leads us to a more complex focus. We believe that the appropriate focus of future research in this area involves addressing the question as to who exhibits what problems under what set of antecedent and consequent conditions. More specifically, antecedent conditions that predate the injury (e.g., family discord) and parental and family reactions (e.g., guilt, support, coping) to the child's injury and during the recovery process likely interact with a variety of child organismic (e.g., personality characteristics), developmental (e.g., age, cognitive level of functioning), and biological (e.g., burn severity) variables to mediate psychological outcome. Of course, psychological adjustment may change over time and is amenable to modification (e.g., via clinical services, reconstructive procedures). The more recent studies employing multivariate methods have enhanced our understanding of this population. However, additional studies are needed that directly assess the utility of various theoretical models (e.g., Daniels, Moos, Billings, & Miller, 1987; Wallander & Varni, 1992) in furthering our understanding of how children and families move from nonimpaired to impaired psychosocial status. Other areas in need of additional research are outlined below.

Given the importance of peer relations, it is surprising that so little effort has been devoted to objectively assessing the status of burned children's social functioning. Along these same lines, although several school reentry programs exist for burned children, there are few data concerning the effectiveness of these programs in assisting children to make the transition from the hospital to home to school environment. Blakeney (this volume) reviews school reentry programs and related community reintegration issues.

Little is known about how marital and family functioning affects children's adjustment both during hospitalization and following discharge (Kaslow, Koon-Scott, and Dingle, this volume). For adult burn victims, there have been reports of increased family interaction and decreased relations with nonfamily members following injury (Andreasen & Norris, 1972; Browne *et al.*, 1985). Unfortunately, for pediatric injuries, data are lacking concerning the near- and long-term effects that the burn event has on marital and family relations. The use of structured diagnostic interview methods with parents of burned children may be an effective means of index premorbid functioning as well as chart changes in symptomatology and adaptive responding as a function of time since child injury. In addition, sibling effects have been entirely neglected in the literature (Breslau, Weitzman, & Messenger, 1981). Finally, although potentially important to child, sibling, marital, and family adjustment, we are lacking empirical data on how the circumstances of injury (e.g., lapsed parental supervision) contribute to psychosocial outcome. Circumstance of injury appears to be a critical variable to include in future investigations given preliminary data from the adult literature suggesting that particular kinds of burn injuries (e.g., electrical) are causally related to the appearance of specific forms of psychopathology [e.g., posttraumatic stress disorder (PTSD)] (Mancusi-Ungaro, Tarbox, & Wainwright, 1986).

In the past decade, there has been increased emphasis on adult and child PTSD (Keane, 1989; Saigh, 1989). Clinically, children may be seen at follow-up who exhibit symptoms consistent with a diagnosis of PTSD (Stoddard, Norman, & Murphy, 1989). Given the life-threatening circumstances under which severe burns occur, the conditions appear optimal for the development of such symptomatology. Maladaptive emotional responses typically evident in patients with PTSD include excessive anxiety, intrusive cognitions or nightmares, sleep disturbance, depression, guilt, and impaired cognitive functioning. In a recent review of the disaster–psychopathology relationship, Rubonis and Bickman (1991) noted that disaster-induced PTSD symptoms tend to improve with the passage of time, a conclusion similar to that noted here for pediatric burn-related psychopathology as well as that determined for adult burn survivors (Patterson *et al.*, 1993). Additional research is needed that assesses the epidemiology, developmental response patterns, and intervention methods applicable to pediatric burn-related PTSD.

Finally, given that the *majority* of burned children have not been found to exhibit *severe* psychopathology at follow-up, a research initiative is needed to identify variables related to stress-resiliency in children (Garmezy, 1986). In this regard, several models of adjustment in pediatric chronic illness have been described and appear to be well suited to this purpose (e.g., Wallander & Varni, 1992). The identification of adaptive resources and protective factors in high-risk stress-resilient children and families may lead to the development of more robust treatment approaches. Patterson *et al.* (1993) have also pointed out that a subset of adult burned patients have reported positive aspects of their injury and that we need to be more attuned to positive patient and family adaptation.

Several general clinical implications follow from the review of findings that have been the focus of this chapter. In essence, the four major treatment implications outlined by Patterson *et al.* (1993) based on their review of the adult literature are pertinent to the pediatric population with minimal adaptation. Specifically, Patterson *et al.* noted that the burn injury can be viewed as a sign of patient dysfunction and that this symptomatology can be targeted for treatment. Although this might include parental psychopathology, such as Axis I disorders or substance abuse, it might also include unstable family relations, marital discord, homelessness, and related social problems. In this instance, one is targeting variables that may have led to the trauma as opposed to solely focusing on the burn injury itself. The intervention strategies discussed in this volume by Brown, Dingle, and Koon-Scott (Chapter 5, Inpatient Consultation and Liaison), Kaslow *et al.* (Chapter 8, Family Considerations), and Jones and Zaharopoulos (Chapter 10, Prevention) are of direct relevance.

A second and obvious focus for intervention concerns the minimization of patient distress during hospitalization. Because the highest rates of psychological disruption occur during the acute phase of treatment, every effort is required to reduce patient suffering during this period. Although data are available concerning the relationship between children's hospitalization experiences and later adjustment (see Thompson & Vernon, 1993), little is known of this relationship specifically for burn-injured children. Specific strategies for management of acute psychosocial issues, pain management, and enhancement of child and family coping are present in detail in Chapters 3, 6, and 8.

A third treatment focus concerns those efforts directed at physical and medical interventions with cosmetic or functional impact. Patterson *et al.* (1993) have noted the complex and cyclical nature of the relationship between moderating and outcome variables for burn-injured patients. They note that the prevention of adverse long-term sequelae will involve, in part, an intense effort to reduce the psychological impact of disability and disfigurement. Such efforts might include efforts to increase patient compliance with physical therapy, wound care, and reconstructive and cosmetic rehabilitation. These topics are addressed in Chapters 3, 5, 6, and 8.

Finally, efforts are needed to refine our predictions of who will evidence long-term suffering. Patterson *et al.* (1993) noted that although patients with premorbid vulnerability (Vitaliano *et al.*, 1987), poor coping strategies (Peterson, 1989), and inadequate social support (Cohen & Wills, 1985) will likely require intensive treatment, we need to appreciate the complexity involved in the "cyclical interplay among social economic, psychological and physical variables" (p. 374). Unfortunately, as evidenced by the present review, we currently possess only a rudimentary understanding of the key variables and have yet to explore the complex interactions that may exist among such variables in efforts to enhance the accuracy of our long-term psychosocial prognosis.

REFERENCES

Achenbach, T. M., & Edelbrock, C. S. (1983). *Manual for the Child Behavior Checklist and Revised Behavior Profile*. Burlington, VT: University Associates in Psychiatry.

American Psychiatric Association. (1980). *Diagnostic and statistical manual of mental disorders* (DSM-III). Washington, DC: Author.

Andreasen, N., & Norris, A. (1972). Long-term adjustment and adaptation mechanisms in severely burned adults. *Journal of Nervous and Mental Disease, 154*, 352–362.

Andreasen, N. J., Norris, A. S., & Hartford, C. E. (1971). Incidence of long-term complications of severely burned adults. *Annals of Surgery, 174*, 785–793.

Beard, S. A., Herndon, D. N., & Desai, M. (1989). Adaptation of self-image of burn-disfigured children. *Journal of Burn Care and Rehabilitation, 10*, 550–554.

Blakeney, P., Herndon, D., Desai, M., Beard, S., & Wales-Seale, M. (1988). Long-term psychosocial adjustment following burn injury. *Journal of Burn Care and Rehabilitation, 9*, 661–665.

Blakeney, P., Portman, S., & Rutan, R. (1990). Familial values as factors influencing long-term psychological adjustment of children after severe burn injury. *Journal of Burn Care and Rehabilitation, 11*, 472–475.

Breslau, N., Weitzman, M., & Messenger, K. (1981). Psychologic functioning of siblings of disabled children. *Pediatrics, 67*, 344–353.

Brezel, B. S., Kassenbrock, J. M., & Stein, J. M. (1988). Burns in substance abusers and in neurologically and mentally impaired patients. *Journal of Burn Care and Rehabilitation, 9*, 169–171.

Brown, G., Chadwick, O., Shaffer, D., Rutter, M., & Traub, M. (1981). A prospective study of children with head injuries: III. Psychiatric sequelae. *Psychological Medicine, 11*, 63–78.

Browne, G., Byrne, C., Brown, B., Pennock, M., Streiner, D., Roberts, R., Eyles, P., Truscott, D., & Dabbs, R. (1985). Psychological adjustment of burn survivors. *Burns, 12*, 28–35.

Bruhn, J. G., Hampton, J. W., & Chandler, B. C. (1971). Clinical marginality and psychological adjustment in hemophilia. *Journal of Psychosomatic Research, 15*, 207–213.

Byrne, C., Love, B., Browne, G., Brown, B., Roberts, J., & Streiner, D. (1986). The social competence of children following burn injury: A study of resilience. *Journal of Burn Care, 7*, 247–252.

Chang, F. C., & Herzog, B. (1976). Burn morbidity: A follow-up study of physical and psychological disability. *Annals of Surgery, 183*, 34–37.

Clarke, A. M., & Martin, H. L. (1978). The effects of previous thermal injuries on adolescent. *Burns, 5*, 101–104.

Cohen, S., & Wills, T. A. (1985). Stress, social support, and the buffering hypothesis. *Psychological Bulletin, 98*, 310–357.

Costello, E., Edelbrock, C., & Costello, A. (1985). Validity of the NIMH Diagnostic Interview for Children: A comparison between psychiatric and pediatric referrals. *Journal of Abnormal Child Psychology, 13*, 579–595.

Daniels, D., Moos, R. H., Billings, A. G., & Miller, J. J. (1987). Psychosocial risk and resistance factors among children with chronic illness, healthy siblings, and healthy controls. *Journal of Abnormal Child Psychology, 15*, 295–308.

Davidson, T. I., & Brown, L. C. (1985). Self-inflicted burns: A 5-year retrospective study. *Burns, 11*, 157–160.

DeWet, B., Cywes, S., Davies, M. R. Q., & Riet, V. S. (1979). Some aspects of post-treatment adjustment in severely burned children. *Burns, 5*, 979–980.

Earls, F., Smith, E., Reich, W., & Jung, K. (1988). Investigating psychopathological consequences of a disaster in children: A pilot study incorporating a structured diagnostic interview. *Journal of the American Academy of Child and Adolescent Psychiatry, 27*, 90–95.

English, R. W., & Palla, D. B. (1971). Attitudes of nondisabled persons toward a photograph of a mildly and severely retarded adolescent. *Training School Bulletin, 68*, 55–63.

Eyles, P., Browne, C., Byrne, B., Pennock, M., Truscott, D., & Dabbs, R. (1984). Methodological problems in studies of burn survivors and their psychosocial prognosis. *Burns, 10*, 427–433.

Garmezy, N. (1986). Developmental aspects of children's responses to the stress of separation and loss. In M. Rutter, C. E. Izard, & P. B. Read (Eds.), *Depression in young people: Developmental and clinical perspectives* (pp. 297–323). New York: Guilford Press.

Giljohann, A. (1979). Adolescents burned as children. *Burns, 7*, 95–99.

Goldberg, R. T. (1974). Adjustment of children with invisible and visible handicaps: Congenital heart disease and facial burns. *Journal of Counseling Psychology, 21*, 428–432.

Goldberg, R. T., Bernstein, N. R., & Crosby, R. (1975). Vocational development of adolescents with burn injury. *Rehabilitation Counseling Bulletin, 18,* 140–146.

Gutterman, E., O'Brien, J., & Young, J. (1987). Structured diagnostic interviews for children and adolescents: Current status and future directions. *Journal of the American Academy of Child and Adolescent Psychiatry, 26,* 621–630.

Heisler, A. B., & Friedman, S. B. (1981). Social and psychological considerations in chronic disease: With particular reference to the management of seizure disorder. *Journal of Pediatric Psychology, 6,* 239–250.

Herjanic, B., & Reich, W. (1982). Development of a structured psychiatric interview for children: Agreement between child and parent on individual items. *Journal of Abnormal Child Psychology, 10,* 307–324.

Herndon, D. N., LeMaster, J., Beard, S., Bernstein, N., Lewis, S. R., Rutan, T. C., Winkler, J. B., Cole, M., Bjarnason, D., Gore, D., Evans, E. B., Desai, M., Linares, H., Abston, S., & Van Osten, T. (1986). The quality of life after major thermal injury in children: An analysis of 12 survivors with ≥80% total body, 70% third-degree burns. *Journal of Trauma, 26,* 609–619.

Hurt, F. J., & Tarnowski, K. J. (1990). Behavioral consultation in the management of pediatric burns. *Medical Psychotherapy, 3,* 117–124.

Jesse, P. O., Strickland, M. P., Leeper, J. D., & Wales, P. (1992). Perception of body image in children with burns, five years after burn injury. *Journal of Burn Care and Rehabilitation, 13,* 33–38.

Katz, E. R., Kellerman, J., & Siegel, S. E. (1980). Behavioral distress in children undergoing medical procedures: Developmental concerns. *Journal of Consulting and Clinical Psychology, 48,* 356–368.

Keane, T. M., (1989). Post-traumatic stress disorder: Current status and future directions. *Behavior Therapy, 20,* 149–153.

Knudson-Cooper, M. S. (1981). Adjustment to visible stigma: The case of the severely burned child. *Social Science Medicine, 15,* 31–44.

Langley, J., McGee, R., Silva, P., & Williams, S. (1983). Child behavior and accidents. *Journal of Pediatric Psychology, 8,* 181–189.

Long, R. T., & Cope, O. (1961). Emotional problems of burned children. *New England Journal of Medicine, 264,* 1121–1127.

Love, B., Byrne, C., Roberts, J., Browne, G., & Brown, B. (1987). Adult psychosocial adjustment following childhood injury: The effect of disfigurement. *Journal of Burn Care and Rehabilitation, 8,* 280–285.

MacDonald, A. P., & Hall, J. (1969). Perception of disability by the nondisabled. *Journal of Consulting and Clinical Psychology, 33,* 654–660.

Maddux, J. E., Roberts, M. C., Sledden, E. A., & Wright, L. (1986). Developmental issues in child health psychology. *American Psychologist, 41,* 25–34.

Malt, U. (1980). Long-term psychosocial follow-up studies of burned adults: Review of the literature. *Burns, 6,* 190–197.

Mancusi-Ungaro, H. R., Tarbox, A. R., & Wainwright, D. J. (1986). Posttraumatic stress disorder in electric burn patients. *Journal of Burn Care and Rehabilitation, 7,* 521–525.

Martin, H. L. (1970). Parents' and children's reactions to burns and scalds in children. *British Journal of Medical Psychology, 43,* 183–191.

Miller, L. C. (1967). Louisville behavior checklist. *Psychological Reports, 21,* 885–896.

Miller, W. C., Gardner, N., & Mlott, S. (1976). Psychological support in the treatment of severely burned patients. *Trauma, 16,* 722–725.

Molinaro, J. R. (1978). The social fate of children disfigured by burns. *American Journal of Psychiatry, 135,* 979–980.

Orr, D. A., Reznikoff, M., & Smith, G. M. (1989). Body-image, self-esteem, and depression in burn-injured adolescents and young adults. *Journal of Burn Care and Rehabilitation, 10,* 454–461.

Patterson, D. R., Everett, J. J., Bombardier, C. H., Questad, K. A., Lee, V. K., & Marvin, J. A. (1993). Psychological effects of severe burn injuries. *Psychological Bulletin, 113,* 362–378.

Peterson, L. (1989). Coping by children undergoing stressful medical procedures: Some conceptual, methodological, and therapeutic issues. *Journal of Consulting and Clinical Psychology, 57,* 380–387.

Quinby, S., & Bernstein, N. R. (1971). How children live after disfiguring burns. *Psychiatric Medicine, 2,* 146–159.

Riss, A., Andersen, M., Pederson, M. B., & Hall, K. W. (1992). Long-term psychosocial adjustment in patients with severe burn injuries: A follow-up study. *Burns, 18,* 121–126.

Rodin, G., & Voshart, K. (1986). Depression in the medically ill: An overview. *American Journal of Psychiatry, 143,* 696–705.

Rubonis, A. V., & Bickman, L. (1991). Psychological impairment in the wake of disaster: The disaster–psychopathology relationship. *Psychological Bulletin, 109,* 384–399.

Rutter, M., Chadwick, O., Shaffer, D., & Brown, G. (1980). A prospective study of children with head injuries: I. Design and methods. *Psychological Medicine, 10,* 633–645.

Saigh, P. A. (1989). The validity of DSM-III posttraumatic stress disorder classification as applied to children. *Journal of Abnormal Psychology, 98,* 189–192.

Salfilios-Rothschild, C. (1970). *The sociology and social psychology of disability and rehabilitation.* New York: Random House.

Sawyer, M. G., Minde, K., & Zuker, R. (1983). The burned child—scarred for life? *Burns, 9,* 205–213.

Seligman, R., Carroll, S., & MacMillan, B. G. (1972). Emotional responses of burned children in a pediatric intensive care unit. *Psychiatric Medicine, 3,* 59–65.

Skipper, J. K., & Leonard, R. C. (1968). Children, stress, and hospitalization: A field experiment. *Journal of Health and Social Behavior, 9,* 275–287.

Stoddard, F. J. (1982). Body image development in the burned child. *Journal of the American Academy of Child Psychiatry, 21,* 502–507.

Stoddard, F. J., & O'Connell, K. G. (1983). Dysphoria in children with severe burns. *Journal of Children in Contemporary Society, 15,* 41–50.

Stoddard, F., Norman, D., & Murphy, M. (1989). A diagnostic outcome study of children and adolescents with severe burns. *Journal of Trauma, 29,* 471–477.

Stoddard, F. J., Norman, D. K., Murphy, J. M., & Beardslee, W. R. (1989). Psychiatric outcome of burned children and adolescents. *Journal of the American Academy of Child and Adolescent Psychiatry, 28,* 589–595.

Sutherland, S. (1988). Burned adolescents' descriptions of their coping strategies. *Heart and Lung, 17,* 150–157.

Tarnowski, K. J., & Brown, R. T. (in press-a). Pediatric burns. In M. C. Roberts (Ed.), *Handbook of pediatric psychology* (2nd ed.). New York: Guilford Press.

Tarnowski, K. J., & Brown, R. T. (in press-b). Psychological aspects of pediatric disorders. In M. Hersen & R. T. Ammerman (Eds.), *Advanced abnormal and child psychology*. Hillsdale, NJ: Lawrence Erlbaum, Inc.

Tarnowski, K. J., & Rasnake, L. K. (1989). Pediatric burns. In A. Gross & R. S. Drabman (Eds.), *Handbook of clinical behavioral pediatrics* (pp. 231–242). New York: Plenum Press.

Tarnowski, K. J., McGrath, M., Calhoun, B., & Drabman, R. S. (1987). Self- versus therapist-mediated debridement in the treatment of pediatric burn injury. *Journal of Pediatric Psychology, 12,* 567–579.

Tarnowski, K.J., Rasnake, L. K., & Drabman, R. S. (1987). Behavioral assessment and treatment of pediatric burn injuries: A review. *Behavior Therapy, 18,* 417–441.

Tarnowski, K. J., Rasnake, L. K., Linscheid, T. R., & Mulick, J. A. (1989a). Ecobehavioral characteristics of a pediatric burn injury unit. *Journal of Applied Behavior Analysis, 22,* 102–109.

Tarnowski, K. J., Rasnake, L. K., Linscheid, T. R., & Mulick, J. A. (1989b). Behavioral adjustment of pediatric burn victims. *Journal of Pediatric Psychology, 14,* 607–615.

Tarnowski, K. J., Rasnake, L. K., Gavaghan-Jones, M. P., & Smith, L. (1991). Psychosocial sequelae of pediatric burn injuries: A review. *Clinical Psychology Review, 11,* 371–398.

Thompson, R. H., & Vernon, D. T. A. (1993). Research on children's behavior after hospitalization: A review and synthesis. *Journal of Developmental and Behavioral Pediatrics, 14,* 28–35.

Vadaro, J. A. (1973). Preadmission anxiety and mother–child relationships. *Children's Health Care, 7,* 8–15.

Vigliano, A., Hart, L. W., & Singer, F. (1964). Psychiatric sequelae of old burns in children and their parents. *American Journal of Orthopsychiatry, 34,* 753–761.

Vitaliano, P. P., Maiuro, R. D., Bolton, P. A., & Armsden, G. C. (1987). A psychoepidemiologic approach to the study of disaster. *Journal of Community Psychology, 15,* 99–122.

Wallander, J. L., & Varni, J. W. (1992). Adjustment of children with chronic physical disorders: Programmatic research on a disability-stress-coping model. In A. M. LaGreca, L. J. Siegel, J. L. Wallander, & C. E. Walker (Eds.), *Stress and coping in child health* (pp. 279–298). New York: Guilford Press.

Watson, E. J., & Johnson, A. M. (1958). The emotional significance of acquired physical disfigurement in children. *American Journal of Orthopsychiatry, 28,* 85–97.

Welner, Z., Reich, W., Herjanic, B., Jung, K., & Amado, H. (1987). Reliability, validity, and parent-child agreement studies of the diagnostic interview for children and adolescents. *Journal of Child and Adolescent Psychiatry, 26,* 649–653.

Woodward, J. (1959). Emotional disturbances of burned children. *British Medical Journal, 1,* 1009–1113.

Woodward, J., & Jackson, D. M. (1961). Emotional reactions in burned children and their mothers. *British Journal of Plastic Surgery, 13,* 316–324.

Wright, L., & Fulwiler, R. (1974). Long range emotional sequelae of burns: Effects of children and their mothers. *Pediatric Research, 8,* 931–934.

5

Inpatient Consultation and Liaison

RONALD T. BROWN, ARDEN D. DINGLE, and KAMELA KOON-SCOTT

OVERVIEW

The contribution of psychological and psychiatric consultation is increasingly recognized as an essential component of comprehensive pediatric health care (Lewis, 1991; Roberts, 1986; Stabler, 1988). Moreover, there has been a realization that psychosocial factors play a significant role in the process and outcome of physical illness and trauma (Lewis, 1991). Consultants collaborate with other health care professionals to directly address the psychological needs and issues of the physically ill. The liaison component of the consultant's role is to advise and educate other medical personnel about psychosocial and psychiatric issues (Lewis, 1991; Roberts, 1986; Stabler, 1988).

This chapter describes the various roles of the consultant on an inpatient pediatric burn unit. Areas included are general models of consul-

RONALD T. BROWN and ARDEN D. DINGLE • Departments of Psychiatry and Behavioral Sciences and Pediatrics, Emory University School of Medicine, Atlanta, Georgia 30322. **KAMELA KOON-SCOTT** • Department of Psychiatry and Behavioral Sciences, Emory University School of Medicine, Grady Memorial Hospital, Atlanta, Georgia 30322; *present address*: Department of Pediatrics, University of Florida College of Medicine, Jacksonville, Florida 32209.

Behavioral Aspects of Pediatric Burns, edited by Kenneth J. Tarnowski. Plenum Press, New York, 1994.

tation with recommendations of application to the burn unit, assessment issues, treatment strategies, and liaison. Given the dearth of empirical research in the area of consultation–liaison with burns, we have drawn from the general pediatric consultation literature as well as our own clinical experience with chronic illnesses and trauma. Finally, recommendations are presented to guide research and clinical endeavors in an area that has received too little attention.

Role of Consultation Liaison with the Burn Unit

Burns combine aspects of trauma and chronic physical illness. The physical stressors and sequelae of burns are varied and multifaceted requiring multidisciplinary care from many specialty areas in pediatrics and surgery (Adler, 1992; Miller, Elliott, Funk, & Pruitt, 1988). Thus, the consultant's role is challenging and encompasses many different aspects of patient care. In a recent survey of pediatric burn centers conducted by these authors, the majority of burn units in this country are housed in tertiary comprehensive teaching hospitals where psychiatric consultation and liaison services are readily available. In this role, the consultant's task may vary from crisis stabilization and psychological assessment to therapeutic recommendations, including individual and family psychotherapy and pain management (Adler, 1992; Knudson-Cooper & Thomas, 1988). In essence, work with the burned child epitomizes the range of skills necessary to successfully function as a consultant with any type of chronic illness or trauma.

Despite the availability and accessibility of psychiatric consultation and liaison services in many tertiary care facilities, there seems to be an inadequate recognition of the psychological sequelae of burns in children (Miller *et al.*, 1988; Tarnowski, Rasnake, Gavaghan-Jones, & Smith, 1991). For example, pediatric residency training programs offer limited training in the area of burns. Miller *et al.* (1988) have pointed out that because of the inherent stressors associated with the arduous nature of burn care, many professionals avoid working on this specialty service. In fact, in the general psychological literature it has been suggested that thermal injuries have been a neglected area of investigation (Miller *et al.*, 1988). Although there has been some increase in the clinical and research literature, only a few empirically sound studies exist regarding the predominant psychological issues that pediatric burn victims may face (Miller *et al.*, 1988; Wisely, Masur, & Morgan, 1983). This inadequacy in the literature mirrors the underutilization of psychiatric consultation services in clinical practice on many burn units.

There are several explanations that may account for the underutilization of burn unit consultation services. On presentation of a pediatric burn patient, the initial focus must necessarily be on the assessment and management of the acute medical needs of the child. The obvious medical priorities may supersede the consideration of the psychological status of the victim and the family (Carvajal & Parks, 1988). Once the child is stabilized, often these psychological needs continue to be overlooked secondary to physical rehabilitation. However, an important consideration is that these rehabilitation needs which include debridement, skin grafting, dressing changes, and physical therapy may pose particularly traumatic stressors which also need to be addressed (Carvajal & Parks, 1988).

Often, those providing medical care have not been educated and trained in identifying and managing psychosocial issues that arise around illness and hospitalization (Lewis, 1991; Miller *et al.*, 1988). Additionally, medically ill children present other challenges that are beyond the typical scope of training of those health care professionals who work with burn patients (Miller *et al.*, 1988; Routh, 1988; Stabler, 1988). As a result, there tend to be limited requests for assistance with psychological needs except when there is an obvious behavioral problem that must be addressed. Surviving a burn injury is a remarkable accomplishment for patient, family, and staff. Often it is difficult to acknowledge that there are subsequent physical and psychological sequelae to this trauma. Those involved prefer to focus on the positive medical outcome of the injury rather than recognize the sometimes more negative psychological ramifications of the child's injury. Thus, even when the consultant has made recommendations for a child with poor psychological adjustment, there may be a reluctance to implement them on the part of the staff (Lewis, 1991). Frequently, psychological interventions are time-consuming and may be difficult to execute, particularly on an intensive care unit where staff have many responsibilities (Lewis, 1991).

Those facilities in which psychiatric consultation services appear to thrive are those in which the consultant is an integral part of the treatment team and all children are referred routinely for evaluation and treatment (Gillman & Mullins, 1991). In these settings the consultant is viewed as a necessity rather than a luxury and is relied on as an integral part of the multidisciplinary team.

Models of Consultation

A theoretical framework for conceptualizing consultation has been proposed by Roberts (1986). Based on the available literature, three distinct models of consultation are presented: the indirect psychological consultation model, the independent function model, and the collaborative team model. According to the indirect consultation model, the consultant serves as a source of information for the treatment team by responding to particular questions that might arise, yet does not directly participate in patient care. An example of such a request is when a general surgeon might consult with a psychiatric consultant regarding pain management in a burned child. In accordance with this model, it would be the surgeon's plan to manage the patient's pain with recommendations from the consultant. Therefore, the consultant does not work directly with the patient. Typically, in this type of consultation request other patient problems are revealed and require more extensive psychological intervention. For this reason, the authors do not believe this to be a viable model for use on a pediatric burn unit.

The independent function model occurs when the consulting clinician takes responsibility for specific aspects of the child's care (Roberts, 1986). These components would include psychosocial care, family issues, pain management, and behavior management issues. The consultant would directly assess and treat the burned child. While working within this framework, it is imperative to maintain effective and clear communication between the primary physician, burn staff, and the consultant. Otherwise, the consultant works in a vacuum and will likely encounter difficulty in implementing a clinical treatment plan.

Finally, the collaborative team model occurs when the psychiatric consultant is an integral member of the treatment team and the members function together bringing their own unique skills to provide optimal care for the patient (Roberts, 1986). Team members should include physicians in charge of the child's medical treatment, nursing staff, physical and occupational therapists, social workers, child life or recreational therapists, nutritionists, and psychiatric consultants. Given that pediatric victims have a wide array of difficulties and require comprehensive care across disciplines, this model is most likely to be appropriate and successful for the unique needs of pediatric burn patients.

In implementing the collaborative team model with a burned child, the primary physician should take responsibility for the child's medical needs. Nurses spend the majority of time with the patients providing medical care and support. For this reason it is important to obtain their observations when developing any type of behavioral management program. Because the loss of motor functioning in these patients is common (Carvajal & Parks, 1988), occupational and physical therapists assist with sustaining functioning and rehabilitation. The child life specialist or recreational therapist provides developmentally appropriate activities while the child is in the hospital. Because nutrition is a vital part of burn rehabilitation, the nutritionist provides a strategy for nutritional requirements. Social workers may assist with obtaining necessary services such as transportation, financial support, housing, and consulting with legal authorities. Finally, the psychological consultant provides therapeutic support to the child and family in dealing with the stressors of hospitalization, implements pain management strategies, and works with staff and parents regarding the behavioral management of the child. Gillman and Mullins (1991) also have suggested that the psychiatric consultant can facilitate case management, coordinate team efforts, and provide education regarding the developmental level of the child as well as family issues which may affect the patient's care.

Critical to the successful implementation of any consultation service regardless of theoretical model is a clear delineation of roles and tasks which are to be performed by the various team members (Gillman & Mullins, 1991). Regardless of the theoretical model employed, careful documentation in the chart is necessary regarding any information that the consultant has learned as well as impending treatment plans and results. Clearly, the need for sustained and productive communication among all members is vital, as well as mutual respect among disciplines, to prevent duplication of efforts, misunderstandings, and territorial disputes (Gillman & Mullins, 1991). Often this ideal is difficult to obtain and requires constant effort and revision over time. However, this does not minimize the importance of striving toward this goal. Unfortunately, the research literature is sparse in the area of consultation and liaison and leaves few empirical data to guide practice efforts (Adler, 1992). As research mounts in the field of burn injuries, greater attention should be focused on delineating and determining relevant consultation issues and their outcomes.

ASSESSMENT ISSUES

The assessment of pediatric burn patients has similarities and differences from that of children with other chronic illnesses and trauma (Lewis, 1991; Roberts, 1986; Stabler, 1988). In the assessment of any chronic illness, it is important to obtain information pertaining to the psychosocial and medical functioning of the child both past and present (Lewis, 1991; Simmons, 1991). In addition to interviewing relevant individuals, the consultant should carefully review the chart for relevant medical data as well as anecdotal observations of behavior. This is particularly critical for burn injuries, as studies have demonstrated significant psychiatric symptomatology found both at the present and lifetime in a postburn pediatric population (Goodstein, 1985; Molinaro, 1978; Stoddard, Norman, & Murphy, 1989; Tarnowski, Rasnake, & Drabman, 1987; Tarnowski, Rasnake, Linscheid, & Mulick, 1989a; West & Schuck, 1978).

Nature and Etiology of the Injury

Specifically, for burn injuries, certain areas of assessment warrant particular attention. First, it is important for the consultant to understand the injury. This would include how the injury occurred, as well as the physical characteristics of the burn, the medical and rehabilitative treatment required, both immediately and in the future. Important in the assessment of a burn injury is an evaluation of the physical parameters of the burn including the location, severity (first-, second-, or third-degree burns), total body surface area (TBSA), and projected course of medical management. Medical interventions may consist of management of respiratory difficulties, pharmacological pain management, hydration, wound care and debridement, need for possible surgery for excision and/or grafting, and nutritional needs (Carvajal & Parks, 1988; Miller *et al.*, 1988). Infection is a significant risk factor for these patients and its control has important implications to the child's course of hospitalization. After the critical needs of the pediatric burn patient are addressed, the child may need significant physical and occupational rehabilitation (Carvajal & Parks, 1988).

A critical component of evaluation is a determination of the etiology of the injury. First, the consultant must determine the cause of the burn injury: scald, flame, heat, electrical, chemical, or friction (Carvajal & Parks, 1988). Injuries then must be classified according to the circumstances surrounding the incident such as abuse, neglect, accidents, or self-injury. Classification of burn injuries is important, as it has implication for the types of services that may be needed from the consultant during the course of hospitalization. For example, children who have been neglected or abused typically come from families where there is significant dysfunction (Kaslow, Koon-Scott, & Dingle, this volume; Long & Cope 1961). To assess the etiology of the burn, vital information includes the burn pattern and location, time course of the burn, persons involved, and their actions (including the response and behavior of the primary caretakers whether present or not during the injury).

Burn injuries that are the result of abuse and neglect occur frequently in infants and toddlers. Abuse should be suspected when the injury pattern and the description of the incident is not consistent with what is usually observed in similar accidents. It has been estimated that approximately 10 to 25% of pediatric burn injuries are deliberately inflicted by adults (Rieg & Jenkins, 1991). Mortality has been found to approach 30% in these types of burns versus 2% in burns that are the result of accidents (Rieg & Jenkins, 1991).

In summary, the determination of abuse is done within a collaborative team model by a thorough evaluation of the physical characteristics of the burn and the circumstances surrounding its occurrence. This investigation typically is conducted by the primary care physician and the social service team associated with the burn unit. Any child with a burn injury where there is suspicion of neglect and/or abuse must be reported to the state agency responsible for the welfare of children. Although it is important for consultants to provide any relevant data regarding the injury, it is essential for them to remain objective and neutral so that they are in a position to work with and provide support for the child's family. Those types of burn injuries that frequently are associated with abuse are scald, flame, and heat burns.

Child and Family

Assessment in the hospital also should include the child and caretaker's understanding of and reaction to the burn and the necessary medical and rehabilitative treatments. This appraisal is important with regard to determining how well the child and caretaker will be able to participate in and comply with the treatment regimen. This assessment should include the level of knowledge that the family and patient have regarding the injury, its sequelae and essential therapies (Adler, 1992; Knudson-Cooper, 1984). Other aspects should include cognitive functioning, psychological reactions, level of guilt and blame, ability to anticipate and care for the needs of the child, and capacity to assist the child in the reintegration of the home and social milieus (Knudson-Cooper & Thomas, 1988; Lewis, 1991; Miller *et al.*, 1988). The children's perceptions and expectations of the treatment outcome as well as their repertoire of coping strategies also need to be identified (Constable & Bernstein, 1979; Doctor, 1992; Rolland, 1987).

Child Functioning

Vital to any assessment is a thorough consideration of the individual child, previous history, current functioning, developmental and cognitive functioning, family context, and cultural environment (Lewis, 1991; Simmons, 1991). This information is best obtained within a collaborative team model from multiple informants including the child, parents, and any other agents involved with the child (i.e., school personnel) (Simmons, 1991).

First, it is necessary to determine the child's premorbid functioning, as this is frequently related to the occurrence of the burn and recovery from the injury (Tarnowski *et al.*, 1991). This involves the collection of data regarding the child's temperament, level and type of activity, school or day care performance, peer interactions, coping strategies, previous medical problems or accidents, hospitalizations, and psychiatric symptoms of externalizing or internalizing behavior problems.

To assess the child's current emotional status, sensorium, and degree of coping and adjustment to injury and hospitalization, comprehension and serial mental status examinations are imperative (Lewis, 1991; Simmons, 1991). Moreover, careful evaluation of mental status is also important because of the associated central nervous system effects that may occur with burn injuries (Carvajal & Parks, 1988). Possibilities include the effects of carbon monoxide inhalation, other hypoxic or anoxic conditions, effects of electrical injury and associated cardiac abnormalities, generalized burn encephalopathies, and other syndromes such as intensive care unit (ICU) psychosis, burn psychosis, and delirium (Miller *et al.*, 1988).

Another area of the child's functioning that needs to be carefully considered is the past and present developmental and cognitive functioning. A complete and detailed history of developmental milestones should be obtained from the child's caretakers that should include physical or motor functioning, language, and social behavior as well as school functioning and peer relationships (Simmons, 1991). This is best assessed by caretakers, as very frequently children are unaware of their very early history and tend to regress in response to an injury or hospitalization (Lewis, 1991). However, it is important to obtain a sense of the child's current developmental functioning and intellectual knowledge about the injury as well as his/her emotional reaction.

Family Functioning

With pediatric populations, it is necessary to understand the child within the context of the family. Since there is an accumulating body of research to suggest that family functioning is integrally related to postinjury sequelae (Miller *et al.*, 1988; Tarnowski *et al.*, 1991), careful evaluation of the family is important for the pediatric burn patient. Important factors are family composition, style of interaction, social support networks, socioeconomic status, prior experience with hospitalizations or trauma, and psychiatric history (Fiese & Sameroff, 1992). Moreover, any other associated losses with the child's burn injury must be carefully evaluated. These might include the death or injury of others, and/or the loss of a home or other property. Additionally, an important predictor of the child's and family's adjustment to the burn injury is their previous experience with medical conditions and/or hospitalizations.

In addition to conducting a careful assessment, it is important for the consultant to remain unbiased so as to effectively function as a support and liaison with the child, family, and staff. The family has been found to be a significant mediating factor throughout the child's hospitalization and postrecovery phase (Blakeney, Herndon, Desai, Beard, & Wales-Seale, 1988; Blakeney, Portman, & Rutan, 1990; Miller *et al.*, 1988; Tarnowski *et al.*, 1991). The literature in pediatric psychology also suggests that siblings are frequently ignored in the recovery phase (Horwitz & Kazak, 1990; Lavigne & Ryan, 1979; Lobato, Faust, & Spirito, 1988) and thus an important role of the consultant is to actively involve the siblings in the assessment process as well as other relevant family members. This conclusion is supported by Tarnowski and associates (Tarnowski *et al.*, 1991) who have found that family adjustment is an important influence on the child's overall resilience.

Hospital Environment

It is important to assess the hospital environment in terms of the unit and staff characteristics. Essential is the knowledge of the type of unit on which the child has been hospitalized, and whether the unit is specifically for children and/or burns. The optimal situation is a pediatric burn unit or hospital. These units are designed and oriented for children with trained staff in pediatrics and are most flexible and accommodating to the child's needs (Cahners, 1979). However, this ideal situation may not be available, and injured youth are often on units with adults and/or on units that are not necessarily for burns. Regardless of the type of unit, a good understanding of the organization and structure of the unit is vital to identifying stressors and possible resources that may be beneficial during the child's stay (Gillman & Mullins, 1991; Gilstrop, 1987).

A major aspect of treatment of the burn injury is the requirement for stringent isolation and sterility to prevent infection (Gilstrop, 1987). This is a primary stressor for the child and the family since separation from caretakers and support systems may be more stressful than the injury itself (Knudson-Cooper & Thomas, 1988; Wisely *et al.*, 1983). The process of burn care which may include isolation, masks and gowns, frequent hand washings, and avoidance of physical contact may be very threatening and confusing, particularly to younger children (Wisely *et al.*, 1983).

A significant component of the unit is the personnel. Each unit has its own unique flavor and style based on staff characteristics and interactive patterns (Brack, LaClave, & Campbell, 1987; Gillman & Mullins, 1991). Thus, the consultant within a collaborative team model needs to be interpersonally skilled as well as diplomatic in working with these various staff members. Because a visitor has difficulty penetrating any system

(Billowitz & Schubert, 1988), the consultant must be a member of the treatment team.

TREATMENT ISSUES

The treatment modalities for pediatric burn patients are fairly similar to those employed with other chronic illness populations; however, the acute nature of the injury adds a component that the consultant also must address. Treatment issues for burn-injured youth include pain management, management of medical interventions, consideration of developmental issues, interventions for abuse and neglect, and support for the children and the family system.

Pain Management

Pain management is an integral part of the consultant's role. It has been well established that pain is a major aspect of a burn injury (Maron & Bush, 1991). Unfortunately, this often is not adequately identified or treated as there are many misconceptions about how children experience pain and how this pain is best managed in children (McGrath, 1990; Tarnowski & Brown, in press). The consultant can be a valuable source of information and an advocate for the child in the assessment and management of pain and in assisting staff and family members to interpret behaviors that may be indicative of pain in children.

Behavioral Symptoms

Pain behaviors in children may include generalized complaints about pain that cannot be localized to a specific area (McGrath, 1990). The type of complaint is typically a function of cognitive ability with older children being able to verbalize the location, intensity, duration, and sensation of pain (Tarnowski & Brown, in press). Younger children are unable to separate pain from other negative affective states (Katz, Kellerman, & Siegel, 1980). Although it has been believed that infants do not experience pain and that children's perception of pain is a milder variant of adult pain because of an immature central nervous system, recent evidence has contradicted these notions (Abu-Saad, 1981; Craig & Grunau, 1991).

Pain in a burned infant can be demonstrated by crying, gazed patterns, postural patterns, characteristic autonomic responses, facial expressions, and specific neurological and endocrinological events (Maron & Bush, 1991; McGrath, 1990). Toddlers typically exhibit teeth clenching, body rocking, clenched fists, physical aggression, and crying, while preschool children may attach special meaning to the pain such as punishment. Finally, pain expression in children is modified by each child's previous history, cognitive development, cultural and family factors, and associated psychological symptoms such as anxiety and fear (Tarnowski & Brown, in press).

Management of Pain

Consistent with the collaborative team model of consultation, the treatment of pain requires a unified and cooperative effort. The psychiatric consultant should encourage the coordination of the various disciplines early in the intervention and apprise the various physicians and staff members of strategies that are viable and realistic (Gillman & Mullins, 1991). Treatment goals should be established early on in the treatment program and should be agreed upon by all team members. The parents and child should be part of this treatment process as appropriate. Engaging the entire family also will be helpful and will encourage compliance in the pain management program (Kazak & Nachman, 1991).

Various modalities for managing pain in the burn-injured are available to the consultant and include behavioral, cognitive, and pharmacological approaches (Maron & Bush, 1991). Behavioral and cognitive techniques have been demonstrated to be effective for these children (Bush & Harkins, 1991; McGrath, 1990). Techniques that have demonstrated particular promise for pediatric burns include relaxation, imagery, modeling, contingency management, distraction, visualization, and hypnotherapy (Tarnowski, Rasnake, & Drabman, 1987). The aforementioned techniques also have been shown to be effective during stressful procedures such as hydrotherapy, debridement, dressing changes, and physical therapy (Tarnowski, Rasnake, & Drabman, 1987). Typically, several techniques are employed simultaneously consistent with the stress-inoculation model (Turk, 1978).

Pharmacological approaches are nearly always used in the management of pain for burn injuries (Gillman & Mullins, 1991). In fact, until the pain is under some control and until the child is medically stable, pharmacotherapy is always the preferred modality of pain management (Carvajal & Parks, 1988; McGrath, 1991; Tarnowski & Brown, in press). Initially, pain management would include the use of narcotics (Carvajal & Parks, 1988; McGrath, 1991). Very frequently, adjunctive and combination medications are used including benzodiazepines, neuroleptics, and tricyclic antidepressants (McGrath, 1991). As the pain begins to diminish in intensity, antipyretics have been demonstrated to be useful (McGrath, 1991). The route of administration in acutely burned children is nearly always intravenous, with gradual progression to oral administration as the burn improves. Children may be reluctant to request intramuscular injections, so the physician must be sensitive to this issue when ordering pain medication on an as-needed basis.

Frequently, the pharmacological management of pain in burn injuries is inadequate. There are several myths concerning children in pain, including that children do not experience the same pain intensity as do adults, that children are at greater risk for addiction and respiratory depression, and that children are unable to communicate their pain (Eland & Anderson, 1977). In recent years, however, these misconceptions have been refuted (McGrath, 1991). Adequate management of pain in children must include both somatic and nonsomatic forms of treatment, as it is not possible to completely eliminate pain with medication in burn injuries. Similarly, nonsomatic approaches are apt to reduce severe pain by only 10% (Gillman & Mullins, 1991). Regardless of whether the consultant is a psychiatrist or psychologist, given the importance of pharmacotherapy in the management of pain, it is imperative that the consultant be familiar with and attuned to the use of pharmacological approaches in the management of pain in burned children.

Management of Medical Interventions

In the rehabilitation of burn injuries, multiple procedures are required which contribute to a great deal of stress in the child. These interventions include dressing changes, hydrotherapy, debridement, surgery and grafting, physical therapy, and rehabilitation (Carvajal & Parks, 1988). Relaxation, distraction, imagery, and contingency management have demonstrated particular efficacy for these stressful procedures (Tarnowski, Rasnake, & Drabman, 1987). Self-control procedures whereby the child is given control in deciding the order of the procedure and/or in performing part of the procedure also have been found to show promise for debridement procedures (Tarnowski, McGrath, Calhoun, & Drabman, 1987).

In attempting to enhance compliance to physical therapy and rehabilitation, operant techniques such as reinforcement and token economy systems have been the techniques of choice in encouraging children to comply with the rehabilitation process (i.e., wearing pressure garments, use of splints, and performing requisite exercises) (Tarnowski, Rasnake, & Drabman, 1987). In the overall rehabilitation program, Tarnowski, Rasnake, & Drabman (1987) have recommended that the hospital environment be predictable and consistent with clear expectations as to what will occur and the timing of these events. Kavanaugh (1983) implemented a program where children were in an environment in which procedures were predictable. For example, nurses wore special aprons when doing aversive procedures in burn care. In addition, the children received maximum control consistent with their developmental level. For example, young children were allowed to remove splints, while older children were allowed to remove dressings. Findings revealed that control patients who were not exposed to these techniques scored higher on measures of depression, anxiety, hostility, and stress analgesia. The study underscores the importance of predictability and control when children receive aversive procedures.

The high calorie needs of pediatric burn patients make nutrition and dietary requirements vital (Carvajal & Parks, 1988). Food refusal and inadequate dietary and fluid intake are common problems and contingency management has been found to be the most successful treatment modality (Tarnowski, Rasnake, & Drabman, 1987). Contingencies ranging from magazines to recreational activities have been demonstrated to be effective reinforcers.

Another stressor on the burn unit is the child's isolation from the rest of the hospital reflecting the need for infection control (Bernstein & Robson, 1988; Carvajal & Parks, 1988). It is important to keep the child as integrated as possible with the environment. This may be accomplished by allowing as many visitors as reasonable, utilizing the parents as support for the child, securing child life services, and keeping the child occupied with age-appropriate activities. Isolation is particularly threatening to younger children because of anxiety about separation from caregivers (Knudson-Cooper & Thomas, 1988) and may best be alleviated by allowing the caretaker to remain with the child throughout the hospital stay. Moreover, familiar objects from home help alleviate this stress. Finally, hospital gowns and masks can exacerbate this problem and hospital staff need to be encouraged to be emotionally supportive and available by holding small children, being particularly sensitive to any child's fears and anxieties, and explaining procedures thoroughly. The consultant within a collaborative team model functions both to provide emotional support to the child and the family, as well as to negotiate with the burn unit staff in mitigating these stressors.

Developmental Issues

One of the major components of children's capacity to cope with any chronic illness including burn injuries is their cognitive and emotional development (Miller *et al.*, 1988). This is important for the consultant and the team as it determines the child's level of understanding of the injury and treatment, as well as the type and extent of explanations given by the staff regarding the injury and procedures. Bibace and Walsh (1980) have expanded on Piaget's theories of cognitive development to conceptualize children's understanding of illness to various stages.

According to Bibace and Walsh (1980), the sensorimotor stage is characteristic of infants; they understand their environment through manipulation and activity. The burned infant is apt to be very restricted in the hospital environment and thus frequent contact with caretakers is critical.

The prelogical thinking of children from ages 2 to 7 years is characterized by phenomenism (attribution of illness to a remote cause) and contagion (attribution of illness to a proximate object) (Bibace & Walsh, 1980). Rather than attributing pain to the actual burn injury, a burned preschooler may attribute the pain experienced to hospital events such as wearing a dressing, seeing staff in gowns and masks, and being separated from their parents.

Concrete logical explanations of illness (7 to 11 years) involve explanation based on contamination (i.e., person, object, or bad behavior) and internalization (looking for the source of the illness inside the body) (Bibace & Walsh, 1980). A burned child in this phase of development may attribute the pain experience as being caused by the staff, or may believe it to be a function of bad character.

Formal logical thinking, which develops after the age of 12 years, involves cause-and-effect relationships that are physiological (Bibace & Walsh, 1980). Adolescents in this phase of development have a more realistic and accurate understanding of the etiology and processes of the burn injury. For example, an adolescent typically can understand the reasons for grafting, why tissue may become scarred, and is able to comprehend the goals of rehabilitation.

Given that children experience illness in accordance with their development (Bibace & Walsh, 1980), it is important to tailor interventions to their developmental level. The stressors associated with burns as in other pediatric diseases are apt to cause children to regress emotionally and cognitively and this phenomenon must be considered by the consultant and team in all phases of treatment.

Family Involvement

Inclusion of families by the team is an essential aspect of treatment. Parents and other relevant family members should be actively involved in decisions and protocols so as to be able to support the child throughout hospitalization (Gywther & Smith, 1980). It has been demonstrated that pediatric burn patients' adaptation to the trauma of the injury and subsequent hospitalization is intimately related to family functioning and reaction to the injury (Tarnowski, Rasnake, Linscheid, & Mulick, 1989b). Thus, it is important to address the needs and concerns of family members including siblings. Hospitalization of the burned child is apt to produce significant stressors resulting in increased familial stress and possible dysfunction (Bowden & Feller, 1973; Knudson-Cooper, 1984). All families will be in need of support during this time, although it should be noted that families with premorbid dysfunction are likely to have significant stress and limited ability to cope (Blakeney *et al.*, 1988, 1990; Kaslow *et al.*, this volume; West & Shuck, 1978). The staff must be attuned to these stressors, tolerant of families' reactions to stress, and maintain a unified effort in developing a plan to deal with these families and their children.

Because the procedures used in the treatment of burned children are extremely stressful, parents often may be a source of support for their children during these demanding and painful procedures. In one innovative pain management protocol with cancer patients, Kazak (1993) demonstrated that integration of behaviorally focused techniques with family involvement assisted children in coping with the stress of painful procedures. That this technique was successful with cancer patients suggests its potential use with other pediatric populations, such as burned children who also experience similar pain and stress. Involving the parents in treatment regimens within the hospital assists in the transition to home care where parents may be responsible for various procedures including dressing changes and assisting with physical therapy exercises. Frequent visitation also is important in helping the burned child cope throughout hospitalization (Knudson-Cooper & Thomas, 1988).

Abuse and Neglect

It has been demonstrated that most parents of abused and neglected children are not seriously emotionally disturbed (Azar & Wolfe, 1989). However, there has been an abundance of research to indicate that these parents frequently have poor coping skills, unrealistic expectations regarding appropriate developmental behavior of their children, limited knowledge and education, and generally low intellectual functioning (Azar & Wolfe, 1989). Often the abuse is a result of frustration and poor management and is not necessarily maliciously intended (Azar & Wolfe, 1989). Frequently, it has been our observation that burned children who have been abused and neglected elicit very strong responses of empathy from the staff with the tendency to blame and be punitive toward the parents. Establishment of a good relationship with these parents is likely to be arduous because abusive parents may be angry, hostile, guilty, and suspicious (Azar & Rohrbeck, 1986). Moreover, abusive parents tend to believe that they do not have a problem and are not particularly motivated for treatment (Azar & Rohrbeck, 1986; Azar & Wolfe, 1989). Thus, it is important that parents perceive the consultant as supportive and encouraging so that effective therapeutic interventions around parenting supervision can be implemented in order to begin modifying poor parenting skills. Consequently, it is the consultant who provides support and is in a position to assist the parents throughout the hospitalization and the legal process (Roberts, 1986). The current emphasis by the courts and social service agencies is to sustain the family unit, and if children are placed outside the home this tends to be only for a limited period of time (Azar & Wolfe, 1989).

Interventions for Parents

The interventions that have been demonstrated to be most efficacious for parents of abused children are behavioral techniques that are problem focused, time limited, and are tailored to the individual needs of the family (Azar & Wolfe, 1989; Gordon & Davidson, 1981). Modeling and role playing of newly acquired behavior including *in vivo* practice of appropriate parenting skills have been demonstrated to be effective and are appropriate for group intervention (Barth, Blythe, Schinke, Stevens, & Schilling, 1983). Continual feedback regarding the parents' newly acquired skills as well as information about inappropriate behaviors are integral components of a parent training program (Azar & Wolfe, 1989).

It should be noted that the consultant's sensitivity is essential so as to foster an alliance between the parent and consultant. One technique that has demonstrated particular promise with these parents has been the use of cognitive restructuring, which is based on the model that irrational beliefs may lead to inappropriate behaviors (Azar, 1986; Azar & Wolfe, 1989). This technique focuses on altering inappropriate cognitions that the parents may have, including a tendency to ascribe negative intentions to normal behaviors and having unrealistic expectations regarding their children's behavior (Azar & Wolfe, 1989). Finally, skills training such as anger control, stress management, and parent training have been demonstrated to be useful adjuncts to the aforementioned techniques (Azar & Wolfe, 1989).

Several studies have addressed predictors of unsuccessful treatment intervention with abusive and neglectful parents which may assist in identifying parents who may be more refractory to psychotherapy. These risk factors include insularity, significant stressors, birth problems, a number of abused children in the family, severity of inflicted injuries, extensive involvement with legal and social agencies, and poor compliance (Azar & Wolfe, 1989). Including the child in this intervention, as well as working with the legal system to garner its cooperation and support, is imperative to ensure the success of any program. Finally, it is essential to work with parents of abused children even if they are not the abusers. For example, it has been demonstrated repeatedly in the literature that abused children have a host of adjustment difficulties (Azar, Barnes, & Twentyman, 1988; Friedman, Sandler, Hernandez, & Wolfe, 1981) and parents may often require assistance in dealing with their child's symptoms, as well as their own feelings of anger, guilt, and inadequacy.

Interventions for Children

Given the history of abused children with adults, the first task of the consultant is to develop a trusting relationship (Azar & Wolfe, 1989). For toddlers and infants, the therapeutic work revolves primarily around parent–child interactions as well as the parents' own response to stress. For older children, in addition to work with their parents, individual treatment addressing the interactions between parent and child as well as the burn injury, the hospitalization, and issues of abuse merit attention. Unique aspects of therapy with these children include difficulty developing trust, aggressive behavior, and a tendency to not disclose abusive behavior for fear of the consequences (Azar & Wolfe, 1989).

On discharge from the hospital, it is the responsibility of the consultant to work collaboratively with the social service agencies to ensure that the child is discharged to a safe environment either with parents or elsewhere. Additionally, adequate supervision should be in place to help the family initiate and maintain treatment and to prevent the recurrence of abuse and neglect. This requires a great deal of effort and discharge planning on the consultant's part as well as careful follow-up and consultation with other involved agencies. Any outside agencies should be involved in the treatment team and consensus should be reached about disposition and treatment that will be in the best interest of the child.

Legal Issues

The burn consultant may be asked to participate in legal proceedings concerning issues of the neglect or abuse. Typically the consultant is asked to be an expert witness to provide expertise on parental psychopathology, competency, recidivism, and treatment as well as the child's psychological and mental status, psychological sequelae of the burn, appropriate treatment, and the most appropriate living situation that will ensure the child's safety (Knudson-Cooper & Thomas, 1988). In this endeavor, it is important for the consultant to be cognizant of current statutes and standards for abuse and neglect, and norms regarding appropriate parenting behavior.

The consultant will be required to submit a number of reports to the court. It has been recommended that these be written in layman's language and be very specific in terms of recommendations (Knudson-Cooper & Thomas, 1988). The consultant should work with the appropriate attorneys in preparing testimony. A particularly important area that the consultant will be asked to address is the parents' potential for future abusive acts. Because every case is unique, the consultant is advised to be very familiar with the clinical aspects of child abuse and neglect, as well as the current child development literature (Knudson-Cooper & Thomas, 1988).

Coping, Adjustment, and Psychopathology

In the general pediatric literature, children with chronic diseases have been shown to have a variable rate of psychopathology associated with their illnesses (Lewis, 1991). The literature concerning the relationship of disease severity and psychopathology has been contradictory and inconclusive (Lewis, 1991) even though associations have been found with the child's premorbid functioning and familial dysfunction (Fiese & Sameroff, 1992). Similarly, the pediatric burn literature is generally reminiscent of the research conducted with chronically ill youth (Tarnowski *et al.*, 1991). However, most of the psychosocial literature has focused on the adjustment in these children at some point after the burn (Tarnowski *et al.*, 1991). Future research efforts need to focus on adjustment during the hospitalization phase of treatment.

During hospitalization, the severity of the illness and intensity of the medical needs and associated procedures render arduous any sound empirical research investigating coping and psychiatric functioning. The available literature has delineated three stages of adaptation which have been hypothesized to present with specific psychological components. These phases include the acute, intermediate, and recuperative stages (Knudson-Cooper & Thomas, 1988; Wisely *et al.*, 1983). Research has been more extensive with adult burn patients (Kiecolt-Glaser & Williams, 1987; Tucker, 1986), and there is a dearth of research with burned children regarding the psychological adjustment and reactions during the hospitalization course. There is a great deal of anecdotal and clinical literature to suggest a course of adaptation characterized by anxiety, depression, grief, and posttraumatic stress symptoms (Bernstein, 1976; Knudson-Cooper & Thomas, 1988; Tucker, 1986; Wisely *et al.*, 1983). Thus, it is important for the consultant to assess over time the psychological status of the injured child and determine the appropriate treatment(s). These may include child and family behavioral and cognitive therapy, supportive counseling, education, and psychopharmacology.

In addition to those psychiatric issues, the team is frequently confronted with behaviors that impede optimal burn care. For example, eating problems, noncompliance with medication and rehabilitation, sleep disturbances, and disruptive behavior problems are commonly reported by burn unit staff (Knudson-Cooper & Thomas, 1988; Tarnowski *et al.*, 1987). Whenever such a problem develops, a careful assessment of desired behaviors and goals is necessary to delineate and implement an effective behavior management program (Tarnowski, Rasnake, & Drabman, 1987). As with any treatment intervention, success is contingent on cooperation and consistency among all team members.

Other significant issues include loss of functioning, disfigurement, and the need for long-term rehabilitation (Bernstein, 1988). The adjustment to these issues occurs primarily after discharge; however, the initial management of these reactions and problems is crucial in determining long-term adjustment (Bernstein, 1976; Constable & Bernstein, 1979). Key events include the family's initial recognition of the extent of disfigurement, the child's first glimpse of the injury, the child's initial exit from the sheltered burn unit, and the child's discharge from the hospital setting. Advanced preparation is paramount with sensitive truthful discussion of possible reactions and ramifications. It is important to assist the child with appropriate coping strategies and to accompany the child when first encountering these situations (Knudson-Cooper, 1984; Knudson-Cooper & Thomas, 1988). Disfigurement may be exacerbated by self-excoriation at the skin graft sites (Tarnowski, Rasnake, & Drabman, 1987) and must be managed expeditiously.

Loss of functional capacity and autonomy also are significant stressors (Goodstein, 1985; Wisely *et al.*, 1983). The affected individual is now unable to perform many daily tasks without assistance and must rely on others for basic needs. The impact of this difficulty varies depending on the child's developmental level. Commonly with adolescents, this is a major stressor because of their developmental need to strive for autonomy (Knudson-Cooper, 1984). Frequently, this issue is compounded by extensive prolonged rehabilitation which includes splints, pressure garments, and additional painful surgical procedures and repetitive physical therapy. The team's role within a collaborative consultation model is to provide supportive psychotherapy and psychoeducation to assist these children in exploring their experiences and in developing effective strategies of coping. After discharge, an important component of continued burn care should be sustained psychological assessment and support.

Liaison refers to the process of educating and training physicians and allied health professionals regarding psychosocial issues pertaining to the patients and themselves. Jellinek, Herzog, and Selter (1981) have delineated major areas of liaison which include formal and informal teaching, participating in social service assessments, and conducting staff support groups. These authors have suggested that two primary goals of the liaison process are to provide information regarding psychosocial stressors and to assist staff in tolerating the stress associated with caring for very ill children. Typically, the liaison work can be difficult because of the significant emotional demands in working with severely ill children and their families and the tendency for nonpsychiatric personnel to underappreciate the value of psychosocial interventions (Lewis, 1991).

Consultants are apt to be most successful when they work within the spirit of a collaborative team model, are a member of the team, and have a long history of involvement with the burn unit (Gillman & Mullins, 1991). It is helpful for the consultant to approach the burn unit systemically and determine the hierarchy of relationships and predominant precepts and biases shared by the staff. It must be recognized that the goals and priorities of the burn unit staff are necessarily different as a result of the variation in disciplines and professions. Typically, these staff are concerned with the acute care of the patient and may believe that the consultant should be involved only when difficulties arise such as problems with behavior and compliance with treatment (Gillman & Mullins, 1991). For this reason it is important for the consultant to acknowledge the expertise and treatment priorities of other team members. The consultant must be a socially skilled diplomat who is able to work within systems frequently characterized by complex boundaries and territorial issues. Further, the consultant within a collaborative team model must be skilled at maintaining relationships with individuals who hold prominent roles on the interdisciplinary team. This permits successful treatment of the child and ensures that the team does not become dysfunctional and exhibit behavior that is incompatible with optimal care (i.e., apathy, negativism, anger, hostility, depression).

One of the vital roles of the consultant on the burn unit is to assist with the organization and implementation of multidisciplinary staffings which should occur frequently. The purpose of such meetings can include discussion of problems related to patient care, design, implementation, and monitoring of a treatment plan, and staff education regarding development and mental health needs of patients and staff. These staffings are likely to be most successful when they are part of the routine schedule and all relevant burn staff are expected to attend and participate.

These meetings are apt to be most productive when there is an agenda and a designated leader. All members should be actively encouraged to participate and share their ideas, knowledge, and concerns. Disagreements should be openly addressed in a structured and amicable fashion with resolution. In our clinical experience, when open communication is encouraged, conflicts do not impact negatively on patient care. Topics of discussion might include a particular patient and associated management problems, dealing with the recent death of a patient, reviewing developmental issues of hospitalization, and helping staff cope with stress and burnout.

A particular staff problem that might arise is a lack of understanding of the developmental issues unique to children and families. Another phenomenon that may occur on the burn unit is that staff may perceive themselves as being responsible for all aspects of the child's care and may view psychological intervention as an indication that their job performance is less than optimal (Gillman & Mullins, 1991). Thus, the consultant also must be cognizant of the fact that the staff are not necessarily being oppositional, but are in need of support and education. It also must be recognized that work on the burn unit is characterized by constant stressors. These include caring for patients who are constantly in pain, working in a specialty area with limited professional contacts and support leading to feelings of isolation, and having patients who require lengthy and intensive treatment (Mendelsohn, 1983). Further, the patients are often disfigured, incapacitated, and seriously medically ill.

While the consultant primarily acts as a clinician, one vital aspect of liaison work is education (Lewis, 1991). Based on our review of relevant issues in this chapter, specific topics with staff should include developmental issues, neglect and abuse, psychological and emotional responses, pain management, behavior management, and fostering compliance. Various modalities of instruction may include informal individual mentorship, seminars and lectures, and formal case presentations (Lewis, 1991). The consultant also educates family members and caretakers regarding physical and psychological issues, hospital and medical procedures and policies, children's and family members' responses to the burn injury, appropriate parenting strategies, and mechanisms to advocate and obtain support and resources for the child and family (Roberts, 1986).

CASE STUDY

To illustrate some of the challenges presented by inpatient psychiatric consultation to a pediatric burn unit and some successful techniques of management as exemplified by the collaborative consultation model, we have included a discussion of a recent patient and his hospital course.

> TC is a 12-year-old male who sustained 54% TBSA second- and third-degree burns to his chest, neck, arms, and anterior legs. The injury occurred

when he had taken his mother's keys and subsequently attempted to drive the family automobile to his grandparents' home after an argument with his mother. En route, he was involved in an automobile accident during which he sustained injuries. He was subsequently rushed by ambulance to the regional burn unit where he was medically stabilized. This ward serves both adults and children; it functions primarily as an adult unit and is managed by the surgery service. None of the burn staff are pediatrically trained. As his mother could not be contacted, his grandfather immediately came to the hospital following notification.

TC lived with his biological mother and younger brother (age 10 years), with frequent contact with his maternal grandfather. TC came to reside with his mother only one year previously, having been raised by his grandparents up to that point, because of the fact that his mother had been incarcerated. This move to his biological mother's home had been fraught with many stressors for TC, as this new home environment was characterized by a great deal of rigidity, strict discipline, and a basic lack of nurturance. Assessment of the family environments revealed that TC's current home was typified by a lack of positive communication, a disregard and a lack of tolerance for personal feelings and individual differences among family members, and conflict between TC's mother and his maternal grandfather. His grandfather's home was characterized by a great deal of nurturance, with no consistent structure, rules and/or responsibilities. Although TC lived with his mother, he continued to spend most weekends and school vacations with his grandparents. An additional stressor included a change in schools and peer groups with the move to his mother's home, and TC had adjustment difficulties, exemplified by poor school performance and social isolation.

Following the initial medical stabilization and a return to normal consciousness, TC began having considerable difficulty with pain coupled with periods of anxiety. When awake, TC was continually preoccupied with his pain and its management; he frequently demanded additional medication specifying the type he preferred. He whined and cried throughout the day, refused to participate in his physical therapy activities because of "excruciating pain," and refused to eat anything except fast foods brought in by his grandfather. His mother's response to TC's behaviors included infrequent and brief visitation with lectures to "grow up and be a man." In contrast, TC's grandfather remained at the hospital, totally agreed with and supported TC's perspective, and criticized the performance of the burn unit staff as unyielding, unempathetic, and inadequate. Initially the burn staff attempted to be understanding and flexible about TC's medication and behaviors. However, they soon became concerned and responded with increased rigidity about administering TC's pain medications exactly on schedule, limiting visitation, and using punitive techniques to manage his behaviors (i.e., threatening to turn the television off if TC did not eat his dinner at the prescribed time).

The psychological consultant was contacted at this point by the staff to address TC's disruptive and noncompliant behavior. After meeting with the primary burn staff to delineate and specify their perspective, the consultant then met with TC and his family individually and conjointly. After a complete assessment had been conducted, the consultant arrived at the conclusion that individual and systematic family and staff issues needed to be addressed. In collaboration with the burn team, the consultant developed a program of pain

> management which included relaxation, imagery, and a routine schedule of analgesic medication. The consultant also performed liaison work with the nursing staff regarding pain behaviors in preadolescents and appropriately involved TC's family in the pain management protocol. At the same time, the consultant educated the family members regarding pain management and their role in the successful implementation of the pain management protocol.
>
> The consultant also identified several other areas of concern which all were related to a lack of structure and clear expectations and consequences regarding behavior. With the team's assistance, the consultant developed a behavior management program that included a specific calorie count with various contingencies for success and expectations for attendance and participation in physical therapy with clear reinforcement for attaining goals. Finally, a daily schedule including hospital-bound education, designated play periods, and family therapy was developed. TC, his family, and staff all were involved in the development of the program.
>
> Additionally, TC participated in individual psychotherapy to assist him in dealing with burn-related issues (e.g., medical care, hospital care, disfigurement, rehabilitation, return to home) and his developmentally appropriate strivings for autonomy and independence. Complementary family therapy was initially started with TC's mother and grandfather to resolve their ongoing familial conflicts and to develop alternative means of problem-solving. Finally, TC was included so that the family could work on developing productive and meaningful relationships among themselves.
>
> TC enthusiastically embraced his behavior management program and eagerly worked toward obtaining rewards. He boasted of his accomplishments and became less preoccupied with his pain and quickly was weaned to an appropriate dosing schedule. His mother and grandfather recognized the negative impact of their conflict and were able to work out an agreement to cooperate. Finally, the burn unit staff became more tolerant of TC's regressive behavior and began to seek additional information on child development.

This case study exemplifies the tremendous variety of clinical difficulties that a consultant may encounter and the variety of skills and techniques that must be utilized. It emphasizes the necessity of an approach utilizing the collaborative team model since the consultant would have been considerably less successful functioning alone.

SUMMARY AND THE CHALLENGE AHEAD

The specialty area of consultation–liaison to pediatric burns is exciting and challenging with many unanswered questions, fascinating clinical work, and a plethora of research opportunities. Similar to other traumas and chronic illnesses in pediatric populations, burned children have demonstrated various levels of successful long-term adjustment and outcome. It is unclear which children have a more successful adjustment to hospitalization and what predicts this positive hospital course. A paucity of research exists regarding adjustment and coping during the acute and initial phase of the injury. This is a promising area of research for mental health consultation personnel because initial responses and treatment may determine the child's long-term outcome.

In reviewing the available literature in the area of consultation–liaison, it is striking that there is a lack of theoretical framework to guide research endeavors. It is important to note that pediatric burn injuries share many similarities to other chronic physical disorders and trauma, and perhaps a conceptualization of burns based on the chronic illness literature will drive more theory-based research. Hopefully, this would improve the assessment and treatment armamentarium of burn-injured youth, as previous clinical efforts with these children have been guided by the adult literature and practical considerations.

Clearly, the consultant has a multifaceted role that can range from using various techniques to diminish children's pain to complex systems negotiations to gain support for the patients and their families. Thus, the consultant must be broadly trained and informed in the essential areas of pediatric psychology and psychiatry as well as having a working knowledge of pediatric medicine and surgery. The consultant needs to be a skilled diplomat who is able to work with a variety of personnel who have different priorities and values.

Frequently, the psychological concerns of the burned child are masked by their overwhelming physical and rehabilitative needs. As there are burgeoning advances in lifesaving medical techniques, quality of life has become a significant issue in the determination of treatment. There has been increasing recognition that quality of life includes psychological well-being. The consultant is in the best position to assess, treat, and advocate for the child and family to promote the optimal quality of life.

Finally, the data regarding liaison work with the staff are sparse even though the clinical lore is that providing support to the staff is beneficial to both staff members and the patients. Obtaining basic information to delineate the successes and impediments regarding optimal delivery of care would be a necessary first step in promoting future liaison research. This basic research could be used as a model for guiding liaison efforts with burn staff and determining a future research agenda.

The literature regarding consultation with children with physical disorders and impairments clearly indicates that these children are underserved psychologically (Lewis, 1991; Roberts 1986; Stabler, 1988). This state of affairs is even worse with burned children. Although the complexity of the medical rehabilitative process in these children may seem overwhelming, it is our belief that this chapter provides a means of organizing and conceptualizing the psychological assessment and treatment needs of these patients. Further, it is our hope that it will stimulate further clinical and research interest in this area.

REFERENCES

Abu-Saad, H. (1981). The assessment of pain in children. *Issues in Comprehensive Nursing, 5,* 327–335.

Adler, R. (1992). Burns are different: The child psychiatrist on the pediatric burns ward. *Journal of Burn Care and Rehabilitation, 13,* 28–32.

Azar, S. T. (1986). A framework for understanding child maltreatment: An integration of cognitive behavior and developmental perspectives. *Canadian Journal of Behavioral Science, 18,* 340–355.

Azar, S. T., & Rohrbeck, C. A. (1986). Child abuse and unrealistic expectations: Further validation of the parent opinion questionnaire. *Journal of Consulting and Clinical Psychology, 54,* 867–868.

Azar, S. T., & Wolfe, D. A. (1989). Child abuse and neglect. In E. J. Mash & R. A. Barkley (Eds.), *Treatment of childhood disorders* (pp. 451–459). New York: Guilford Press.

Azar, S. T., Barnes, K. T., & Twentyman, C. T. (1988). Developmental concerns in abused children: Consequences of parental abuse or a more general breakdown in caregiver behavior? *The Behavior Therapist, 11,* 27–32.

Barth, R. P., Blythe, B. J., Schinke, S. P., Stevens, P., & Schilling, R. F. (1983). Self-control training with maltreating parents. *Child Welfare, 62,* 313–324.

Bernstein, N. R. (1976). Medical tragedies in facial burn disfigurement. *Psychiatric Annals, 6,* 475–483.

Bernstein, N. R. (1988). Coping with disfigurement. In N. R. Bernstein, A. J. Breslau, & J. A. Graham (Eds.), *Coping strategies for burn survivors and their families* (pp. 3–15). New York: Praeger.

Bernstein, N. R., & Robson, M. C. (1988). *Comprehensive approaches to the burned person.* New York: Medical Examination Publishing Company.

Bibace, R., & Walsh, M. E. (1980). Development of children's concepts of their illness. *Pediatrics, 66,* 912–917.

Billowitz, A., & Schubert, D. S. P. (1988). Reverse liaison rounds with a burn unit case. *General Hospital Psychiatry, 10,* 67–73.

Blakeney, P., Herndon, D., Desai, M., Beard, S., & Wales-Seale, P. (1988). Long-term psychosocial adjustment following burn injury. *Journal of Burn Care and Rehabilitation, 9,* 661–665.

Blakeney, P., Portman, S., & Rutan, R. (1990). Familial values as factors influencing long-term psychological adjustment of children after severe burns. *Journal of Burn Care and Rehabilitation, 11,* 472–475.

Bowden, M., & Feller, I. (1973). Family reaction to a severe burn. *American Journal of Nursing, 73,* 317–319.

Brack, G., LaClave, L. J., & Campbell, J. (1987). A survey of attitudes of burn unit nurses. *Journal of Burn and Comprehensive Rehabilitation, 8,* 299–306.

Bush, J. P., & Harkins, S. W. (1991). *Children in pain: Clinical and research issues from a developmental perspective.* Berlin: Springer-Verlag.

Cahners, S. S. (1979). A strong hospital–school liaison: A necessity for good rehabilitation planning for disfigured children. *Scandinavian Journal of Plastic and Reconstructive Surgery, 13,* 167–168.
Carvajal, H. F., & Parks, D. H. (Eds.). (1988). *Burns in children.* Chicago: Year Book Medical Publishers.
Constable, J. D., & Bernstein, N. R. (1979). Public and professional reactions to the facially disfigured which interfere with rehabilitation. *Scandinavian Journal of Plastic and Reconstructive Surgery, 13,* 181–183.
Craig, K. D., & Grunau, R. V. E. (1991). Developmental issues: Preschool and school-age children. In J. P. Bush & S. W. Harkins (Eds.), *Children in pain: Clinical and research issues from a developmental perspective* (pp. 171–193). Berlin: Springer-Verlag.
Doctor, M. E. (1992). Helping the burned child to adapt. *Clinics in Plastic Surgery, 19,* 607–614.
Eland, J. M., & Anderson, J. E. (1977). The experience of pain in children. In A. K. Jacox (Ed.), *Pain: A source book for nurses and other health professionals* (pp. 453–471). Boston: Little, Brown.
Fiese, B. H., & Sameroff, A. J. (1992). Family context in pediatric psychology: A transactional perspective. In M. C. Roberts & J. L. Wallander (Eds.), *Family issues in pediatric psychology* (pp. 239–260). Hillsdale, NJ: Lawrence Erlbaum.
Friedman, R., Sandler, J., Hernandez, M., & Wolfe, D. (1981). Child abuse. In E. J. Mash & L. G. Terdal (Eds.), *Behavioral assessment of childhood disorders* (pp. 221–255). New York: Guilford Press.
Gillman, J. B., & Mullins, L. L. (1991). Pediatric pain management: Professional and pragmatic issues. In J. P. Bush & S. W. Harkins (Eds.), *Children in pain: Clinical and research issues from a developmental perspective* (pp. 117–148). Berlin: Springer-Verlag.
Gilstrop, H. T. (1987). Management of the burn unit. *Issues in Comprehensive Pediatric Nursing, 10,* 51–54.
Goodstein, R. K. (1985). Burns: An overview of clinical consequences affecting patient, staff, and family. *Comprehensive Psychiatry, 26,* 43–57.
Gordon, S. B., & Davidson, N. (1981). Behavioral parent training. In A. F. Verman & D. P. Kniskern (Eds.), *Handbook of family therapy* (pp. 517–555). New York: Brunner/Mazel.
Gywther, O. A., & Smith, J. (1980). Social work with burn patients. *Physiotherapy, 66,* 188–191.
Horwitz, W., & Kazak, A. (1990). Family adaptation to childhood cancer: Siblings and family systems variables. *Journal of Clinical Child Psychology, 19,* 221–228.
Jellinek, M. S., Herzog, D. B., & Selter, L. F. (1981). A psychiatric consultation service for hospitalized children. *Psychosomatics, 22,* 29–33.
Katz, E. R., Kellerman, J., & Siegel, S. E. (1980). Distress behavior in children with cancer undergoing medical procedures: Developmental considerations. *Journal of Consulting and Clinical Psychology, 48,* 356–365.
Kavanaugh, C. (1983). Psychological intervention with the severely burned child: Report of an experimental comparison of two approaches and their effects on psychological sequelae. *Journal of the American Academy of Child and Adolescent Psychiatry, 22,* 145–156.
Kazak, A. E. (1993). *Family adaptation related to procedural distress in childhood leukemia.* Paper presented at the annual meeting of the American Psychological Association, Toronto, Canada.
Kazak, A. E., & Nachman, G. S. (1991). Family research on childhood chronic illness: Pediatric oncology as an example. *Journal of Family Psychology, 4,* 462–483.
Kiecolt-Glaser, J. K., & Williams, D. A. (1987). Self-blame, compliance, and distress among burn patients. *Journal of Personality and Social Psychology, 53,* 187–193.

Knudson-Cooper, M. S. (1984). The antecedents and consequences of children's burn injuries. *Advances in Developmental and Behavioral Pediatrics, 5*, 33–74.

Knudson-Cooper, M., & Thomas, C. M. (1988). Psychosocial care of the severely burned child. In H. F. Carvajal & D. H. Parks (Eds.), *Burns in children* (pp. 345–362). Chicago: Year Book Medical Publishers.

Lavigne, J. V., & Ryan, M. (1979). Psychologic adjustment of siblings of children with chronic illness. *Pediatrics, 63*, 616–627.

Lewis, M. (1991). Introduction to hospital child and adolescent psychiatry consultation-liaison in pediatrics. In M. Lewis (Ed.), *Child and adolescent psychiatry: A comprehensive textbook* (pp. 941–944). Baltimore: Williams & Wilkins.

Lobato, D., Faust, D., & Spirito, A. (1988). Examining the effects of chronic disease and disability on children's sibling relationships. *Journal of Pediatric Psychology, 13*, 389–407.

Long, R. T., & Cope, O. (1961). Emotional problems of burned children. *New England Journal of Medicine, 264*, 1121–1127.

McGrath, P. J. (1990). *Pain in children: Nature, assessment and treatment*. New York: Guilford Press.

McGrath, P. J. (1991). Intervention and management. In J. P. Bush & S. W. Harkins (Eds.), *Children in pain: Clinical and research issues from a developmental perspective* (pp. 83–115). Berlin: Springer-Verlag.

Maron, M., & Bush, J. P. (1991). Burn injury and treatment pain. In J. P. Bush & S. W. Harkins (Eds.), *Children in pain: Clinical and research issues from a developmental perspective* (pp. 275–295). Berlin: Springer-Verlag.

Mendelsohn, I. E. (1983). Liaison psychiatry and the burn center. *Psychosomatics, 24*, 235–243.

Miller, M. D., Elliott, C. H., Funk, M., & Pruitt, S. D. (1988). Implications of children's burn injuries. In D. K. Routh (Ed.), *Handbook of pediatric psychology* (pp. 426–447). New York: Guilford Press.

Molinaro, J. R. (1978). The social fate of children disfigured by burns. *American Journal of Psychiatry, 135*, 979–980.

Rieg, L. S., & Jenkins, M. (1991). Burn injuries in children. *Pediatric Trauma, 3*, 457–469.

Roberts, M. C. (1986). *Pediatric psychology: Psychological interventions and strategies for pediatric problems*. New York: Pergamon Press.

Rolland, J. S. (1987). Chronic illness and the life cycle: A conceptual framework. *Family Process*, 203–221.

Routh, D. K. (Ed.). (1988). *Handbook of pediatric psychology*. New York: Guilford Press.

Simmons, J. E. (1991). *Psychiatric examination of children* (5th ed.). Philadelphia: Lea & Febiger.

Stabler, B. (1988). Pediatric consultation and liaison. In D. K. Routh (Ed.), *Handbook of pediatric psychology* (pp. 538–566). New York: Guilford Press.

Stoddard, F., Norman, D., & Murphy, M. (1989). A diagnostic outcome study of children and adolescents with severe burns. *Journal of Trauma, 29*, 471–477.

Tarnowski, K. J., & Brown, R. T. (in press). Pediatric pain. In R. T. Ammerman & M. Hersen (Eds.), *Handbook of child behavior therapy in the psychiatric setting*. New York: Wiley.

Tarnowski, K. J., McGrath, M., Calhoun, B., & Drabman, S. (1987). Self- versus therapist-mediated debridement in the treatment of pediatric burn injury. *Journal of Pediatric Psychology, 12*, 567–579.

Tarnowski, K. J., Rasnake, L. K., & Drabman, R. S. (1987). Behavioral assessment and treatment of pediatric burn injuries: A review. *Behavior Therapy, 18*, 417–441.

Tarnowski, K. J., Rasnake, L. K., Linscheid, T. R., & Mulick, J. A. (1989a). Behavioral adjustment in pediatric burn victims. *Journal of Pediatric Psychology, 14*, 607–615.

Tarnowski, K. J., Rasnake, L. K., Linscheid, T. R., & Mulick, J. A. (1989b). Ecobehavior characteristics of a pediatric burn injury unit. *Journal of Applied Behavior Analysis, 22,* 101–109.

Tarnowski, K. J., Rasnake, L. K., Gavaghan-Jones, M. P., & Smith, L. (1991). Psychosocial sequelae of pediatric burn injuries; A review. *Clinical Psychology Review, 11,* 371–398.

Tucker, P. (1986). The burn victim—a review of psychosocial issues. *Australian and New Zealand Journal of Psychiatry, 20,* 413–420.

Turk, D. C. (1978). Cognitive behavioral techniques in the management of pain. In J. P. Foreyt & D. P. Rathjen (Eds.), *Cognitive behavior therapy* (pp. 199–232). New York: Plenum Press.

West, D. A., & Shuck, J. M. (1978). Emotional problems of the severely burned patient. *Surgical Clinics of North America, 58,* 1189–1204.

Wisely, D. W., Masur, F. T., & Morgan, S. B. (1983). Psychological aspects of severe burn injuries in children. *Health Psychology, 2,* 45–72.

6

Pain Management

JOSEPH P. BUSH and MARLENE T. MARON

INTRODUCTION

Adequate management of children's pain during the treatment of severe burns remains an important but too rarely achieved goal despite significant recent conceptual and technical innovations. Many of the greatest barriers to further improvements are associated with the extremely intensive and lengthy nature of treatment procedures, marked negative emotional responses in patients, the dearth of developmentally specific research on behavioral and pharmacological pain management techniques in this population, staff problems associated with working in hospital burn units and inflicting pain on children during treatments, and the technical and attitudinal complications of administering sufficient narcotic analgesic drugs to children.

A number of pain management approaches are nevertheless available for children undergoing burn treatment procedures. A key element in many of the most promising of these approaches, both pharmaceutical and psychological, seems to involve maximizing the child's perceptions that he/she has some degree of control over the pain.

This chapter begins by discussing the unique characteristics of burn treatment pain and continues with a consideration of the responses of burn unit staff to their patients' pain management needs. This culminates in a

---

JOSEPH P. BUSH • Graduate School of Clinical Psychology, Fielding Institute, Santa Barbara, California 93105. **MARLENE T. MARON** • Otter Creek Associates, Burlington, Vermont 05401.

Behavioral Aspects of Pediatric Burns, edited by Kenneth J. Tarnowski. Plenum Press, New York, 1994.

presentation of current conceptualizations of pain as related to coping and cognitive control perceptions. Burn treatment pain poses particular challenges to the development of control-enhancing interventions, as do several common areas of interpersonal difficulty in working with these children. This is followed by a review of goals and techniques appropriate in the assessment of pain and other variables pertinent to optimizing pain management. The current state of the art of psychological interventions is reviewed, followed by a brief review of current practice and recent innovations in pharmaceutical approaches. The chapter concludes with recommendations for future research and practice.

CHARACTERISTICS OF BURN PAIN AND TREATMENT

The profound aversiveness and intensity of pain associated with treatment for severe burn injuries is apparent to anyone who has worked in a burn unit, as are the difficulties in managing it adequately. Only recently, however, has evidence begun to accrue concerning the clinical significance of undermanaged pain in children. Practice often continues to reflect the assumption that the effects of pain are less significant or that the costs of managing it adequately are not well justified in children (Bush & Harkins, 1991; Kavanaugh, 1983; Osgood & Szyfelbein, 1989). Researchers and clinicians are beginning to document acute and long-term developmental effects that support the importance of changing these practices (Anand, Hansen, & Hickey, 1990; Anderson & Brill, 1992; Atchison, Osgood, Carr, & Szyfelbein, 1991; Gaukroger, Chapman, & Davey, 1991).

A survey of nurses working in a burn unit revealed that 100% consider dressing changes, including debridement of adhesions and necrotic tissue, as the most painful procedure their patients must undergo (Atchison, Guerico, & Monaco, 1986). Most agreed that, contrary to a common past misconception, manipulations involving third-degree burns are severely painful because of sensations arising in surrounding or intermixed tissues (partial-thickness burns) (Kinsella & Booth, 1991). Severe pain may also be experienced at donor graft sites (Osgood & Szyfelbein, 1989).

Problems associated with undermanaged burn treatment pain in children include distress resulting in uncooperativeness during procedures and negative interactions between children and nurses (Atchison *et al.*, 1986; Kelley, Jarvie, Middlebrook, McNeer, & Drabman, 1984; McGrath & Vair, 1984). Long-term problems include increased likelihood of developing chronic pain (Atchison *et al.*, 1991; Stoddard, 1982), exacerbated anorexia (Elliott, 1985), and withdrawal and other emotional and behavioral difficulties associated with feelings of helplessness (Gaukroger *et al.*, 1991; Kavanaugh, 1983). It has also been observed clinically (Kinsella & Booth, 1991; Maron, 1991; Maron & Bush, 1991), but not yet verified by empirical research, that children whose pain is better managed recover more quickly, cope better with posthospital adjustment, and comply better with prescribed exercises and with wearing pressure garments.

Nociception and Hyperalgesia

Kinsella and Booth (1991) summarized the neurophysiological processes involved in burn pain sensation. Three types of nociceptors are involved: mechanoreceptors respond to physical pressure, thermoreceptors to heat, and polymodal receptors to both of these, as well as to chemical stimuli. Chemicals involved in inflammatory responses include histamine, serotonin, prostaglandins, and leukotrienes. Nonmyelinated C-fibers carry polymodal and thermoreceptive impulses to the substantia gelatinosa (lamina II) of the dorsal horn, leading to the experience of nonspecific pain. Faster-conducting myelinated A-delta fibers carry impulses from mechanoreceptors and thermoreceptors to laminae I and V, leading to pain experienced as specific to site and type. Nociceptive impulses are then transmitted by interneurons to contralateral ascending spinothalamic and spinoreticular tracts. Pain localization and intensity are processed in the thalamus, while the reticular formation is involved in deep diffuse pain, fear, distress, arousal, and suffering. Pain transmission is modulated via synaptic inhibition of primary afferents by descending tracts in the dorsolateral columns from the periaqueductal gray, the reticular formation, and the thalamus. Neurotransmitters at these sites are endorphins and enkephalins which act on opioid receptors.

Hyperalgesia involves peripheral sensitization as well as central hyperexcitability. Peripheral sensitization (tenderness) occurs when inflammatory chemicals sensitize nociceptors, while increases in opioid peptide levels lead to hyperexcitability of dorsal horn neurons (Dubner, 1991). Both processes are likely to be associated with lowered pain threshold, exacerbating the painfulness of procedures such as debridement.

The Repetition of Painful Procedures

Pain and distress suffered by children during burn treatment procedures is often worsened by anticipatory anxiety and feelings of helplessness (Atchison *et al.*, 1986; Kavanaugh, 1983; Maron & Bush, 1991). Painful treatment procedures may be conducted twice daily for up to several months, and data indicate that observed behavioral distress increases over successive treatment episodes (Elliott & Olson, 1983; Kelley *et al.*, 1984).

This is presumably attributable to aversive conditioning as well as to increasing sensitivity caused by regeneration of damaged nerve endings (Elliott, 1985; Kelley *et al.*, 1984). Anticipatory anxiety is likely to be particularly marked when pain has been inadequately managed during previous treatment sessions (Kinsella & Booth, 1991).

A number of problems result from the fact that treatment pain is inflicted by burn unit staff. Young children may develop anxiety-provoking misconceptions, such as believing that the pain is intended either as punishment deserved by the child or as cruelty on the part of the caregiver (Maron & Bush, 1991; Miller, Elliott, Funk, & Pruitt, 1988). Many staff members, as well, have a difficult time adjusting not only to the child's aversive responses to them (Kavanaugh, 1983; Miller *et al.*, 1988), but also to the conflict between the roles of caregiver and paingiver (Lasoff & McEttrick, 1986; McGrath & Vair, 1984; Miller *et al.*, 1988). A majority of nurses surveyed in one burn unit (Atchison *et al.*, 1986) reported that the patient's response to pain sometimes affects their ability to provide optimal care, and that they find this difficult to cope with.

The Burn Wound

Burn wound healing may seem paradoxical in several respects. As full-thickness wounds heal and damaged nerve endings regenerate, sensitivity increases, and therefore, treatment procedures involving manipulation of these sites become more painful (Kelley *et al.*, 1984). Third-degree are often mixed with or proximal to partial-thickness burns, in which intact nerve endings may be exposed (Kinsella & Booth, 1991). And once the eschar is excised, the nerve fibers in underlying tissue become pain-sensitive (Atchison *et al.*, 1991).

Second, therapeutic procedures may be seen by many children, particularly those of preschool age, as damaging (Maron & Bush, 1991). Piaget's theory of cognitive development may help to explain why this is the case. Children of this age are usually in the preoperational stage, during which they are highly prone to perceptual centration. This perceptual tendency is vividly illustrated in the classic conservation tasks. The most perceptually salient characteristic for this child is its defining characteristic, and other (perhaps contradictory) information is not taken into account. Pain is usually the perceptually most salient aspect of burn treatment procedures. And because pain is associated with injury and harm, that which hurts is seen as harmful (Miller *et al.*, 1988). The same logic may lead the child to see burn dressing changes as harmful simply because they expose the gruesome-appearing wound, which looks much worse than the bandaged site.

Coping and the Experience of Pain

The experience of pain is only partly determined by the nature and intensity of nociceptive stimuli. The involvement of descending neural pathways in modulating the propagation of nociceptive impulses has already been described. As is the case with other stressors, the experience of pain is significantly influenced by the manner in which the individual copes with it (McGrath & Vair, 1984).

Coping may be seen as serving the general goal of control (Bush & Harkins, 1991). Effective coping serves to avoid, escape, or minimize undesired experiences. An aversive experience may be desired because it is seen as justified by some ultimate benefit. Thus, for example, restorative dental work may be willingly submitted to because it is seen as instrumental in avoiding loss of teeth and more painful future procedures. A sense of control is, then, maintained by cognitive attribution of a benign meaning to the painful sensations. This is facilitated by gaining information (accurate or otherwise) about the reasons for the pain, and by avoiding catastrophizing cognitions. Coping may also help to control aversive experience through minimization. Attentional distraction and relaxation, for example, are likely to reduce anxious arousal and to focus the individual on less aversive simultaneous experiences. When the pain experience is seen as uncontrollable, unavoidable, and unbearable, coping efforts are stymied and catastrophizing responses become likely.

Several authors have noted that children often experience burn treatment procedures in precisely this manner (Kavanaugh, 1983; Maron & Bush, 1991). Beales (1992) observed and interviewed 60 children undergoing burn treatment at multiple points during their hospitalizations. Their beliefs about their injuries and treatment appeared to be a principal source of anxious anticipation prior to procedures. Many reported seeing treatment as retarding healing and were, thus, unable to rationalize the experience as benign. It is not surprising, then, that their primary means of coping involved attempts at escape and avoidance (e.g., begging their caretakers not to initiate treatment procedures). This generates conflict between patients and staff, often culminating in physical resistance and the use of restraint. Restraint in turn exacerbates the feeling of being out of control, resulting in increased anxious arousal, catastrophizing cognitions, diminished coping, and what is reported by many children to be a "worst pain" experience.

Interventions to enhance child coping with painful procedures should be developmentally appropriate. Developmental specificity applies both to particular vulnerabilities and to intervention choice (Maron & Bush, 1991). Children of this age are unlikely to have the cognitive capacity to rationalize painful procedures as acceptable for any ultimate benefits (Bush & Harkins, 1991), and they may have difficulty understanding reassurances that the pain will be brief because of their poor understanding of time (Miller *et al.*, 1988). Spontaneous strategies for coping with fear and pain appear at a very early age (Anderson & Brill, 1992), usually oriented toward escape, attempts to increase control, and distraction or withdrawal. Interventions should target specific vulnerabilities and should, wherever possible, build on the child's preferred coping style.

ASSESSMENT

Goals of Assessment

Assessment of children undergoing inpatient burn treatment may be undertaken for a number of reasons. These include evaluation of risk for developing adjustment problems, compliance with posthospitalization treatment recommendations, and the family environment in which burns associated with abuse or inadequate supervision occurred. Although important, the current chapter will not deal with these but will instead focus on assessment that is directly relevant to inpatient pain management (though in many cases assessment agenda and techniques may overlap substantially). Specific goals of assessment procedures include: pain intensity and other characteristics of the pain experience; the child's coping style and competencies in the burn unit environment; cognitions and attitudes about his/her pain and injury as well as about treatment procedures and personnel; anxiety and behavioral distress associated with treatment procedures; cognitive developmental status and cognitive functioning; depression and withdrawal in response to lengthy hospitalization and treatment; and the functioning of the family as it affects the child's inpatient adjustment. In addition, assessment should be undertaken to evaluate the functioning of the burn unit and its personnel with respect to effectiveness and impediments to providing optimal pain management.

Pain Assessment

It is now well established that pain is a complex psychological construct and that pain assessment should correspondingly be undertaken in a multidimensional manner (Anderson & Brill, 1992; Bush, 1987; Manne, Jacobsen, & Redd, 1992; Tarnowski, Rasnake, & Drabman, 1987). While the development of psychometrically adequate instruments for the multidimensional assessment of pain in children is incomplete, several such measures are now available (Walco & Varni, 1991). Assessment of self-reported pain intensity may be primary, but assessment of pain quality and location, physiological arousal, and affective responses should also be standard. Unit staff may be trained to perform some aspects of pain assessment, but the services of a pediatric psychologist or a children's pain service are likely to be invaluable (Bush & Harkins, 1991; Osgood & Szyfelbein, 1989).

The child's self-report should be considered the single most important pain index, except in unusual cases (Manne *et al.*, 1992), such as when the child appears to be concealing pain in order to avoid an injection (Atchison *et al.*, 1986). The Visual Analog Scale (VAS), of which several forms have been developed, is quickly and easily administered to most children and has been shown to be a reliable and valid measure of self-reported pain intensity (Bush, 1987; Szyfelbein, Osgood, & Carr, 1985). The VAS consists of one or more visually presented scales (e.g., a line, a "thermometer" with variable levels of "mercury," a series of faces with varying expressions, a ladder). It may be continuous or discrete but generally ranges along a linear dimension from no pain to "the worst pain imaginable." Self-report using a structured interview (Johnston, Abbott, Gray-Donald, & Jeans, 1992) or a multidimensional questionnaire (Walco & Varni, 1991) is appropriate for assessing pain quality, affective and cognitive components, and interference with normal activities. Wilkie *et al.* (1990) have developed and validated a 56-item word list from which children select terms that apply to them. Results indicate adequate psychometric properties across children of different ages, genders, and ethnicities for scales measuring sensory, affective, evaluative, and overall dimensions of pain. Body outline charts are useful for assessing pain location (Walco & Varni, 1991). Based on a survey of nurses in one burn unit (Atchison *et al.*, 1986), however, pain is usually informally assessed by simply asking the child.

In children under about 4 years of age, self-report may be impractical, and observational measures must be more heavily relied on (McGrath & Vair, 1984). Crying is often used as an indicator of pain, but this is difficult because the child may cry for many reasons. There is some evidence to indicate that certain experienced mothers and nurses can distinguish pain cries from other types of crying (Craig & Grunau, 1991), but at this time there does not appear to be any way of making this determination objectively. Nevertheless, this indicator is heavily relied on by burn unit nurses (Atchison *et al.*, 1986). Likewise, behavioral distress and reduction of play activities may indicate pain but may also be attributable to other causes. The absence of obvious pain behaviors often leads to the erroneous conclusion that the child is pain free (Bush & Harkins 1991; McGrath & Vair, 1984), and unit staff should be educated about this.

A number of recent studies have documented significant discrepancies between children's self-report of pain and ratings obtained from others

(Kelley *et al.*, 1984; LaMontagne, Johnson, & Hepworth, 1991; Manne *et al.*, 1992; Van der Does, 1989). Studies have indicated that such discrepancies usually are in the direction of staff underestimation relative to patient self-report (Choiniere, Melzack, Girard, Rondeau, & Paquin, 1990; Schneider & LoBiondo-Wood, 1992). Problems in negotiating analgesic needs between nurses and children are widely acknowledged (Gaukroger *et al.*, 1991), and disputing the child's self-report may seriously erode his/her trust in the clinician (Miller *et al.*, 1988).

Considerable evidence has been reported documenting undermanagement of pain when analgesic administration is delivered by means of PRN prescriptions, which rely heavily on nurse estimates of child pain (Bush & Holmbeck, 1987; Ross, Bush, & Crummette, 1991). One survey of U.S. burn units (Perry & Heidrich, 1982) revealed that analgesic and anesthesia use varies widely, with many units using no opiates whatsoever with children despite their being rated as suffering pain equivalent to adults. Degree of discrepancy between nurse and self-report of pain does not appear to be related to child age, socioeconomic status, or burn severity, nor to whether the child is undergoing a procedure or is at rest. On the other hand, discrepancy is related to nurse experience, with more experienced nurses underestimating and less experienced nurses overestimating relative to child self-report (Choiniere *et al.*, 1990).

Ethnic and cultural influences on pain expression must also be taken carefully into account (Anderson & Brill, 1992). Although it appears that significant ethnocultural differences do exist, methodological problems and the potential for bias in treatment decisions make it dangerous to rely on broad generalizations in clinical assessment (Reid & Bush, 1990; Streltzer & Wade, 1981). It is widely believed that individuals of Latin and African descent express pain more emphatically and have lower pain thresholds than do Caucasians, while Asians seem to be more stoic (Atchison *et al.*, 1986; Bates, Edwards, & Anderson, 1993), but research findings supporting these generalizations have not been conclusive.

Coping, Cognition, Beliefs, and Attitudes

Assessment of cognitive variables can help with understanding the determinants of a child's pain as well as in configuring appropriate interventions. If the child expects pain to be excruciating and uncontrollable, s/he should be helped to learn otherwise. If the child sees procedural pain as punishment or as attributable to provider hostility, or if procedures are seen as hampering rather than furthering healing, altering these cognitions should facilitate the effectiveness of conventional pain management techniques (Osgood & Szyfelbein, 1989). To the greatest extent possible, pain management interventions should address the child's particular beliefs, be appropriate to his/her cognitive developmental level, and work with his/her preferred coping style (Anderson & Brill, 1992; Bush, 1987).

Developmentally specific vulnerabilities are often important in children at various ages. In particular, the assessment of young children should address separation concerns and cognitive distortions as described previously, while in older children, fears of peer rejection and problems with loss of personal autonomy associated with prolonged hospitalization are frequently sources of significant additional distress (Maron & Bush, 1991). Considerable interviewing skill may be needed to evaluate these cognitions, especially in younger children whose verbal capacity is limited by developmental factors (McGrath & Vair, 1984). Some interview schedules have been developed, which may be helpful in ascertaining the child's preferred coping style (Peterson & Toler, 1986; Siegel & Smith, 1991). Other useful instruments which are not, however, specific to pain, include the Children's Health Locus of Control Scale (Perrin & Shapiro, 1985) and the Children's Health Care Attitudes Questionnaire (Bush & Holmbeck, 1987).

Anxiety and Depression

Useful observational measures of behavioral distress during treatment procedures have been developed (reviewed in Tarnowski, Rasnake, & Drabman, 1987), including several based on the Procedure Behavior Rating Scale (Katz, Kellerman, & Siegel, 1980), such as the Burn Treatment Distress Scale, which has been shown to have adequate interrater reliability and validity (Elliott & Olson, 1983), and an adaptation developed by Kelley and her colleagues (Kelley *et al.*, 1984). These may be valuably supplemented with self-report of fear (Knudson-Cooper, 1981) and measures of autonomic arousal. "Excess" behavioral distress or anxiety that is determined to be primarily attributable to sources other than pain should be addressed by appropriate direct interventions, which in turn is likely to allow for superior pain management effectiveness (Kinsella & Booth, 1991). Care should be taken, however, in identifying behavioral distress as excessive relative to pain. Inadequate pain management may result if nurses attribute a child's distress behaviors as related to anxiety rather than pain (Atchison *et al.*, 1986). On the other hand, low levels of behavioral distress should not be assumed to indicate that the child is pain-free (McGrath & Vair, 1984).

Depression is similarly common in children undergoing burn treatment (Elliott, 1985), and assessment should be undertaken to evaluate its sources and manifestations. Amelioration of depression is likely to help the child cope much more effectively with painful procedures and to improve response to pain management interventions (McGrath & Vair, 1984).

INTERVENTION

Psychological interventions for pediatric pain management seek to minimize pain and procedural distress, maximize long-term adjustment, and facilitate treatment compliance and wound healing. Modalities can include elements of supportive psychotherapy, behavior modification, relaxation training (with hypnosis and stress management components), and cognitive-behavioral interventions. It is proposed that, regardless of theoretical orientation, interventions informed by an accurate developmental understanding are most likely to be effective with children. A number of promising treatments are increasingly being reported in the pediatric burn literature.

Kelley *et al.* (1984) evaluated the effects of contingent cartoon viewing and the use of a star feedback chart for two burned children undergoing painful physical therapy. Using a single subject reversal design, replicated with a second subject, the authors observed that distraction (cartoon viewing) along with reinforcement resulted in a marked decrease in pain behavior. In addition, therapist and maternal ratings of children's pain, anxiety, and cooperativeness were correlated significantly with observational data. From this report, it is suggested that relatively simple procedures can be employed that have the potential to considerably alter the burned child's pain experience. In addition, such techniques can be used in the context of a variety of painful procedures, including physical therapy and debridement.

Behavioral contracting for bolstering treatment compliance, increasing appropriate pain expression, and decreasing pain behaviors have also been reported (Simons *et al.*, 1978; Varni, Bessman, Russo, & Cataldo, 1980; Zide & Pardoe, 1976). Although sample sizes have frequently been small in studies of such interventions, behavioral techniques do appear to have a place in pediatric burn care. For example, in the Varni *et al.* (1980) study, pain behaviors were reduced and coping was enhanced in a 3-year-old girl, using a multiple baseline across settings with a reversal design. Delayed reinforcement effectively improved on-unit behavior in a severely burned hyperactive 13-year-old, using a point system in combination with peer modeling (Zide & Pardoe, 1976). Presumably, with these interventions successfully managing problematic patient behaviors, burn care can be facilitated and pain reduction can be anticipated.

Knudson-Cooper (1981) reported lower manifest anxiety and pain in

7- to 16-year-olds ($N = 27$) who received biofeedback or relaxation training compared with children matched on age, sex, and extent of burn who received only pharmaceutical intervention. Similarly, LaBaw (1973) found "adjunctive trance therapy" to be useful for combatting appetite problems and encopresis in 23 severely burned 6-month-old to 14-year-old children. Elliott and Olson (1983) reported substantial reductions in treatment-related distress in four 5- to 12-year-olds who received a stress management package of distraction, breathing exercises, emotive imagery, and/or reinterpretation of the context of pain and reinforcement. However, these reductions in distress were evident only with the psychologist present. This raises the question of which treatment components were effective, e.g., relaxation, cognitive reframing, presence of a benign and caring adult. Greater clarity regarding therapeutic elements and efforts to maximize generalizability of treatment gains are warranted.

Using a learned helplessness paradigm, Kavanaugh (1983) reasoned that unpredictable and uncontrollable aspects of burn care contribute to the child's experience of pain and distress. In a sample of nine severely burned 2- to 12-year-olds, Kavanaugh compared interventions that maximized predictability and control to standard hospital procedures. Intervention strategies included warning patients that a painful procedure was upcoming by means of nurses wearing red aprons and encouraging children to participate in treatment by asking them to remove splints, hold bandages, and so forth. Experimental group children displayed significantly fewer maladaptive behaviors during the first 2 weeks of hospitalization, less nonresponsiveness to noxious stimuli, and less depression at discharge.

Similar findings were reported by Tarnowski, McGrath, Calhoun, and Drabman (1987) using a single-subject reversal design with a severely burned 12-year-old. Observed behavioral distress was significantly less when this child was allowed to debride himself than during standard procedures. In addition, the child reported a marked preference for self-mediated debridement which was rated by the therapist as having been performed satisfactorily. Possible problems with this procedure included its time intensiveness and an apparent reactivity effect in which heightened distress followed the child's relinquishing the debriding task to the therapist.

Tobiasen (1985) found that children who received information about burn care and were taught strategies for coping with treatment procedures reported a greater sense of control over injuries than did children who spent equivalent time with the investigator but were not given specific coping instructions. In addition, children in the experimental group left the hospital significantly sooner than did controls.

Further research is particularly needed regarding techniques for enhancing perceived control and predictability in accordance with varying developmental levels and coping repertoires. In addition to assessing the child's developmental level, the preferred coping style should also be assessed to facilitate appropriate treatment planning. For example, as children mature and develop their ability to inhibit behavioral responses to pain, their tendency to cope via information seeking or avoidance can be determined. Children who make use of an information-seeking coping style may benefit maximally from interventions that enhance perceptions of personal control. These may include preprocedural information to enhance predictive control, patient-mediated debridement, and patient-controlled analgesia, to cite a few examples. On the other hand, these approaches may exacerbate overwhelming anxiety in children preferring more avoidant coping, who might benefit more from relaxation and distraction-based strategies.

How the family mobilizes its resources and engages the challenge of facilitating a child's recovery is likely to affect child adjustment. Social support, marital integrity, an atmosphere of open discussion, family participation in intellectual, cultural, and recreational activities, communication of a sense of hopefulness, and the opportunity for parents to mourn along with their children have been implicated as contributors to positive outcomes for burned children (Browne *et al.*, 1985; Clarke, 1980; Davidson, Bowden, & Feller, 1981; Galston, 1972; Giljohann, 1980; Love, Byrne, Roberts, Browne, & Brown, 1978; Seligman, MacMillan, & Carroll, 1971).

Parental visiting has also been found to relate to adjustment in hospitalized children. Benians (1974) reported a statistically significant relationship between severe psychological disturbance and irregular parental visiting. In his study, children whose parents did not visit daily showed poor physical and emotional in-hospital adjustment. Benians, consistent with Jackson (1974), noted that reinstatement of daily visiting was associated with improved psychological functioning in the burned child.

The nature of the physical environment of the burn unit, the degree to which the burn center welcomes family involvement in treatment, staff levels of communication skills with children and psychological mindedness, and other child-centered factors are rarely subjected to empirical assessment for their relationship to postburn adjustment in children. Yet, clinical observations suggest that such factors do, in fact, play a significant role in the child's hospital experience and overall adjustment.

A recent positive trend in pediatric burn care involves the use of a multidisciplinary team approach. In this model, physicians, nurses, psychologists, social workers, physical and occupational therapists may cooperate to develop comprehensive evaluation and treatment plans for burned children and their families. Clinical observation suggests that such collaboration can be especially valuable. Unfortunately, multidisciplinary teams are not employed at many burn centers. Perhaps with more empirically demonstrated support of their value, more widespread acceptance of multidisciplinary treatment packages will ensue.

PHARMACOLOGICAL APPROACHES

Though often underutilized with children (Anderson & Brill, 1992; Bush, Holmbeck, & Cockrell, 1989; Choiniere *et al.*, 1990), opioids remain the primary treatment of choice for painful burn treatment procedures (Kinsella & Booth, 1991; Osgood & Szyfelbein, 1989). In addition to other centrally and peripherally acting agents, pharmacological management of burn treatment pain makes use of topical and regional analgesics, inhalation and general anesthesia, sedatives, and other psychoactive drugs.

Analgesic Drugs

In most cases opioids are needed to control severe pain during treatment procedures, and continuous infusion may be necessary at times (Kinsella & Booth, 1991). Percocet is usually inadequate except for low to moderate pain. Oral morphine often works well for children undergoing burn dressing changes, though fentanyl may be preferred because it is shorter-acting and causes less subsequent sedation. Because fentanyl is effective for about 20 min, however, repeated doses may be needed during prolonged procedures. Children receiving this usually remain sufficiently alert to cooperate while enjoying superior analgesic effects (Osgood & Szyfelbein, 1989). Unfortunately, fentanyl is expensive and tolerance to it may develop rapidly, so it might be reserved for only the most painful procedures to be endured by a particular child. Atchison and colleagues' (1986) survey of burn unit nurses revealed that many prefer morphine–Valium combinations for procedural pain during burn treatment. Adding Valium allows lower doses of morphine to be administered, therefore providing potent analgesia while minimizing postprocedural sedation.

Continuous pain may respond well to oral or intravenous methadone. Meperidine is problematic for use over long periods because of its toxic metabolite, normeperidine (Osgood & Szyfelbein, 1989). Aspirin is contraindicated because of its anticoagulant and gastric side effects; acetaminophen is preferred for mild pain relief and fever control.

Close individual monitoring of analgesic response and complications is essential when using opioids with children (Anderson & Brill, 1992;

Kinsella & Booth, 1991). While doses can often be reduced during late stages of inpatient treatment, as pain decreases, tolerance may develop to particular agents. Tolerance, which must be distinguished from addiction, may develop quite rapidly in children with massive burns requiring frequent procedures. At least one study of analgesics administered to children undergoing burn treatment (Atchison *et al.*, 1991) revealed minimal variation in dosages administered across individuals and within individuals over time. This was interpreted by the investigators as indicating inadequate individualization of the regimen and failure to compensate for tolerance. Addiction, on the other hand, is rare in children undergoing burn treatment (Osgood & Szyfelbein, 1989); physical dependence when it does occur can be managed relatively easily by careful dosage reductions. Another serious complication of opioids is respiratory depression; this must be monitored carefully and is quickly reversed by administration of naloxone.

The literature is inconsistent with respect to opioid pharmacokinetics in burn treatment. Kinsella and Booth (1991) argue that pharmacokinetics are only trivially different in burn patients relative to others, while Osgood and Szyfelbein (1989) caution that distribution and elimination time are markedly curtailed in burned children. Clearly the dearth of studies in this area (Atchison *et al.*, 1991) indicates a need for further research into this important question.

Patient-Controlled Analgesia

The disadvantages of PRN and intramuscularly injected analgesics have been widely discussed elsewhere (Bush & Harkins, 1991; Gaukroger *et al.*, 1991; McGrath & Vair, 1984), including grossly inadequate analgesic delivery, problems in nurse–patient interactions, and the aversiveness of injections. Patient-controlled analgesia (PCA) is being widely adopted in increasing numbers of applications and has been shown to be effective and advantageous in pediatric burn pain management.

Gaukroger *et al.* (1991) conducted an outcome evaluation study of PCA in 4- to 14-year-olds ($N = 11$) undergoing inpatient treatment. Burn severity ranged from 9 to 65% of total body surface area. PCA using intravenous morphine was begun following the initial debridement session and was continued for as long as patients were determined to require opiate analgesics. The bolus was set at 1 ml with a lockout interval of 5 min and a background infusion of 1 ml/hr, with bolus level and infusion rate adjusted as needed. Pulse rate, respiration, volume of drug used, level of sedation, emesis, adequacy of pain relief, and incidence of other problems were monitored. Supplemental analgesia during procedures was provided using self-administered Entonox (50% nitrous oxide in oxygen), limited to 1 hr daily.

Morphine requirements were found to vary considerably across patients and were unrelated to burn severity, indicating the unsuitability of using standard dosages based on body weight or nurses' estimates of pain based on burn severity. PCA use ranged from 2 to 131 days, with three of the longest-period children showing evidence of tolerance (defined as occurring when morphine requirements more than doubled). Five children stopped the use of morphine before PCA availability ceased. No withdrawal symptoms were observed. Ninety-two percent of pain self-reports were in the acceptable range (mild or less pain intensity), and in no case were patients found to be excessively sedated. Nursing staff strongly favored PCA because it decreased their work load. Nausea and vomiting were not found to be problems, and few other problems were identified. One child was removed from PCA because his arm burned at the infusion sites and he became frustrated with difficulties encountered in operating the PCA button. Another patient who had trouble using the button because of hand and arm injuries was able successfully to employ a foot-operated pneumatic trigger (free of electric components and therefore usable during hydrotherapy). Findings indicated that PCA resulted in superior analgesia and that children benefited from an increased sense of control over pain.

Currently available techniques allow PCA to be administered intravenously or subcutaneously (Anderson & Brill, 1992). Numerous investigators have reported that patients using PCA consistently self-medicate to tolerable pain levels, avoiding excessive sedation (Anderson & Brill, 1992; Gaukroger *et al.*, 1991; Perry, 1984). PCA reportedly works best when set up with an initially higher bolus dose (Anderson & Brill, 1992). Other parameters to be set include dose bolus size, lockout interval, and background basal infusion level. Lockout periods may be set to accelerate and basal infusion level to vary periodically. There is a need for research evaluating possible enhancement of children's perceptions of pain controllability as a function of PCA use (Bush & Harkins, 1991; Gaukroger *et al.*, 1991).

Anesthesia

General anesthesia, while problematic, may be useful in low doses during painful procedures. Total anesthesia may be the only viable alternative for major procedures such as early stage burn dressing change following massive burns or split skin grafting, but repeated use should be avoided because of high risk of toxic side effects, risk of aspiration, tolerance, and the possibility of hallucinations (Osgood & Szyfelbein,

1989). When necessary, propofol has been found to be relatively free of adverse side effects (Kinsella & Booth, 1991), but prolonged use is problematic because of pre- and postprocedural interruptions of food intake. Preinduction psychological preparation should be used routinely when total anesthesia is employed (McGill & Hannallah, 1992).

Regional anesthetics are regaining popularity in pediatric applications (Anderson & Brill, 1992). These may be administered via single injection or catheter for long-term use at skin donor sites and may be particularly desirable in young children because of their fear of needles. Possible complications include sepsis and the development of coagulopathies. A variety of nerve blocking approaches are discussed by Kinsella and Booth (1991). Subtotal inhalant anesthesia using Entonox has been recommended because of its effectiveness, ease of use, and amenability to patient control (Gaukroger *et al.*, 1991; Kinsella & Booth, 1991), but prolonged use of this and other nitrous oxide agents is contraindicated because of the possibility of adverse effects on bone marrow. Topical anesthetics such as lignocaine and EMLA (a lidocaine–prilocaine eutectic mixture) have been used with some success in conjunction with catheterization and grafting (Anderson & Brill, 1992; Kinsella & Booth, 1991) and with partial-thickness burns. Absorption is affected by burn depth, and a high dose may be needed for significant effect.

Inadequate Treatment of Children's Burn Treatment Pain

Substantial inadequacies in the management of children's pain have been widely documented (Atchison *et al.*, 1991; Bush & Harkins, 1991; Denyes, Neuman, & Villaruel, 1991; Gaukroger *et al.*, 1991; Johnston *et al.*, 1992; Kinsella & Booth, 1991; Lavies, Hart, Rounsefell, & Runciman, 1992; Perry & Heidrich, 1982). A number of reasons for this have been explored, including inadequate assessment of burned children's pain, attitudinal and emotional factors, and educational and skill deficits in burn unit personnel.

The tendency of many burn unit personnel to deny or underrecognize children's pain has been noted by a number of researchers (Anderson & Brill, 1992; Atchison *et al.*, 1986). This has been interpreted as avoiding felt responsibility for reducing children's pain (Bush & Harkins, 1992), negative attitudes toward narcotics (Ross *et al.*, 1991), unconscious countertransference against regressive impulses to fuse with the patient (Perry, 1984), and anger at the child for uncooperative behavior or perceived pain exaggeration (Miller *et al.*, 1988).

There is some evidence documenting an association between staff skill and educational deficits and undermedication. Withholding of adequate doses of analgesics has been linked repeatedly to unrealistically high fears of addiction and other complications (Anderson & Brill, 1992; Kavanaugh, 1983; Kinsella & Booth, 1991). Many burn unit staff are inadequately trained in assessing children's pain, fail to recognize it, or misattribute pain behaviors to anxiety (Bush, 1987; Choiniere *et al.*, 1990; Kinsella & Booth, 1991).

These attitudinal barriers should be addressed through in-service training and provision of supportive counseling where needed for staff stress and responses to difficult child patients (Kinsella & Booth, 1991). Training in the rudiments of assessing children's pain should be supplemented by frequent access to appropriately skilled psychological consultants or to a pediatric pain service (Bush & Harkins, 1991).

FUTURE DIRECTIONS

Systematic investigation is necessary to determine the relative efficacy of one psychological intervention approach over another. However, systematic comparative treatment response studies are unwieldy for many burn units. Selecting appropriate outcome variables, ethical constraints, and limited resources all contribute to difficulties in designing and carrying out quality studies. Perhaps the most promising avenue for evaluating treatment effectiveness lies in multiple baseline single case research with sufficiently long-term follow-up. Research should also evaluate the usefulness of assessment data for determining optimal psychological intervention approaches. Cognitive developmental status, specific pain-related fears, preferred coping style and competencies, and beliefs and attitudes have all been proposed (but are essentially unproven) as guidelines to intervention choice. Further work is also warranted with regard to refining techniques for assessing the pediatric patient's experiences of pain, coping with pain experiences, and posttreatment psychological adjustment. Researchers, as well as clinicians, should make use of state-of-the-art instruments for assessing multiple treatment outcome variables.

Programs and policies that enhance parental availability and interventions to support optimal parental functioning as well as facilitating the child's return to developmentally normal activities, should be made responsive to problems arising from developmentally specific challenges. It is imperative that information for patients be provided in language appropriate to their developmental levels, taking into consideration, for example, characteristic misperceptions and cognitive distortions in young children. With adolescents, opportunities to deal with cosmetic and peer concerns will be as important as promoting autonomy during wound care.

Carefully assessing the meaning for the child of his or her pain, the circumstances surrounding injury and treatment, and ideas about the future are recommended. It is important to elicit the child's understanding so that this may be used as a point of departure for provision of more accurate and corrective explanations. In addition, tailoring explanations about treatment to children's cognitive levels is strongly urged. Repetition of age-appropriate explanations is particularly useful with preschool and young school-age children, and may be facilitated by the use of puppets, dolls, and drawings. For example, a preschooler can be told that the silver sulfadiazine, which was applied to affected areas after debridement, will work like magic and make the wound shrink. A somewhat older, concrete operational child might benefit from more factual information coupled with an analogy (e.g., a skin graft is like a patch on clothing).

Avoidance of PRN prescriptions has been suggested to assure adequate provision of analgesics and to avoid inappropriately reinforcing pain behaviors. Intervention attempts should incorporate anxiety and depression management, maximize predictability and control, utilize relaxation and distraction, and target the responses of family members and caregivers. For example, staff members can be encouraged to consider the likelihood that they offer inordinate sympathy to a physically attractive child or that they tend to avoid the badly disfigured child in considerable pain (McGrath & Vair, 1984). We concur with Beales's (1992) recommendations against use of physical restraint, exposing patients to other patients' discussion of the gruesome aspects of burn care, unnecessary visual exposure to treatment instruments in advance of wound care or to wounds during debridement or bandaging, and interruption of the child's attention to distracting media such as stories, television, music, and the like during wound care.

Efforts to increase staff members' sensitivity to developmental aspects of children's experience and expression of pain will be invaluable. Ongoing continuing education and in-service training to improve and maintain sensitivity to treatment aspects unique to pediatric burn patients are also recommended for nursing staff and surgery residents.

Current knowledge suggests that burned children should be admitted to pediatric burn units or burn care sections of the pediatric ward where the staff are trained pediatric health care workers. Inpatient peer interaction could facilitate children's coping with disfigurement and post-hospitalization peer reactions. Parental involvement could mediate separation problems that are so salient for younger children. Mental health support for siblings and parents throughout the child's hospitalization and continuing beyond discharge might enhance families' coping. Because, for some families, the burn event is merely one crisis in a series of dysfunctional or chaotic family experiences, support and guidance during admission and discharge can be an important step toward improved family functioning.

Intervention should serve to optimize pain management. Although behavioral regulation may be related to the pain, interventions that serve to shorten the time involved in the painful procedure and minimize the intensity of pain during the procedure should be strongly encouraged It is not recommended that children in extreme distress be taught to minimize the expression of real pain or that pain should be borne silently and stoically.

To the extent possible, psychological interventions should be guided by empirical validation and should be flexible enough to integrate findings from approaches which have been found to be effective for other pediatric pain populations as well as adults. For example, studies on the effects of hypnosis in adults (Patterson, Questad, & de Lateur, 1989; Van der Does & Van Dyke, 1989; Wakeman & Kaplan, 1978) are increasingly instructive for facilitating children's cognitive control, and enhancement of coping and relaxation in pediatric burn care. Some of the most promising approaches currently being investigated include patient-mediated debridement and patient-controlled analgesia for those children for whom predictability and control are important, and psychological interventions that assist children with reinterpretation and reframing cognitive distortions and catastrophizing. Stories, videos, hypnosis, breathing exercises, and other methods that facilitate distraction and disassociation should also be vigorously investigated, particularly for those children who tend to use more avoidant or emotionally focused coping. For these children, pain-related anxiety may be so great that enlisting their participation and their attention to painful procedures and paraphernalia would be overwhelming.

REFERENCES

Anand, K. J. S., Hansen, D. D., & Hickey, P. R. (1990). Hormonal–metabolic stress responses in neonates undergoing cardiac surgery. *Anesthesiology, 73*, 661–670.

Anderson, C. T. M., & Brill, J. E. (1992). Advances in pediatric pain management. *Seminars in Anesthesia, 9*, 158–171.

Atchison, N., Guerico, P., & Monaco, C. (1986). Pain assessment in the pediatric burn patient: Nursing assessment and perception. *Issues in Comprehensive Pediatric Nursing, 9*, 399–409.

Atchison, N., Osgood, P. F., Carr, D. B., & Szyfelbein, S. K. (1991). Pain during burn dressing change in children: Relationship to burn area, depth and analgesic regimens. *Pain, 47*, 41–45.

Bates, M. S., Edwards, W. T., & Anderson, K. O. (1993). Ethnocultural influences on variation in chronic pain perception. *Pain, 52*, 101–112.

Beales, J. G. (1992). Factors influencing the expectation of pain among patients in a children's burn unit. *Burns, 9*, 187–192.

Benians, R. C. (1974). A child psychiatrist looks at burned children and their families. *Guy's Hospital Reports, 123*, 149–154.

Browne, G., Byrne, C., Brown, B., Pennock, M., Streiner, D., Roberts, R., Eyles, P., Truscott, D., & Dabbs, R. (1985). Psychosocial adjustment of burn survivors. *Burns, 12*, 28–35.

Bush, J. P. (1987). Pain in children: A review of the literature from a developmental perspective. *Psychology and Health, 1*, 215–236.

Bush, J. P., & Harkins, S. W. (1991). Conceptual foundations: Pain and child development. In J. P. Bush & S. W. Harkins (Eds.), *Children in pain: Clinical and research issues from a developmental perspective* (pp. 1–30). Berlin: Springer-Verlag.

Bush, J. P., & Holmbeck, G. N. (1987). Children's attitudes about heath care: Initial development of a questionnaire. *Journal of Pediatric Psychology, 12*, 429–443.

Bush, J. P., Holmbeck, G. N., & Cockrell, J. L. (1989). Patterns of PRN analgesic drug administration in children following elective surgery. *Journal of Pediatric Psychology, 14*, 433–448.

Choiniere, M., Melzack, R., Girard, N., Rondeau, J., & Paquin, M. (1990). Comparisons between patients' and nurses' assessment of pain and medication efficacy in severe burn injuries. *Pain, 40*, 143–152.

Clarke, A. (1980). Thermal injuries: The care of the whole child. *Journal of Trauma, 20*, 823–829.

Craig, K. D., & Grunau, R. V. E. (1991). Developmental issues: Infants and toddlers. In J. P. Bush & S. W. Harkins (Eds.), *Children in pain: Clinical and research issues from a developmental perspective* (pp. 171–193). Berlin: Springer-Verlag.

Davidson, T., Bowden, M. L., & Feller, I. (1981). Social support and postburn adjustment. *Archives of Physical Medicine and Rehabilitation, 62*, 274–278.

Denyes, M. J., Neuman, B. M., & Villaruel, A.M. (1991). Nursing actions to prevent and alleviate pain in hospitalized children. *Issues in Comprehensive Pediatric Nursing, 14*, 31–48.

Dubner, R. (1991). Pain and hyperalgesia following tissue injury: New mechanisms and new treatments. *Pain, 44*, 213–214.

Elliott, C. H. (1985, August). *The reaction of children to burn injuries*. Presented to the American Psychological Association, Los Angeles.

Elliott, C. H., & Olson, R. A. (1983). The management of children's distress in response to painful medical treatment for burn injuries. *Behaviour Research and Therapy, 21*, 675–683.

Galston, R. (1972). The burning and healing of children. *Psychiatry, 35*, 57–66.

Gaukroger, P. B., Chapman, M. J., & Davey, R. B. (1991). Pain control in pediatric burns: The use of patient-controlled analgesia. *Burns, 17*, 396–399.

Giljohann, A. (1980). Adolescents burned as children. *Burns, 7*, 95–99.

Jackson, D. (1974). The psychological effects of burns. *Burns, 1*, 70–74.

Johnston, C. C., Abbott, F. V., Gray-Donald, K., & Jeans, M. E. (1992). A survey of pain in hospitalized children aged 4–14 years. *The Clinical Journal of Pain, 8*, 154–163.

Katz, E. R., Kellerman, J., & Siegel, S. E. (1980). Behavioral distress in children with cancer undergoing medical procedures: Developmental considerations. *Journal of Consulting and Clinical Psychology, 48*, 356–365.

Kavanaugh, C. (1983). Psychological intervention with the severely burned child: Report of an experimental comparison of two approaches and their effects on psychological sequelae. *Journal of Child Psychiatry, 22*, 145–156.

Kelley, M., Jarvie, G., Middlebrook, J., McNeer, M., & Drabman, R. (1984). Decreasing the burned child's pain behavior: Impacting the trauma of hydrotherapy. *Journal of Applied Behavior Analysis, 17*, 147–158.

Kinsella, J., & Booth, M. G. (1991). Pain relief in burns. *Burns, 17,* 391–395.

Knudson-Cooper, M. S. (1981). Relaxation and biofeedback training in the treatment of severely burned children. *Journal of Burn Care and Rehabilitation, 2,* 102–110.

LaBaw, W. (1973). Adjunctive trance therapy with severely burned children. *International Journal of Child Psychotherapy,* 2, 80–92.

LaMontagne, L. L., Johnson, B. D., & Hepworth, J. T. (1991). Children's ratings of postoperative pain compared to ratings by physicians and nurses. *Issues in Comprehensive Pediatric Nursing, 14,* 241–247.

Lasoff, E. M., & McEttrick, M. A. (1986). Participation versus diversion during dressing change: Can nurses' attitudes change? *Issues in Comprehensive Pediatric Nursing, 9,* 391–398.

Lavies, N., Hart, L., Rounsefell, B., & Runciman, W. (1992). Identification of patient, medical and nursing staff attitudes to postoperative opioid analgesia: Stage 1 of a longitudinal study of postoperative analgesia. *Pain, 48,* 313–319.

Love, B., Byrne, C., Roberts, J., Browne, G., & Brown, B. (1987). Adult psychosocial adjustment following childhood injury: The effect of disfigurement. *Journal of Burn Care and Rehabilitation, 8,* 280–285.

McGill, W. A., & Hannallah, R. S. (1992). Parental presence during induction of anesthesia in children. *Seminars in Anesthesia, 11,* 259–264.

McGrath, P. J., & Vair, C. (1984). Psychological aspects of pain management of the burned child. *Children's Health Care, 13,* 15–19.

Manne, S., Jacobsen, P. B., & Redd, W. H. (1992). Assessment of acute pediatric pain: Do child self-report, parent ratings, and nurse ratings measure the same phenomenon? *Pain, 48,* 45–52.

Maron, M. T. (1991). Psychological adjustment of children and adolescents following burn injuries (Doctoral dissertation, Virginia Commonwealth University, 1991). *Dissertation Abstracts International, 52,* 1728B.

Maron, M. T., & Bush, J. P. (1991). Burn injury and treatment pain. In J. P. Bush & S. W. Harkins (Eds.), *Children in pain: Clinical and research issues from a developmental perspective* (pp. 275–295). Berlin: Springer-Verlag.

Miller, M. D., Elliott, C. H., Funk, M., & Pruitt, S. D. (1988). Implications of children's burn injuries. In D. K. Routh (Ed.), *Handbook of pediatric psychology* (pp. 426–447). New York: Guilford Press.

Osgood, P. F., & Szyfelbein, S. K. (1989). Management of burn pain in children. *Pediatric Clinics of North America, 36,* 1001–1013.

Patterson, D. R., Questad, K. A., & de Lateur, B. J. (1989). Hypnotherapy as an adjunct to narcotic analgesia for the treatment of pain for burn debridement. *American Journal of Clinical Hypnosis, 31,* 156–163.

Perrin, E., & Shapiro, E. (1985). Health locus of control beliefs of healthy children, children with a chronic physical illness, and their mothers. *Journal of Pediatrics, 107,* 627–633.

Perry, S. W. (1984). Undermedication for pain on a burn unit. *General Hospital Psychiatry, 6,* 308–316.

Perry, S. W., & Heidrich, G. (1982). Management of pain during debridement: A survey of US burn units. *Pain, 13,* 267–280.

Peterson, L., & Toler, S. M. (1986). An information seeking disposition in child surgery patients. *Health Psychology, 5,* 343–358.

Reid, V., & Bush, J. P. (1990). Ethnic factors influencing pain expression: Implications for clinical assessment. In T. W. Miller (Ed.), *Chronic pain* (Vol.1, pp. 117–145). New York: International Universities Press.

Ross, R. S., Bush, J. P., & Crummette, B. D. (1991). Factors affecting nurses' decisions to

administer PRN analgesic medication to children after surgery: An analog investigation. *Journal of Pediatric Psychology, 16,* 151–167.
Schneider, E. M., & LoBiondo-Wood, G. (1992). Perceptions of procedural pain: Parents, nurses, and children. *Children's Health Care, 21,* 157–162.
Seligman, R., MacMillan, B., & Carroll, S. (1971). The burned child: A neglected area of psychiatry. *American Journal of Psychiatry, 128,* 52–57.
Siegel, L. J., & Smith, K. E. (1991). Coping and adaptation in children's pain. In J. P. Bush & S. W. Harkins (Eds.), *Children in pain: Clinical and research issues from a developmental perspective* (pp. 149–170). Berlin: Springer-Verlag.
Simons, R., McFadd, A., Frank, H., Green, L., Malin, R., & Morris, J. (1978). Behavioral contracting in burn care facility: A strategy for patient participation. *Journal of Trauma, 18,* 257–260.
Stoddard, F. (1982). Coping with pain: A developmental approach to treatment of burned children. *American Journal of Psychiatry, 139,* 736–740.
Streltzer, J., & Wade, T. C. (1981). The influence of cultural group on the undertreatment of postoperative pain. *Psychosomatic Medicine, 43,* 397–403.
Szyfelbein, S. K., Osgood, P. F., & Carr, D. B. (1985). The assessment of pain and plasma beta-endorphin immunoactivity in burned children. *Pain, 22,* 173–182.
Tarnowski, K. J., McGrath, M., Calhoun, B., & Drabman, R. S. (1987). Pediatric burn injury: Self- versus therapist-mediated debridement. *Journal of Pediatric Psychology, 12,* 567–579.
Tarnowski, K. J., Rasnake, L. K., & Drabman, R. S. (1987). Behavioral assessment and treatment of pediatric burn injuries: A review. *Behavior Therapy, 18,* 417–441.
Tobiasen, J. M. (1985, August). *Adjustment to burn injury: Effects of information and control.* Presented to the American Psychological Association, Los Angeles.
Van der Does, A. J. W. (1989). Patients' and nurses' ratings of pain and anxiety during burn wound care. *Pain, 39,* 95–101.
Van der Does, A. J. W., & Van Dyck, R. (1989). Does hypnosis contribute to the care of burn patients? *General Hospital Psychiatry, 11,* 119–124.
Varni, J. W., Bessman, C., Russo, D., & Cataldo, M. (1980). Behavioral management of chronic pain in children: A case study. *Archives of Physical Medicine and Rehabilitation, 61,* 375–378.
Wakeman, R. J., & Kaplan, J. Z. (1978). An experimental study of hypnosis in painful burns. *American Journal of Clinical Hypnosis, 21,* 3–12.
Walco, G. A., & Varni, J. W. (1991). Chronic and recurrent pain: Hemophilia, juvenile rheumatoid arthritis, and sickle cell disease. In J. P. Bush & S. W. Harkins (Eds.), *Children in pain: Clinical and research issues from a developmental perspective* (pp. 297–335). Berlin: Springer-Verlag.
Wilkie, D. J., Holzemer, W. L., Tesler, M. D., Ward, J. A., Paul, S. M., & Savedra, M. C. (1990). Measuring pain quality: Validity and reliability of children's and adolescents' pain language. *Pain, 41,* 151–159.
Zide, B., & Pardoe, R. (1976). The use of behavior modification therapy in a recalcitrant burned child. *Plastic and Reconstructive Surgery, 57,* 378–382.

7

Body Images and Pediatric Burn Injury

THOMAS PRUZINSKY and MARION DOCTOR

Body image is a critical variable in understanding children and adolescent's adjustment to burn injury (Bernstein, 1976; Stoddard, 1982). The primary goal of this chapter is to provide a broad theoretical, clinical, and empirical overview of the influence of body-image factors in children and adolescents' adjustment to burn injury. However, when considering body-image adjustment we must also consider the total socioemotional adjustment of the patient and family to the burn injury; including such critical variables as social support, child temperament, existence of psychopathology, and the family's socioeconomic status (Bernstein, 1976, 1990; Tarnowski, Rasnake, Gavaghan-Jones, & Smith, 1991).

However, while we must not forget the importance of these other variables, we believe much can be gained by focusing on body image. Body-image experiences have the potential to deeply affect quality of life, self-concept, self-esteem, peer relations, and social/sexual competence (Cash & Pruzinsky, 1990; Fisher, 1986). We concur with Fisher (1986, 1989), who has provided us with the most comprehensive empirical reviews of the voluminous literature on body image (Fisher, 1986), when he states that

THOMAS PRUZINSKY • Department of Psychology, Quinnipiac College, Hamden, Connecticut 06518. **MARION DOCTOR** • Children's Hospital Burn Center, University of Colorado School of Medicine, Denver, Colorado 80218.

Behavioral Aspects of Pediatric Burns, edited by Kenneth J. Tarnowski. Plenum Press, New York, 1994.

"[it] is difficult to exaggerate the importance of body attitudes in human conduct" (Fisher, 1989, p. 1).

CHAPTER GOALS

Despite some important progress (e.g., Cash & Pruzinsky, 1990; Fisher, 1986; Offman & Bradley, 1992; Thompson, 1990), we are still at a relatively early stage in our understanding of body image, especially with respect to children and adolescents. There also has not been a great deal of research specific to body image and burn injury. Therefore, in this chapter it is not possible to provide definitive answers about the body-image effects of burn injury. However, it is possible to provide a conceptual framework for understanding the many important dimensions of body image in relation to burn injury. For example, throughout the chapter we emphasize the need to understand the effects of the "external" (i.e., social) responses to human appearance (e.g., Adams, 1985; Alley, 1988; Bull & Rumsey, 1988; Patzer, 1985) and facial deviance in children (Hill-Beuf, 1990) as well as the "internal" (i.e., body image) experience of disfigurement. We will also discuss specific factors which may influence the body-image effects of pediatric burn injury; including size and location of the injury, the developmental stage and gender of the burn survivor, and the response of the family to the injury. Finally, we will provide suggestions regarding body-image rehabilitation for children and adolescents.

BODY-IMAGE DEFINITIONS

When we think of body image, we often think about self-perception of physical appearance. However, body image is composed of much more than our perception and evaluation of our physical appearance (Cash & Pruzinsky, 1990; Fisher, 1986). Body image refers to the thoughts, feelings, and attitudes that one has toward one's body as a whole (Fisher, 1986; Pruzinsky & Cash, 1990). In addition to thoughts and feelings about appearance, we may also focus on feelings about our sexuality, the degree to which we feel safe in our bodies, the size of various body parts, the overall strength of our bodies, the manner in which we experience physical sensations, including emotions, and the experience of body boundaries (Fisher, 1986, 1989); that is, body image is multidimensional (Pruzinsky & Cash, 1990). Furthermore, our body-image experience can influence our self-concept, behavior, and perceptions of the world (Pruzinsky & Cash,

1990). To reinforce the idea that body image is multidimensional and cannot be understood as a unitary concept, we often refer to the body-image concept in the plural form—body images (Cash & Pruzinsky, 1990).

That body image is a multidimensional experience has direct relevance to understanding the body-image adaptation of the child or adolescent burn survivor. For example, the child or adolescent who has sustained a burn injury may be concerned with the appearance of their body and how others will see them. However, they also may have lost some physical function (e.g., range of motion), they have likely experienced a significant amount of pain, and may also have experienced changes in skin sensation (e.g., skin tightness, itching, loss of ability to moderate temperature) which can contribute to body-image experience (Bernstein, 1976; Fisher, 1986). The pediatric burn survivor may also feel that their body is more vulnerable to harm (Giljohann, 1979). Each of these body experiences may impact the youngster's body image (Fisher, 1986) and can influence their thoughts, feelings, and behaviors. Therefore, when addressing the psychosocial adjustment of pediatric and adolescent burn survivors, we attempt to consider the full spectrum of body-image variables. However, by necessity we will devote much of our attention to the social and psychological response to disfigurement.

SOCIAL RESPONSE TO HUMAN APPEARANCE: THE "EXTERNAL" PERSPECTIVE

There are two perspectives to approach our understanding of the impact of burn injury on body image: the "external" and the "internal" (Cash, 1990a; Shontz, 1990). The external (social) perspective focuses on the social response to human appearance and disfigurement. The internal (body image) perspective focuses on how individuals interpret these social messages and how they subjectively experience their body. It is important to emphasize that there is no necessary correlation between external (objective) appearance and body image (Albino & Tedesco, 1988).

Social Perception of Physical Appearance and Disfigurement

One's physical appearance has a very powerful impact on social perception (Alley, 1988; Bull & Rumsey, 1988; Cash, 1990a; Hildebrandt, 1982; Jackson, 1992). A large body of scholarly literature documents the negative social response to individuals who are disfigured (Bernstein, 1976; Bull & Rumsey, 1988; Hill-Beuf, 1990; Macgregor, 1979, 1991). Facial deformities are among the most negatively perceived stigmatizing conditions (Hill-Beuf & Porter, 1984). These observations are true for "appearance-impaired" children (Hill-Beuf, 1990) and for adults.

> Nearly twenty years of reading questionnaires, interviewing children and parents, and observing activities in treatment centers . . . have created in me a painful awareness of the social stigmatization of appearance-impaired children in the United States, the burdensome social consequences of this stigmatization for its victims, and the psychological price such stigmatization exacts. [Hill-Beuf, 1990, p. 6]

Highest on the list of concerns among young burn survivors is the nature of the social response of peers and members of the opposite sex (Knudson-Cooper, 1981, 1984). A particularly difficult aspect of disfigurement is the experience of being stared at in public (Knudson-Copper, 1984; Macgregor, 1979, 1990). Staring entails an invasion of one's privacy and a loss of control over one's social environment (Bull & Rumsey, 1988; Macgregor, 1979, 1990). The experience of the person with disfigurement is often one of feeling like an object instead of a person (Hill-Beuf, 1990; Macgregor, 1990). Another social concern in the lives of individuals with visible disfigurement is that of teasing (Gerrard, 1991). There is a growing awareness of the potential long-term negative effects of teasing on body image (Thompson, 1990).

In addition to the constant social strain of having to cope with staring or teasing, there is also the potential for negative social stereotyping based on appearance (Bull & Rumsey, 1988). That is, the existing literature on the social perception of unattractive individuals is that negative judgments are often made about their personal characteristics or abilities (e.g., they may be viewed as less intelligent, able, or likable) on the basis of appearance alone (Bull & Rumsey, 1988; Hill-Beuf, 1990). These judgments can lead to prejudicial treatment of the appearance-impaired individuals by peers, teachers, or potential employers (Bull & Rumsey, 1988; Hill-Beuf, 1990).

The negative social reaction to burn-induced disfigurement is not surprising given the existing negative cultural stereotypes of the burn-injured (Petro, 1993; Petro & Salzberg, 1992). The representation of burn-injured individuals in the popular culture reveals that "there are no positive images of burn survivors within popular culture . . ." (Petro & Salzberg, 1992, p. 619). Burn victims are often portrayed as "evil personified" (as in the "Friday the 13th" series of movies as well as the "Nightmare on Elm Street" films) (Petro & Salzberg, 1992). These movies are particularly popular with children and adolescents. Petro and Salzberg (1992) point out that "the public's image of a burn survivor as evil or as victim or even as tragic figure must . . . unconsciously and negatively influence the public and the professional's attitude" (p. 621).

Internalization of Appearance Standards: Physical Appearance and Self-Concept

When considering the social perspective on human appearance, we must ask: To what degree does the individual with disfigurement internalize the social response? Currently, we do not know the answer to this question. However, we do know that children internalize society's standards for physical appearance very early in life (Fisher, 1986), and that there is a strong relationship between self-concept, self-esteem, and body image (Lerner & Jovanovic, 1990; Pruzinsky & Cash, 1990). For example, Lerner and colleagues have found that ". . . those male and female late adolescents who see their bodily characteristics as less interpersonally attractive, or less instrumentally effective, have lower self-esteem than is the case for late-adolescent males and females whose body images are more favorable . . ." (Lerner & Jovanovic, 1990, pp. 117–118). We also know that self-perception of physical appearance makes the largest contribution to global evaluations of self-esteem and self-worth for children in grades three through eight (Harter, 1987).

However, we still do not have a clear way of predicting if a child with residual disfigurement resulting from a burn injury will internalize negative social perceptions. Individuals differ in terms of the emphasis they place on the importance of physical appearance (Cash, 1992). Furthermore, some mechanisms may exist to provide a measure of psychological self-protection, thus allowing children with disfigurement to maintain a positive self-concept despite social stigmatization (Crocker & Major, 1989; Tobiasen, 1992).

FACTORS INFLUENCING BODY-IMAGE ADJUSTMENT

There is no question that the pain, loss of function, changes in skin sensation, and disfigurement of a burn injury require adjustment of the individual's body image. It is important to note the special role of the skin in body image development (Montague, 1978; Pruzinsky, 1990a). Damage to the skin results in disfigurement, disability, and threatens the individual's psychological integrity (Solnit & Priel, 1975). Therefore, the pediatric burn survivor may experience changes in many levels of body image.

However, these observations do not help us to predict the nature or extent of the body-image effect of burn injury. That is, to what degree will a child's body image be changed by a burn injury? Just as it is difficult to specify variables which predict the general social–emotional response to burn injury (Bernstein, 1976; Tarnowski *et al.*, 1991), it is also difficult to identify variables which predict the body-image effects of body injury in children and adolescents (Fisher, 1986). We are also hampered by the small number of studies specifically evaluating body image in the pediatric burn population as well as the lack of psychometrically sound body-image measures (Pruzinsky & Doctor, in preparation).

Therefore, given our current level of understanding, we cannot provide definitive answers regarding the body-image effects of burn injury. However, we can begin by examining four critical factors which may influence body-image adjustment: (1) location and degree of disfigurement, (2) the youngster's developmental stage, (3) gender differences, and (4) family influence.

Location and Degree of Disfigurement

We intuitively assume that the more extensive the burn injury (including the extent of residual scarring, loss of function, and visibility of burn disfigurement), the greater the degree of body-image disturbance an individual will experience. However, it is very clear from the study of body image, disfigurement, and disability that there is no necessary relationship between the degree of body damage and the degree of psychological response to that body damage (e.g., Bernstein, 1976; Lansdown, Lloyd, & Hunter, 1991; Macgregor, 1979; Pruzinsky, 1993; Shontz, 1990). Similar to the cosmetic impact of limb loss in children (Tyc, 1992; Varni, Setoguchi, Rappaport, & Talbot, 1992), some pediatric patients with major body damage appear not to experience negative body-image effects (Fisher, 1986), whereas others with relatively minor forms of body damage have tremendous difficulty coping.

This same pattern of findings is evident in the burn literature. Tarnowski and colleagues summarized the data regarding the relationship between the extent of a burn injury and psychological adjustment by concluding that there were "mixed results" (Tarnowski *et al.*, 1991, p. 380):

> Several studies found disfiguring burns to be associated with depression, vague career plans, increased psychopathology, and lower vocational aspirations (Chang & Herzog, 1976; Giljohann, 1979; Goldberg, 1974; Love *et al.*, 1987; Salfilios-Rothschild, 1970; Stoddard *et al.*, 1989), while other studies did not find injury visibility to be a significant factor in adjustment (Blakeney *et al.*, 1988; Bowden *et al.*, 1980; Knudson-Cooper, 1981; Molinaro, 1978; Tarnowski *et al.*, 1989). Six studies failed to identify a significant relationship between burn

severity and psychosocial adjustment (Blakeney *et al.*, 1988; Giljohann, 1979; Goldberg, 1974; Goldberg *et al.*, 1975; Love *et al.*, 1987; Molinaro, 1978).

However, when noting these conclusions we must emphasize the important difference between assessment of disfigurement and extent of injury (i.e., degree/location/visibility of burn injury) and body image. These "external" variables are very important to consider, but should not be construed as body-image measures *per se*.

With respect to studies specifically measuring body image, Jessee, Strickland, Leeper, and Wales (1992) reported no relationship between the location or severity of the burns and body image as measured by the Human Figure Drawing. Orr, Reznikoff, and Smith (1989) reported that body image scores (as measured with the semantic differential technique) were not correlated with size or location of burn. Furthermore, Knudson-Cooper (1981), utilizing the Burn-Related Supplement to assess body image, reported a lack of relationship between this measure and the size or degree of burn injury. Therefore, it appears that for those studies specifically evaluating body image, no relationship was found between degree of body damage and body-image adjustment.

In some instances there may be an inverse relationship between the degree of disfigurement and general psychological coping. For example, one investigation found that a greater degree of burn severity (though not degree of disfigurement or disability as rated by a parent) was a predictor of positive social competence (Byrne *et al.*, 1986). This is similar to the finding of Macgregor and colleagues (Macgregor *et al.*, 1953), who noted that individuals with severe facial deformities appeared to cope *better* than individuals with moderate disfigurement.

Similarly, it has been noted that a "hidden burn" (i.e., burn disfigurement sustained in childhood which can be hidden) can apparently have a very negative impact on quality of life and psychological functioning (Breslau, 1989; Cahners, 1992; Willis-Helmrich, 1992), including limiting involvement in intimate social relationships or other situations (e.g., beach activities) where scar exposure is imminent. Although we could appreciate the dramatic effect of "hidden burns" involving breasts or genitals, it is important to note that many of these individuals sustained leg burns (Breslau, 1989).

There are a number of explanations for why the hidden burn may result in high levels of psychological distress. Cahners (1992) in her description of adapting to breast burn states: "The patient with facial and hand scars that show clearly is forced to deal with his or her disfigurement. Patients who have body scars that are hidden by clothes and who fear exposure may never deal with the reality of their damaged selves and thus suffer from low self-esteem and accompanying depression and anxiety" (p. 44).

The lack of correlation between degree/location of disfigurement can perhaps be explained by noting the important role defense mechanisms play in adapting to body damage (Fisher, 1986), including facial deformity (Macgregor, 1979) and burn injury (Jessee *et al.*, 1992; Stoddard, 1982). Fisher (1986) makes some very important points regarding body-image adaptation to body damage:

> Perhaps the major impression to emerge is that the body image is a sturdy structure. People seem to adapt well to extreme forms of body disablement, disfigurement, and change. It is difficult to detect body image alterations even in persons with crippling body defects. Denial and repression seem to be major defenses in restoring body image equilibrium after severe body damage has occurred. Use of denial has been particularly well documented in the case of patients with disfiguring burns. [pp. 263–264]

In summary, it appears that the location or size of the burn injury is not an accurate predictor of the extent of body-image effect. The burn team must take care to treat each burn survivor as an individual. Some individuals with small injuries that can be hidden from view may be just as psychologically affected by the body change as the individual with facial, hand, genital, or breast burns.

Developmental Stage and Body Image

Is it more damaging to body-image development and experience to sustain a burn injury in infancy, early childhood, or adolescence? This is a very difficult question. Assessing the effect of developmental stage on body image in the pediatric burn survivor requires considering the child's developmental stage at the time of injury and evaluation, as well as comparing these assessments to "normal" body-image functioning. Such an assessment also requires developmentally sensitive measures which take into account the child's level of cognitive functioning (e.g., age-related norms for body-image scores). Currently, our evaluation methods and data are quite limited, and only an initial answer to the question of developmental stage effects of burn injury is available.

Stoddard (1982), in a descriptive evaluation of body image and pediatric burn injury, provides much insight into developmental stage-specific body image issues. He describes how the pediatric burn survivor may experience guilt regarding body damage, a pervasive theme in the literature on body-image development in children (Fisher, 1986). Guilt feelings are likely related to the pediatric burn survivor's "distortion of meaning of the damage" (Stoddard, 1982), and may be related to the child's perception that others have sustained injuries greater than their own. They may believe that they are being punished for something they have done wrong (Stoddard, 1982). The experience of guilt seems to occur in children and adolescents despite whether or not they played an active role in sustaining their injury (Fisher, 1986) and may be associated with the cooccurrence of depressed affect (Stoddard, 1982). Additionally, body-image concerns may emerge during sleep (e.g., as "recurrent night terrors of annihilation," Stoddard, 1982, p. 506). Overall, the pediatric burn survivor experiences and expresses their body-image concerns in many more ways than concern regarding appearance.

Stoddard (1982) and others (Giljohann, 1979) have observed that the child burned before the age of 2 requires minimal body-image adaptation because the injury becomes a part of their "normal" body image. This is consistent with the developmental literature on body image which documents that it is at approximately the end of the second year that children develop a relatively well-solidified sense of body-self (Fisher, 1986). However, the fact that the child incorporates body damage into their body image is no guarantee that there will not be an emotional response to the body damage later in life.

The experience of body image and body damage is quite different for the school-age child (Stoddard, 1982), a period in which dramatic progress in body-image development occurs (i.e., around 4 to 5 years of age) (Fisher, 1986). Though children at this age have a relatively clear conception of their body-self, they also may have some misconceptions about body functioning (Fisher, 1986; Stoddard, 1982). Additionally, these children are aware of cultural standards of appearance, standards similar to those held by adults (Fisher, 1986). Furthermore, the school-age child will have at least some memory of the preinjury appearance, and therefore is likely to have to mourn the losses sustained (Stoddard, 1982). Each of these factors can influence the child's experience and expression of body-image concerns.

The literature on "normal" body-image development in adolescence fails to document any critical developmental issues (Fisher, 1986), though Fisher does note a ". . . heightening of concern about the security of the body" (Fisher, 1986, p. 104) during this period. Within the burn literature, there appears to be a general concern that adolescence is an especially challenging time with respect to body-image adjustment (e.g., Bernstein, 1976; Giljohann, 1979; Sawyer, Minde, & Zuker, 1982; Stoddard, 1982), and that some children may evidence problems at this stage of development even if they have not done so earlier in life (Sawyer *et al.*, 1982).

In summary, it seems that there are some developmental trends evident in body-image adjustment to burn injury. However, in the future it will be important to assess the changes in body image with psychometrically sound and developmental stage-specific measures which take into account the child's changing cognitive, social, and physical development.

Gender Differences and Body Image

Fisher's (1986) extensive review of the literature on body image concluded that males and females consistently demonstrate very different ways of perceiving and experiencing their bodies, and that though some differences may be biologically based, most appear to be related to socialization. There is little question that our culture places greater value on the physical appearance of females and that females internalize this cultural standard (Jackson, 1992).

This emphasis on the importance of appearance-related variables can lead to the conclusion that, as a result of burn injury, females are at greater risk for body-image dysphoria than are males. However, Fisher (1986) clearly states that ". . . it is apparent from the available evidence that the male child is *not* superior, and probably is *inferior*, to the female child in attaining a sense of body security and adequacy" (p. 106; emphasis added). It appears that despite being consistently more critical of their physical appearance, females are generally more comfortable with their bodily experiences (including body change) than are males (Fisher, 1986).

This set of observations may lead one to conclude that males would be more threatened by sustaining disability as a result of burn injury than would be females, and that females would be more threatened by disfigurement (Fisher, 1986; Jackson, 1992). However, one investigation (Brown *et al.*, 1988) specifically focusing on gender differences in adult burn survivors, found that issues regarding body function were critical for both males *and* females, and that the impact of disfigurement for the females was not particularly critical.

At least one study specifically evaluating body image and burn injury in a younger group of subjects documented that males had a more positive body image (as measured by the Semantic Differential Technique) than females (Orr *et al.*, 1989). However, no gender differences in body image were found in the study of Knudson-Cooper (1981), when using the Burn Related Supplement (as the measure of body image), nor were there gender differences found in the evaluation of body image via Human Figure Drawings (Jessee *et al.*, 1992). This pattern of "mixed results" is consistent with the findings regarding the general influence of gender on the psychosocial response to burn injury (Tarnowski *et al.*, 1991). Therefore, it is not currently possible to draw conclusions regarding the differential impact of gender on body-image adjustment to burn injuries.

Parental Influence on Body-Image Adaptation

Parents are instrumental in children's body-image development (Fisher, 1986; Fisher & Cleveland, 1968). Therefore, it logically follows that the body-image adaptation of the pediatric burn survivor must be influenced by the response of the parents to the child's injury (Bernstein, 1976; Tarnowski *et al.*, 1991). To provide the most positive "mirroring" for their child, parents may have to mourn the loss of the child they once knew (Clarke & Martin, 1978), and they may have to come to terms with any real or imagined responsibility that they have had for the injury.

Parents can have many possible reactions to the child's change in appearance or functioning, including acceptance, denial, anger, anxiety, guilt, promotion of overcompensation, pursuit of perfection in surgical reconstruction, or an avoidance of surgical reconstruction in an attempt to accept the child "as they are." Some parents may attempt to hide the child. Each of these responses may have a body-image effect on the child, depending on the child's developmental stage, preinjury body image, peer support, and a host of other factors.

One common type of parental reaction is that of overprotection, especially as a response to the teasing that "appearance-impaired" children experience (Hill-Beuf, 1990). The possible negative ramifications of parental overprotection are many and include delaying the development of critical social skills. Parental overprotection may also have a body-image effect. Fisher (1986) notes that the literature on body image reveals that fostering weakness or dependency in a child can ". . . induce feelings of body vulnerability . . ." (p. 644). Therefore, in their efforts to protect their child, parents may undermine body-image development.

Parents can also influence their child's adaptation to body damage very directly by providing social support (Orr *et al.*, 1989). The attitude taken by the parents toward the child's disfigurement or disability is likely to be modeled by the child (Stoddard, 1982). If the parent is anxious and overconcerned, it is more likely that the child will respond similarly. Anxiety regarding the disfigurement may also lead to repression or avoidance of these concerns, thus decreasing the chances that adaptive solutions to these challenges are developed (Giljohann, 1979). Therefore, anything that can be done to help parents adapt to the child's injury will ultimately be of value to the child.

Summary and Conclusions

We have considered the influence of four factors on body image adaptation, including the size and location of the burn injury, the developmental stage and gender of the burn survivor, as well as parental factors. On the basis of this selective review, it is apparent that the relationship between body damage and body-image adjustment is complex. A more thorough review would consider such issues as the special body-image concerns for children of ethnicity (e.g., African-American children) who may undergo particularly stressful changes in appearance, and the effect of the mechanism of burn injury (e.g., if it was the result of abuse or self-inflicted) on body-image adaptation. Progress in addressing these complex issues requires more systematic approaches to body-image assessment (Pruzinsky & Doctor, in preparation). However, we do not need definitive answers regarding the adaption process before we can facilitate body-image rehabilitation.

PHYSICAL INTERVENTIONS IN BODY-IMAGE REHABILITATION

Total body-image rehabilitation requires that equal attention be given to the physical and psychological recovery of the pediatric burn survivor. The rehabilitation process begins with maximizing the degree to which reconstructive surgery can bring about positive changes in appearance. Many practical issues arise during the course of reconstructive surgery including (1) addressing the child's or adolescent's need for some control over the process of surgical reconstruction; (2) the need to shape the patient's and family's expectations regarding what can be surgically accomplished; and (3) considering the use of cosmetics in body-image rehabilitation.

During the process of undergoing reconstructive surgery many body-image issues emerge. As one burn survivor astutely observes: "Visits to the plastic surgeon for consultation about scar revisions reopen emotional wounds. These visits can be painful; the injury is once again a major focus, and even though some improvement may be offered, the permanency of the disfigurement must be faced" (Cahners, 1992, p. 44). This is just as true for children and adolescents as it is for adults. The plastic surgery team should be acutely aware of the emotions and body-image concerns stirring in their patient during "routine" consultations.

Control and Surgical Reconstruction

Whenever possible, the child or adolescent should be allowed to choose the surgical procedure which is done next in the course of undergoing reconstruction (Lefebvre & Arndt, 1988). That is, whenever possible (i.e., when there is some discretion without any harm coming to the patient), the child or adolescent should be allowed to define, from their subjective body-image perspective, the part of the body that is of greatest concern to them (Pruzinsky, 1990b). This choice allows them to regain some measure of control over their lives and their bodies; a sense of control undermined by being injured, undergoing burn treatment, and being subjected to negative social responses to their disfigurement.

Bjarnason *et al.* (1992) documented that the reconstructive surgery goals for the patient, parents, and treatment team often differ. Family members and the treatment team must be cautious about the messages given to the child when conversing, in front of them, regarding their "deformities" and what needs to be done to modify them. How does the child interpret the parent's or surgeon's desire to "fix" them? The challenge is to convey a loving acceptance of the child, no matter how they appear, while supporting surgical interventions to improve the child's appearance.

Setting Expectations for Outcome of Surgical Reconstruction

Setting realistic patient and family expectations regarding the ultimate outcome of the program of reconstructive surgery is essential (Pruzinsky, 1992). From a body-image perspective, *expectations* regarding the surgical outcome can play as important a role as the *actual* surgical change in the patient's ultimate satisfaction with the outcome (Pruzinsky & Edgerton, 1990). Furthermore, there is always the potential for differences between what the patient (from their "internal" perspective), family, and surgeon (from their "external" perspectives) might expect regarding the surgical outcome. Of course, there is always a degree of uncertainty in knowing the ultimate surgical outcome (Pruzinsky, 1992). However, the surgeon's experience allows for some reasonable understanding of the youngster's eventual appearance-related outcome. This needs to be communicated to the patient and the family with great care, compassion, and honesty. When setting surgical expectations, a crucial task is to facilitate the patient's cognitive *and* emotional understanding of the distinction between "I want to look the way I did before" and "I want to look the best that I can." The emotional and body-image ramifications of this distinction are critical.

The burn-care team must maintain a balance between hope for future reconstruction and the reality of the expected surgical outcome. The reality is that there is almost always residual disfigurement, no matter how skilled the surgeon and no matter how many reconstructive surgical procedures are conducted. At some point the treatment team, family, and patient may need to address the question: "When is enough, enough?" (Marsh, 1990). That is, how does one weigh the risks and costs (emotional and financial) of operations that have minimal returns? In some instances the patient will insist on continued surgical intervention in the face of diminishing returns. This may be evidence for nonacceptance of the disfigurement. In other instances, it may be the surgeon or the parent who pursues more surgical reconstruction when the risks and costs appear to outweigh the benefits. Each of these scenarios has their own body-image implications.

Cosmetic Rehabilitation

There is a growing awareness of the importance of cosmetics in burn rehabilitation (Graham, 1985, 1988; Phoenix Society, 1993; Seidel, 1988; Westmore, 1991). This field has been referred to as "esthetic rehabilitation," "cosmetic camouflage," and the use of "rehabilitative makeup." These techniques have been used extensively with children (Seidel, 1988). Cosmetic rehabilitation adds an important dimension to the patient's total rehabilitation program. Graham (1985) has developed "appearance training programs" which include ". . . advice and training on all aspects of appearance, hairstyles, color sense, all aspects of nonverbal communication and self-presentation, with training in effective cosmetic care as a central feature . . ." (p. 33).

Use of cosmetics has proven helpful during the surgical reconstruction process and is also of value when the limits of surgical reconstruction are reached. The use of cosmetic camouflage allows the individual greater access to and greater control over social interactions. Ideally, cosmetic rehabilitation would be integrated as one component in the total treatment process. Not only do these interventions provide direct body-image benefit, the use of the rehabilitative cosmetic consultation may also provide a unique opportunity for the burn survivor to voice appearance-related concerns (Graham, 1985). That is, the nature of the relationship between the burn survivor and the makeup consultant, which includes close physical proximity (when applying the makeup), camaraderie, touching, and conveying feelings of hope, may provide a unique opportunity for discussing appearance-related concerns not previously addressed (Graham, 1985).

The use of rehabilitative makeup clearly holds great promise and has been used with success. However, more research on the body-image effects should be conducted. For example, we need to know more about the degree to which children, especially males, are compliant with regimens of cosmetic camouflage. We also need to know about the balance of negative and positive effects of makeup. That is, is the fear of exposure of the camouflaged disfigurement a part of the process of using rehabilitative makeup, and how does this balance out with the positive effects? We already know that everyday cosmetic usage in individuals who are not disfigured is associated with positive changes in social perception (Cash, 1990a), and self-perception, including improved body image, and social confidence (Cash, 1990a). Can we document these effects for individuals with disfigurement? If we can empirically document these findings, then perhaps the use of rehabilitative cosmetics would receive even greater acceptance. Certainly such research will shed light on the body-image adaptation of burn-injured patients.

PSYCHOSOCIAL APPROACHES TO BODY-IMAGE INTERVENTION

In this section, we address the goals and methods of psychosocial intervention to change body image in children and adolescents. The general goals of psychosocial interventions are to prevent body-image problems or to ameliorate existing body-image problems. The specific goals of psychosocial body-image intervention are (1) to provide the youngster with social skills, (2) modify the cognitive interpretation of body and appearance-related experiences, and (3) facilitate development of alternative areas of physical competence.

There are many unanswered questions regarding how to psychologically facilitate body-image adjustment. For example, a frequently asked question is: When should the patient be allowed to see their scars? When should they be encouraged or discouraged from viewing their disfigurement? What should they be told when they ask what they look like? What (and when) should they be told about what can honestly be expected from reconstructive surgery? Unfortunately, there are no clear answers to these important questions. Each patient and clinical situation is different. Perhaps the most constructive approach to caring for the body-image needs of our patients is expressed in the following quotation:

> Honest, sensitive discussion of wounds and healing, availability of mirrors, interaction with other acute patients as well as graduate patients and their families, participation in the hospital community and chaperoned outings prior to discharge are all useful tools that can be employed to achieve the goal of education and beginning integration of the new body image. [Doctor, 1992b, p. 612]

In addition to these interventions, youngsters adjusting to body changes may benefit from social skills training, cognitive-behavioral forms of therapy, and/or involvement in programs which facilitate the development of physical competence (e.g., through sports). It is important to note that not all individuals with residual disfigurement or dysfunction require or desire psychosocial services. Many have the emotional resilience and/or family and peer support which allows them to develop positive coping strategies without formal intervention.

Social Skills Training

The major goals of social skills training for individuals who have some type of disfigurement are to reduce the frequency and intensity of the negative social messages they receive, increase their positive social interactions, and provide them with a means of gaining some control over their social environments (e.g., Bull & Rumsey, 1988; Kapp-Simon & Simon, 1991; Macgregor, 1990). Furthermore, it is also clear that peer support is one of the most important factors in predicting the development of a positive body image in young burn survivors (Orr *et al.*, 1989). The basic premise of social skills training is that the attitudes and behaviors of the youngster with disfigurement can help to modify their social experiences, and can result in improvements in social support. For example, through the use of school reentry programs, children are greeted into the school environment with immediate acceptance and for a time may enjoy "hero" status. However, the long-term social acceptance of the child is determined by the child's self-acceptance and his/her ability to interact with peers.

The effectiveness of social skills training for individuals with many types of disabilities has been well documented (Dunn, 1987; Dunn & Herman, 1982). Social skills programs for children with facial deformities exist (Kapp-Simon & Simon, 1991). Parents of young children with facial deformities can be taught how to help their children cope with teasing and staring (Gerrard, 1991). Such programs have also been developed for children experiencing changed appearance resulting from cancer (Walco & Varni, 1991). In these programs ". . . children are taught specifically how to cope with the verbal and physical teasing and name calling associated with changes in their personal appearance. . . . Strategies such as extinguishing inappropriate peer responses through lack of behavioral response, giving age-appropriate explanations for physical changes, as well as going to an authoritative adult for support and assistance are emphasized" (Walco & Varni, 1991, p. 236). These same interventions can be implemented for children and adolescents with burn injuries. The essence of the social skills approach is to teach the youngsters "social-cognitive problem-solving strategies" (Walco & Varni, 1991, p. 231), so that they can learn to relate more effectively to peers and others.

Cognitive-Behavioral Coping Techniques

A primary goal of this section is to advocate for integrating cognitive-behavioral therapy (CBT) methods (Kendall, 1991a,b; Pope, McHale, &

Craighead, 1988) into the psychosocial care programs of children and adolescents with residual disfigurement resulting from burn injury. The CBT approach offers promise to those individuals requiring psychosocial interventions to cope with body-image problems (Cash, 1992) and can be used in combination with the social skills training.

The essence of the CBT approach to body-image therapy is an understanding that negative body-image-related emotions, and maladaptive body-image-related behaviors are associated with maladaptive cognitive processes (Cash, 1992; Freedman, 1990). For example, the youngster with residual facial scarring may say to themselves "I am ugly." This may lead them to the erroneous cognitive conclusion that "No one wants to be around me." These thoughts may be associated with negative affects, including self-consciousness, anger, anxiety, or depression. Additionally, these thought patterns and emotions may be associated with specific behavioral patterns (e.g., acting out or social withdrawal). CBT is designed to break these maladaptive connections between cognition, emotion, and behavior, and to replace them with more adaptive thought and behavioral patterns (Cash, 1992).

CBT is increasingly being used to treat a wide range of childhood problems (Kendall, 1991a; Pope *et al.*, 1988), including internalizing (Kendall *et al.*, 1991; Stark, Rouse, & Livingston, 1991) and externalizing disorders (Kendall *et al.*, 1991). CBT is a short-term, problem-solving form of intervention. The role of the practitioner is that of "consultant, diagnostician, and educator" (Kendall, 1991b, p. 6). Kendall (1991b) refers to the practitioner of CBT as ". . . a person who does not have all of the answers, but one who has some ideas worthy of trying out . . ." (p. 6). This is an ideal posture to take when working with children and families learning to cope with bodily disfigurement. In my work with families and individuals with disfigurement (T.P.), I have often referred to myself as a "coach," i.e., someone who has some experience and strategies that have worked for others and may work for them. Taking this approach addresses the resistance that some patients and families have to seeing a mental health professional (Pruzinsky, 1993).

Cognitive-behavioral interventions have proven effective in the treatment of body-image-related problems in adults (e.g., Butters & Cash, 1987; Cash, 1990b, 1992; Freedman, 1990; Rosen, Saltzberg, & Srebnik, 1989). However, these specific techniques have not been directly applied to coping with facial disfigurement in adults or children, though some initial steps in this direction have been proposed (Cash, 1992; Pruzinsky, 1993). Therefore, what is currently needed is specific application of these techniques to children with burn injuries, that is, development of programs similar to the ones already available in cancer care (Walco & Varni, 1991). It is only a matter of time before an integrated and formalized approach to body-image rehabilitation program integrating CBT techniques is developed.

Physical Competence

As we have emphasized throughout the chapter, there are many different modes of body experience other than physical appearance. One method of improving body image is to provide these youngsters with alternative means of developing body competency. Harter (1987) has documented the importance of physical competence in contributing to overall self-concept. One method by which children and adolescents can learn to enhance their overall sense of physical competence is through sports (Danish, Petitpas, & Hale, 1990). Additionally, it is important that children and adolescents have the opportunity to talk about their developing sexuality (Whitehead, 1993).

Perhaps one of the most important arenas for the development and integration of many of these approaches is through the burn camp experience (Doctor, 1992). Burn camps are widely accepted as a source of pleasure and recreation as well as a means of providing for the ongoing rehabilitation needs of burn-impaired children and adolescents. A quality camp program is able to provide an opportunity for participants to develop physical competence and social skills, both of which are crucial ingredients in building self-image and social acceptance (Doctor, 1992). In the safety of a camp environment, children are able to benefit from guidance and practice in the social graces as well as in the art of living harmoniously with others. The extent of counseling varies according to the goals and philosophy of the camp. Universally, however, a milieu is established to foster improved body image and social acceptance. The effectiveness of meeting this important goal is yet to be empirically documented. Clinically, however, there remains little doubt that camps provide self-esteem building experiences that have important residual effects in the real world of home and school.

In summary, therefore, there are many possible ways to facilitate body-image rehabilitation. It appears clear that programs of body-image rehabilitation can be developed which address the physical, social, and psychological aspects of body-image experience. However, it is essential that we develop programs of body-image intervention which can be evaluated for their efficacy and cost-effectiveness. In this era of cost-consciousness, outcome data are essential for ensuring that we can provide these valuable clinical services so that we can continue to make strides toward improving the quality of life of pediatric burn survivors.

SUMMARY AND CONCLUSION

In this review of the body-image effects of burn injury we have considered the importance of the social response to human disfigurement as well as factors influencing the body-image adaptation to burn injury. Not many definitive statements can be made about which social and psychological factors will influence the body-image adaptation of this population. However, we are certain that body image is a critical factor influencing the quality of life of children and adolescents who have sustained burn injuries. We also know that each individual child and family will respond in their own unique way. Hopefully, in the future we will make progress in empirically evaluating the validity and reliability of body-image measurement and the efficacy of body-image interventions.

REFERENCES

Adams, G. R. (1985). Attractiveness through the ages: Implications of facial attractiveness over the life cycle. In J. A. Graham & A. M. Kligman (Eds.), *The psychology of cosmetic treatments* (pp. 133–151). New York: Praeger.

Albino, J. E., & Tedesco, L. A. (1988). The role of perception in treatment of impaired facial appearance. In T. R. Alley (Ed.), *Social and applied aspects of perceiving faces* (pp. 217–237). Hillsdale, NJ: Lawrence Erlbaum.

Alley, T. R. (Ed.). (1988). *Social and applied aspects of perceiving faces*. Hillsdale, NJ: Lawrence Erlbaum.

Bernstein, N. R. (1976). *Emotional care of the burned and the facially disfigured*. Boston: Little, Brown.

Bernstein, N. R. (1990). Objective bodily damage: Disfigurement and dignity. In T. F. Cash & T. Pruzinsky (Eds.), *Body images: Development, deviance, and change* (pp. 131–148). New York: Guilford Press.

Bjarnason, D., Phillips, L. G., McCoy, B., Murphy, L., McCauley, R. L., Desai, M., Herndon, D. N., & Robson M. C. (1992). Reconstructive goals for children with burns: Are our goals the same? *Journal of Burn Care and Rehabilitation*, *13*, 389–390.

Blakeney, P., Herndon, D., Desai, M., Beard, S., & Wales-Seale, M. (1988). Long-term psychosocial adjustment following burn injury. *Journal of Burn Care and Rehabilitation*, *9*, 661–665.

Bowden, M. L., Feller, I., Tholen, D., Davidson, T. N., & James, M. H. (1980). Self-esteem of severely burned patients. *Archives of Physical Medicine and Rehabilitation*, *61*, 449–452.

Breslau, A. J. (1989). The hidden burn. *The Icarus File*, *7*(4), 1.

Brown, B., Roberts, J., Browne, G., Byrne, C., Love, B., & Streiner, D. (1988). Gender differences in variables associated with psychosocial adjustment to a burn injury. *Research in Nursing and Health*, *11*, 23–30.

Bull, R., & Rumsey, N. (1988). *The social psychology of facial appearance*. Berlin: Springer-Verlag.

Butters, J. W., & Cash, T. F. (1987). Cognitive–behavioral treatment of women's body-image dissatisfaction. *Journal of Consulting and Clinical Psychology*, *55*, 889–897.

Byrne, C., Love, B., Browne, G., Brown, B., Roberts, J., & Streiner, D. (1986). The social competence of children following burn injury: a study of resilience. *Journal of Burn Care and Rehabilitation, 7*, 247–252.

Cahners, S. S. (1992). Young woman with breast burns: A self-help "Group by mail." *Journal of Burn Care and Rehabilitation, 13*, 44–47.

Cash, T. F. (1990a). The psychology of physical appearance: Aesthetics, attributes, and images. In T. F. Cash & T. Pruzinsky (Eds.), *Body images: Development, deviance and change* (pp. 51–79). New York: Guilford Press.

Cash, T. F. (1990b). *Body image therapy: A program for self-directed change*. New York: Guilford Press.

Cash, T. F. (1992, November). Body image therapy for persons with facial disfigurement: A cognitive-behavioral approach. Presentation to The National Foundation for Facial Reconstruction conference on "Special faces: An understanding of facial disfigurement," New York.

Cash, T. F., & Pruzinsky, T. (Eds.). (1990). *Body images: Development, deviance and change*. New York: Guilford Press.

Chang, F. C., & Herzog, B. (1976). Burn morbidity: A follow-up study of physical and psychological disability. *Annals of Surgery, 183*, 34–37.

Clarke, A. M., & Martin, H. L. (1978). The effects of previous thermal injury on adolescents. *Burns, 5*, 101–104.

Crocker, J., & Major, B. (1989). Social stigma and self-esteem: The self-protective properties of stigma. *Psychological Review, 96*, 608–630.

Danish, S. J., Petitpas, A. J., & Hale, B. D. (1990). Sport as a context for developing competence. In T. P. Gullotta, G. R. Adams, & R. Montemayor (Eds.), *Developing social competency in adolescence* (pp. 169–194). Beverly Hills: Sage Publications.

Doctor, M. E. (1992a). Burn camps and community aspects of burn care. *Journal of Burn Care and Rehabilitation, 13*, 68–76.

Doctor, M. E. (1992b). Helping the burned child to adapt. *Clinics in Plastic Surgery, 19*, 607–614.

Dunn, M. (1987). Social skills and rehabilitation. In B. Caplan (Ed.), *Rehabilitation psychology desk reference* (pp. 345–364). Rockville, MD: Aspen Publishers.

Dunn, M. E., & Herman, S. H. (1982). Social skills and physical disability. In D. M. Doleys, R. L. Meredith, & A. R. Ciminero (Eds.), *Behavioral medicine: Assessment and treatment strategies* (pp. 117–144). New York: Plenum Press.

Fisher, S. (1986). *Development and structure of the body image*. Hillsdale, NJ: Lawrence Erlbaum.

Fisher, S. (1989). *Sexual images of the self: The psychology of erotic sensations and illusions*. Hillsdale, NJ: Lawrence Erlbaum.

Fisher, S. (1990). The evolution of psychological concepts about the body. In T. F. Cash & T. Pruzinsky (Eds.), *Body images: Development, deviance, and change* (pp. 3–20). New York: Guilford Press.

Fisher, S., & Cleveland, S. E. (1968). *Body image and personality* (rev. ed.). New York: Dover Press.

Freedman, R. (1990). Cognitive–behavioral perspectives on body-image change. In T. F. Cash & T. Pruzinsky (Eds.), *Body images: Development, deviance, and change* (pp. 272–295). New York: Guilford Press.

Gerrard, J. (1991). Beating the teasing syndrome. In E. P. Caronni (Ed.), *Craniofacial surgery: Proceedings of the Second International Conference of the International Society of Cranio-Maxillo-Facial Surgery* (pp. 429–432). Bologna, Italy: Monduzzi Editore.

Giljohann, A. (1979). Adolescents burned as children. *Burns, 7*, 95–99.

Goldberg, R. T. (1974). Adjustment of children with invisible and visible handicaps: Congenital heart disease and facial burns. *Journal of Counseling Psychology, 21*, 428–432.

Goldberg, R. T., Bernstein, N. R., & Crosby, R. (1975). Vocational development of adolescents with burn injury. *Rehabilitation Counseling Bulletin, 18,* 140–146.

Graham, J. A. (1985). Overview of psychology of cosmetics. In J. A. Graham & A. M. Kligman (Eds.), *The psychology of cosmetic treatments* (pp. 26–36). New York: Praeger.

Graham, J. A. (1988). The psychology of cosmetic treatments for the disfigured patient. In N. R. Bernstein, A. J. Breslau, & J. A. Graham (Eds.), *Coping strategies for burn survivors and their families* (pp. 89–96). New York: Praeger.

Harter, S. (1987). The determinants and mediational role of global self-worth in children. In N. Eisenberg (Ed.), *Contemporary topics in developmental psychology* (pp. 219–242). New York: Wiley.

Hildebrandt, K. A. (1982). The role of physical appearance in infant and child development. In H. E. Fitzgerald, B. M. Lester, & M. W. Yogman (Eds.), *Theory and research in behavioral pediatrics* (Vol. 1, pp. 181–220). New York: Plenum Press.

Hill-Beuf, A. (1990). *Beauty is the beast: Appearance-impaired children in America.* Philadelphia: University of Pennsylvania Press.

Hill-Beuf, A., & Porter, J. D. R. (1984). Children coping with impaired appearance: Social and psychologic influences. *General Hospital Psychiatry, 6,* 294–301.

Jackson, L. A. (1992). *Physical appearance and gender: Sociobiological and sociocultural perspectives.* Albany: State University of New York Press.

Jessee, P. O., Strickland, M. P., Leeper, J. D., & Wales, P. (1992). Perception of body image in children with burns, five years after burn injury. *Journal of Burn Care and Rehabilitation, 13,* 33–38.

Kapp-Simon, K. A., & Simon, D. J. (1991). *Meeting the challenge: A social skills training program for adolescents with special needs.* Chicago: University of Illinois at Chicago Press.

Kendall, P. C. (Ed.). (1991a). *Child and adolescent therapy: Cognitive–behavioral procedures.* New York: Guilford Press.

Kendall, P. C. (1991b). Guiding theory for therapy with children and adolescents. In P. C. Kendall (Ed.), *Child and adolescent therapy: Cognitive–behavioral procedures* (pp. 3–22). New York: Guilford Press.

Kendall, P. C., Chansky, T. E., Freidman, M., Kim, R., Kortlander,E., Sessa, F. M., & Siqueland, L. (1991). Treating anxiety disorders in children and adolescents. In P. C. Kendall (Ed.), *Child and adolescent therapy: Cognitive–behavioral procedures* (pp. 131–164). New York: Guilford Press.

Knudson-Cooper, M. S. (1981). Adjustment to visible stigma: The case of the severely burned. *Social Science and Medicine, 15B,* 31–44.

Knudson-Cooper, M. S. (1984). The antecedents and consequences of children's burn injuries. *Advances in Developmental and Behavioral Pediatrics, 5,* 33–74.

Lansdown, R., Lloyd, J., & Hunter, J. (1991). Facial deformity in childhood: Severity and psychosocial adjustment. *Child Care Health Development, 17,* 165–171.

Lefebvre, A. M., & Arndt, E. M. (1988). Working with facially disfigured children: A challenge in prevention. *Canadian Journal of Psychiatry, 33,* 453–458.

Lerner, R. M., & Jovanovic, J. (1990). The role of body image in psychosocial development across the life-span. In T. F. Cash & T. Pruzinsky (Eds.), *Body images: Development, deviance, and change* (pp. 110–127). New York: Guilford Press.

Love, B., Byrne, C., Roberts, J., Browne, G., & Brown, B. (1987). Adult psychosocial adjustment following childhood injury: The effect of disfigurement. *Journal of Burn Care and Rehabilitation, 8,* 280–285.

Macgregor, F. C., Abel, T. M., Byrt, A., Lauer, E., & Weissmann, S. (1953). Facial deformities and plastic surgery: a psychosocial study. Springfield, IL: Charles C. Thomas Publishers.

Macgregor, F. C. (1979). *After plastic surgery: Adaptation and adjustment*. New York: Praeger.

Macgregor, F. C. (1990). Facial disfigurement: Problems and management of social interaction and implications for mental health. *Aesthetic Plastic Surgery, 14*, 249–257.

Marsh, J. L. (1990). When is enough enough? Secondary surgery for cleft lip and palate patients. *Clinics in Plastic Surgery, 17*, 37–47.

Molinaro, J. R. (1978). The social fate of children disfigured by burns. *American Journal of Psychiatry, 135*, 979–980.

Montague, A. (1978). *Touching: The human significance of the skin* (2nd ed.). New York: Harper & Row.

Offman, H. J., & Bradley, S. J. (1992). Body image of children and adolescents and its measurement: An overview. *Canadian Journal of Psychiatry, 37*, 417–422.

Orr, D. A., Reznikoff, M., & Smith, G. M. (1989). Body image, self-esteem, and depression in burn-injured adolescents and young adults. *Journal of Burn Care and Rehabilitation, 10*, 454–461.

Patzer, G. L. (1985). *The physical attractiveness phenomena*. New York: Plenum Press.

Petro, J. A. (1993, May). Contemporary popular culture and the burn victim. *Proceedings of National Symposium on the Psychosocial Aspects of Plastic Surgery*, Columbia–Presbyterian Medical Center, New York.

Petro, J. A., & Salzberg, C. A. (1992). Ethical issues of burn management. *Clinics in Plastic Surgery, 19*, 615–621.

Phoenix Society. (1993) *Cosmetology for burn survivors*. Phoenix Society, 11 Rust Hill Rd., Levittown, PA 19056.

Pope, A. W., McHale, S. M., & Craighead, W. E. (1988). *Self-esteem enhancement with children and adolescents*. New York: Pergamon Press.

Pruzinsky, T. (1990a). Somatopsychic approaches to psychotherapy and personal growth. In T. F. Cash & T. Pruzinsky (Eds.), *Body images: Development, deviance, and change* (pp. 296–315). New York: Guilford Press.

Pruzinsky, T. (1990b). Collaboration of plastic surgeon and medical psychotherapist: Reconstructive surgery for congenital craniofacial deformities. *Medical Psychotherapy: An International Journal, 3*, 103–116.

Pruzinsky, T. (1992). Social and psychological effects of major craniofacial deformity. *Cleft Palate and Craniofacial Journal, 29*, 578–584.

Pruzinsky, T. (1993, May). Adapting to facial disfigurement: Multiple perspectives, clinical interventions, and unanswered questions. *Proceedings of National Symposium on the Psychosocial Aspects of Plastic Surgery*, Columbia–Presbyterian Medical Center, New York.

Pruzinsky, T., & Cash, T. F. (1990). Integrative themes in body-image development, deviance, and change. In T. F. Cash & T. Pruzinsky (Eds.), *Body images: Development, deviance, and change* (pp. 337–349). New York: Guilford Press.

Pruzinsky, T., & Doctor, M. (in preparation). Body image measurement in pediatric burn survivors.

Pruzinsky, T., & Edgerton, M. T. (1990). Body-image change in cosmetic plastic surgery. In T. F. Cash & T. Pruzinsky (Eds.), *Body images: Development, deviance, and change* (pp. 217–236). New York: Guilford Press.

Rosen, J. C., Saltzberg, E., & Srebnik, D. (1989). Cognitive behavior therapy for negative body image. *Behavior Therapy, 20*, 393–404.

Salfilios-Rothschild, C. (1970). *The sociology and social psychology of disability and rehabilitation*. New York: Random House.

Sawyer, M. G., Minde, K., & Zuker, R. (1983). The burned child—scarred for life? A study of the psychosocial impact of a burn injury at different developmental stages. *Burns, 9*, 205–213.

Seidel, L. (1988). Corrective cosmetics for disfigurement. In N. R. Bernstein, A. J. Breslau, & J. A. Graham (Eds.), *Coping strategies for burn survivors and their families* (pp. 97–102). New York: Praeger.

Shontz, F. C. (1990). Body image and physical disability. In T. F. Cash & T. Pruzinsky (Eds.), *Body images: Development, deviance, and change* (pp. 149–169). New York: Guilford Press.

Solnit, A., & Priel, B. (1975). Psychological reactions to facial and hand burns in young men: Can I see myself through your eyes? *Psychoanalytic Study of the Child, 30*, 549–566.

Stark, K. D., Rouse, L. W., & Livingston, R. (1991). Treatment of depression during childhood and adolescence: Cognitive–behavioral procedures for the individual and the family. In P. C. Kendall (Ed.), *Child and adolescent therapy: Cognitive–behavioral procedures* (pp. 165–206). New York: Guilford Press.

Stoddard, F. J. (1982). Body image development in the burned child. *Journal of the American Academy of Child Psychiatry, 21*, 502–507.

Stoddard, F. J., Norman, D. K., Murphy, J. M., & Beardslee, W. R. (1989). Psychiatric outcome of burned children and adolescents. *Journal of the American Academy of Child and Adolescent Psychiatry, 28*, 589–595.

Tarnowski, K. J., Rasnake, L. K., Linscheid, T. R., & Mulick, J. A. (1989). Behavioral adjustment of pediatric burn victims. *Journal of Pediatric Psychology, 14*, 607–615.

Tarnowski, K. J., Rasnake, K. L., Gavaghan-Jones, M. P., and Smith, L. (1991). Psychosocial sequelae of pediatric burn injuries: A review. *Clinical Psychology Review, 11*, 371–398.

Thompson, J. K. (1990). *Body image disturbance: Assessment and treatment*. Elmsford, NY: Pergamon Press.

Tobiasen, J. M. (1992). *Facial appearance and self-perception*. Paper presented at the 49th Annual Meeting of the American Cleft Palate–Craniofacial Association, Portland, Oregon.

Tyc, V. L. (1992). Psychosocial adaptation of children and adolescents with limb deficiencies: A review. *Clinical Psychology Review, 12*, 275–291.

Varni, J. W., Setoguchi, Y., Rappaport, L. R., & Talbot, D. (1992). Psychological adjustment and perceived social support in children with congenital/acquired limb deficiencies. *Journal of Behavioral Medicine, 15*, 31–44.

Walco, G. A., & Varni, J. W. (1991). Cognitive–behavioral interventions for children with chronic illnesses. In P. C. Kendall (Ed.), *Child and adolescent therapy: Cognitive–behavioral procedures* (pp. 209–244). New York: Guilford Press.

Whitehead, T. L. (1993). Sexual health promotion of the patient with burns. *Journal of Burn Care and Rehabilitation, 14*, 221–226.

Willis-Helmich, J. J. (1992). Reclaiming body image: The hidden burn. *Journal of Burn Care and Rehabilitation, 13*, 64–67.

8

Family Considerations and Interventions

NADINE J. KASLOW, KAMELA KOON-SCOTT, and ARDEN D. DINGLE

Family functioning is an important aspect of the care and psychosocial adjustment in burned children and adolescents. There is a paucity of data addressing family factors associated with positive adjustment in pediatric burn victims and delineating optimum family treatment. Any discussion is complicated by the fact that some burns are unrelated to the family environment; others are associated with problematic family dynamics (e.g., abuse, neglect, psychopathology) (e.g., Andreasen, Noyes, Hartford, & Proctor, 1972; Cahners & Bernstein, 1979; Noyes, Frye, Slymeh, & Canter, 1979).

Comprehensive health care must take into account a variety of factors in the assessment and intervention process. A useful model for conceptualizing risk and resistance factors associated with the child's adjustment to a physical condition was proposed by Wallander, Varni, Babani, Banas, and Wilcox (1989). This disability-stress-coping model (Wallander *et al.*, 1989; Wallander & Varni, 1992) addresses child variables and social ecologi-

---

NADINE J. KASLOW, KAMELA KOON-SCOTT, and ARDEN D. DINGLE • Department of Psychiatry and Behavioral Sciences, Emory University School of Medicine, Grady Memorial Hospital, Atlanta, Georgia 30335; *present address for K.K.-S.*: Department of Pediatrics, University of Florida College of Medicine, Jacksonville, Florida 32209.

Behavioral Aspects of Pediatric Burns, edited by Kenneth J. Tarnowski. Plenum Press, New York, 1994.

cal factors that may impact the child's coping. The model provides a useful framework for understanding variables that are prognostic indicators for the adjustment of pediatric burn sufferers.

This chapter focuses on the social–ecological variables that serve as risk and resistance factors for both incurring and adjusting to a burn injury. Intervention strategies for working with pediatric burn-injured youth and their families are articulated. These strategies address the child's risk and resistance factors and physical and psychosocial adaptation within a family context.

DISABILITY-STRESS-COPING MODEL

Family dynamics, which are both risk and resistance factors, must be considered in the context of injury-related parameters, individual child variables, and the sociocultural environment. To provide a framework, a brief review of the variables associated with this model follows.

Disease/disability parameters, functional independence, and psychosocial stressors comprise the three major risk factors in this model. Disease/disability parameters refer to burn size, location, and severity. Functional independence is related to the child's daily living skills, prior and subsequent to the burn. Injury- and treatment-related difficulties, daily stressors, and major life events and changes, either predating or following the child's burn, are key psychosocial stressors. Resistance factors encompass intrapersonal dimensions (child's temperament, competence, motivation, problem-solving ability), stress processing cognitive appraisal, coping strategies), and social–ecological factors (family environment, family member's adaptation, social support systems, utilitarian resources). A burned child's adaptation is mediated by the interaction of these factors, and is reflected in his/her psychological presentation, social reintegration and functioning, and rehabilitative outcome.

Family Risk Factors Associated with Incurring Injury

Personal health, personality, and social factors predispose individuals to burn injury (Tucker, 1986). Certain social factors (e.g., life events and stresses, utilitarian resources, social networks) are associated with increased risk for burns in children and adults. Individuals with major life events and changes are vulnerable to the occurrence of injury (e.g., Andreasen *et al.*, 1972). Insufficient utilitarian resources (e.g., low income, parental unemployment) commonly have been reported among burn victims (e.g., Noyes *et al.*, 1979). Individuals who reside in families characterized by instability and disorganization, parental psychopathology, single-parenthood, and limited social support also are at risk (Andreasen *et al.*, 1972; Cahners & Bernstein, 1979; Noyes *et al.*, 1979).

Family Resistance Factors

Good Adjustment

Family variables have been associated with a child's long-term psychosocial adjustment following burn injury. Family environment accounts for up to 50% of the variance associated with the child's psychosocial adjustment (e.g., Blakeney, Portman, & Rutan, 1990; Tarnowski, Rasnake, Gavaghan-Jones, & Smith, 1991). Positive postburn adjustment is seen in children who perceive their families as cohesive and committed to one another (e.g., Blakeney *et al.*, 1990). This closeness provides an environment in which conflicts can be expressed and resolved. Family members also are supported in attaining age-appropriate autonomy and mastery over the environment (Blakeney *et al.*, 1990). Children are encouraged to resume previous roles and activities as soon as possible, with families who have realistic expectations regarding the rehabilitation process and outcome, demonstrate better postburn adjustment (Shenkman & Stechmiller, 1987). High levels of perceived social support from family and friends predict positive self-esteem following burn injury (e.g., Beard, Herndon, & Desai, 1989; Bowden, Feller, Tholen, Davidson, & James, 1980; Orr, Reznikoff, & Smith, 1989). It has been argued that social support is the best predictor of psychological adjustment following a burn injury (e.g., Blakeney *et al.*, 1990; Knudson-Cooper & Thomas, 1988). Finally, a large family size of higher socioeconomic status (SES) is associated with positive postburn adjustment (Tarnowski *et al.*, 1991).

Poor Adjustment

Child burn victims residing in economically deprived environments often evidence more problematic adjustment than their more affluent counterparts (e.g., Cahners & Bernstein, 1979; Tucker, 1986). Infrequent family visitation during hospitalization, and a perception of a noncohesive family unit that is not supportive of independence, also have been correlated with poor child adjustment (e.g., Blakeney, Herndon, Desai, Beard, & Wales-Seale, 1988; Blakeney *et al.*, 1990; Browne *et al.*, 1985). These youth may find themselves in a passive and dependent role, which conflicts with their strivings for age-appropriate independence (Blakeney *et al.*, 1990). This stance renders them susceptible to feeling helpless and hopeless, and having low self-esteem (Blakeney *et al.*, 1988), cognitions associated with the development and maintenance of depression in youth.

Children from families with poor coping in stressful situations are at risk for maladaptive coping with their burn and evidencing emotional problems (West & Shuck, 1978). Some researchers have shown that children whose mothers have difficulty adjusting to the injury, themselves evidence impaired psychosocial adjustment (Browne *et al.*, 1985; Cahners & Bernstein, 1979). Not all studies, however, have revealed an association between maternal and child adjustment (Byrne *et al.*, 1986; Knudson-Cooper, 1981).

Unrealistic expectations regarding the course, process, and prognosis of hospitalization and rehabilitation are another family variable placing a burned youth at increased risk for poor psychological adjustment (Constable & Bernstein, 1979; Constable, Bernstein, & Sheehy, 1979; Shenkman & Stechmiller, 1987). Expectations are problematic when the goals of the family and the child are discrepant (Shenkman & Stechmiller, 1987). The child's adjustment is a function of both individual and family coping abilities and resources (Browne *et al.*, 1985).

Only a minority of burn survivors (10–15%) manifest serious psychological difficulties. A minority of families (e.g., 24%) evidence the problematic family interaction patterns associated with depression, risk factors for burn injury, and poor psychosocial outcome in their burn-injured youth (Blakeney *et al.*, 1988; Browne *et al.*, 1985).

Stress and Emotional Reactions

Innumerable acute and chronic stresses are associated with burns due to the trauma of the injury, hospitalization, medical procedures, rehabilitation, reintegration, and short- and long-term sequelae. Indecision, intensification of preexisting problems, denial, and feelings of guilt, anxiety, depression, helplessness, fear, and anger are common family reactions to severe burns (e.g., Bowden & Feller, 1973; Tucker, 1986). Stresses and associated emotional reactions originate with the burn and persist throughout all phases of treatment. Although these responses are normal, they may become problematic and interfere with optimum recovery if the patient, family, and social systems lack adequate coping strategies and resources.

The Burn Injury

Family members, particularly parents, experience guilt about the burn incident, regardless of actual culpability (Knudson-Cooper &

Thomas, 1988). Parents typically are preoccupied with thoughts that they should have prevented the burn and that they have failed in their role as protector (Knudson-Cooper & Thomas, 1988). This guilt is compounded by feelings of powerlessness and helplessness because parents cannot eliminate their child's suffering and possible disfigurement and impairment. Family members often experience shock and grief, feelings of loss, fears that the child may die, and anger that the injury occurred (e.g., Tucker, 1986).

Acute Phase

Parents' feelings of guilt, helplessness, anger, and fear may intensify as they consent to painful procedures for their child (Miller, Elliott, Funk, & Pruitt, 1988). Attempts to relieve this guilt, anger, and sense of powerlessness may be manifested in demanding behavior toward the staff (Miller *et al.*, 1988). They may displace their anger onto their child or other family members (Miller *et al.*, 1988). During this acute phase, relatives may be frightened about their child's physical distress and psychological state (Tucker, 1986), and may develop symptoms and/or an intensification of preexisting problems (Knudson-Cooper & Thomas, 1988).

With time, family members increasingly may feel frustrated about treatment duration, recovery time, and uncertainty regarding the future (e.g., Goodstein, 1985). Requirements of burn care can exacerbate the child's and family's psychological distress (Bernstein, 1976; Knudson-Cooper & Thomas, 1988). The burned child may evidence more behavior problems, which result in increased conflict between the child, family members, and the staff (Knudson-Cooper & Thomas, 1988; Vanderplate, 1984).

Numerous practical considerations increase the burden that family members experience during hospitalization. These include the financial cost of burn care, travel expenses, and loss of income related to the need to care for the child (Knudson-Cooper & Thomas, 1988). This financial drain is most problematic for families whose property also has been damaged or destroyed. Further, having a burned child in the hospital interferes with the family's normal functioning, as one or both parents must spend extended periods of time at the hospital leaving siblings feeling unattended to when they may be experiencing distress, anxiety, and fear (Knudson-Cooper & Thomas, 1988). These difficulties are compounded for those families who must travel considerable distances for their child to receive optimal care.

Intermediate and Rehabilitative Phases

After the acute phase, the child and family must face the stresses associated with a rehabilitation program that includes physical and occupational therapy protocols, return to home and school, and possible returns to the hospital for further surgery. These requirements stress the burned child and family members, since family members must assist the child with treatment protocols and promote compliance. Additionally, both the child and the family may develop unrealistic expectations regarding the rehabilitative outcome that may be detrimental to the postburn adaptation process. The rehabilitation phase is marked by slow progress and uncertainty regarding the future, requiring the child and family to be patient and understanding (Goodstein, 1985).

Close to the child's discharge, the focus centers on reintegrating into home and school (Goodstein, 1985). The child may need additional reassurance and acceptance, and may begin to acknowledge fears and expectations of rejection (Goodstein, 1985; Tarnowski, Rasnake, & Drabman, 1987; Wisely, Masur, & Morgan, 1983). As Goodstein relates (1985), the family must confront the "misconception of healing" and realize that going home does not indicate wellness. Since most burns still will require additional care, the child and family must face the realization that others may or may not accept the changed body form and disfigurement (Bernstein, 1976; Goodstein, 1985; Knudson-Cooper & Thomas, 1988; Wisely *et al.*, 1983). Leaving the relatively "safe" environment of the hospital is a significant stressor for most children and families.

Resocialization Phase

The process of reintegration into the social and familial milieu is extremely problematic for children and adolescents (e.g., Blumenfield & Reddish, 1987; Knudson-Cooper & Thomas, 1988; Miller *et al.*, 1988; Molinaro, 1978). During this period, family support and encouragement of autonomy has been demonstrated as instrumental in facilitating successful social reentry (Blakeney *et al.*, 1990). However, even with high levels of familial support, the stigmatization of disfigurement can be overwhelming and negatively impact adjustment (Cahners, 1979; Knudson-Cooper & Thomas, 1988). The success of the parents in adapting to the "changed" child, grieving appropriately, and facilitating the reintegration process depends on the extent and permanence of disfigurement, available social support networks, and the unique personality traits and coping styles of the parents (Bernstein, 1976).

Disability-Stress-Coping Model: Implications for Assessment and Intervention

The literature regarding family risk and resistance factors associated with a child's and family's positive or negative adjustment to a burn injury can serve as a useful guide for assessment and intervention with burn-injured youth and their families. Sensitive assessment and intervention can be accomplished when the family therapist is attuned to the expected family stresses and emotional reactions associated with burn injury and rehabilitation. Optimal intervention maximizes individual and family resistance factors and reduces risk factors, fostering adaptive coping with the disabilities and stresses associated with a child or adolescent's burn injury.

RECOMMENDED FAMILY ASSESSMENT AND INTERVENTION

The literature regarding pediatric burn injuries underscores the importance of family treatment, but contains little information about specific intervention techniques and strategies for this population. Psychological services to medically ill children typically include treating the family, as family support is associated with positive psychosocial adjustment and optimal recovery (Tucker, 1986), and the family is an important mediator of change (Fiese & Sameroff, 1992). Mental health professionals need to engage families to facilitate their ability to support and care for their burn-injured child. Supportive and sensitive contacts enhance the family's commitment and active involvement in their child's burn care and their trust in the health care providers (Blakeney *et al.*, 1988; Cahners & Bernstein, 1979).

Families require support and psychological intervention to handle optimally the stresses and strains associated with their child's burn injury. The extent of the services offered and the specific strategies used depend on the family's characteristics and previous level of functioning. However, regardless of the approach utilized, family-based interventions should begin when the child enters the hospital and continue throughout the recovery and rehabilitation process (Blakeney *et al.*, 1988; Cahners & Bernstein, 1979; Knudson-Cooper & Thomas, 1988).

A child must be considered within the context of the family system, and therefore, a thorough assessment of both the child and the family is necessary to determine the optimal intervention. Conceptualization of the family should include the impact of the child's medical condition on the family, as well as that of the family on the child's medical problems, recovery, and rehabilitation (Fiese & Sameroff, 1992). Thus, crisis intervention, assessment, education of the patient and family regarding the medical and psychological aspects of burns, and interventions must consider the medical problem and associated physical sequelae, stages in the life cycle, and individual and family dynamics (Rolland, 1987).

Joining

Prior to the family assessment, the therapist must "join" with the family to understand the family's view in order to enable them to cope effectively with the crisis at hand (Minuchin & Fishman, 1981). To facilitate this process, the therapist must support the existing family structure (maintenance), follow the content of the family's communication with minimal intervention (tracking), and adopt the style and affective experience of the family (mimesis). Given the crisis experienced by the family in response to a child's burn injury, joining is a cyclical process that often overlaps with the assessment and intervention phases.

Crisis Intervention

Beginning with the initial contact, the therapist needs to assess the family's current state and use a crisis intervention approach to stabilize the family unit. Immediate attention should be directed toward delineating the family's current level of functioning, identifying existing and/or potential support systems, helping the family to mobilize and implement effective coping strategies, and assisting family members with the negotiation of a complex hospital superstructure. The primary goal is stabilization so that family members can deal constructively with the effects of the burn injury and can support their child through a difficult process. The therapist, an advocate for the family and child, may help the family understand medical options and make appropriate choices.

During the emergency and acute periods, death may be a realistic possibility. Grief counseling can become a major component of the intervention. Often death is a predominant concern for the family, even when it is unlikely. In these latter cases, treatment needs to provide education and reassurance, focusing on realistic medical outcomes and sequelae. However, mourning for the losses associated with the burn accident (e.g., child's health, loss of persons or property) remains a major aspect of the family's emotional response.

Throughout the crisis intervention and subsequent phases of treatment, the therapist serves as the liaison between the child, family, and staff. This role includes helping the burn team provide the family with frequent and clear verbal and written information regarding the child's condition, prognosis, and treatment (Goodstein, 1985; Knudson-Cooper & Thomas, 1988). Additionally, information should be provided to the burn team about family background, resources, level of functioning, and the psychosocial impact of the injury on the family unit (Knudson-Cooper & Thomas, 1988). This information may be gleaned from contacts with the individual child, nuclear and extended family, other involved individuals (e.g., child protective services, school personnel), and when possible and indicated, home visits (e.g., Goodstein, 1985). Reframing child and family reactions and behaviors as normal to the staff also is critical (West & Shuck, 1978). The therapist also should share information with the family, as well as the burn team, regarding the child's unique reactions to the burn trauma, general developmental considerations, and specific recommendations about behavioral and psychopharmacological interventions, and discharge plans (Knudson-Cooper & Thomas, 1988).

Assessment

Following the resolution of the initial shock and crisis and the development of a working alliance, a more intensive evaluation of the family can be performed. This assessment, conducted within the framework of the disability-stress-coping model, delineates those factors within each family that can help or hinder successful adaptation to the burn injury. The data gleaned from this comprehensive assessment guide the psychosocial interventions provided during the recovery process.

Risk Factors

As noted earlier, risk factors consist of disease/disability parameters, functional independence, and psychosocial stressors. The disease/disability parameters focus on the extent, nature, and severity of the burn injury and its sequelae. Although all burns have an acute onset, they differ in terms of their course, outcome, and degree of associated impairments. These differences, combined with the developmental stage of the child and family, influence the child's and family's adaptation to the injury and the psychosocial interventions that need to be undertaken (Rolland, 1987).

Assessment of the child's functional independence should focus on the child's pre- and postburn abilities to perform daily living skills and to effectively communicate and socialize. The greater the discrepancy between the child's pre- and postburn functional independence and between expected developmental and actual postburn abilities, the greater is the risk for difficulties in adaptation.

The third risk factor to be assessed is those major life events and daily stressors that placed the child at risk for the injury (e.g., neglect or abuse, poverty, single-parent home) or may impede postburn adjustment (presence of other children in the home, limited support network, few utilitarian resources, other significant losses). Children are at greater risk for poor adjustment and/or for future injury if they reside in social environments characterized by negative life events and high levels of chronic stress. Assessment of these risk factors should include the physical, medical, and realistic considerations, as well as the psychological responses and beliefs of the child and family. Assessment foci might include level of guilt, willingness of family members to participate actively in treatment protocols, and child and family beliefs about the injury and its prognosis.

Resistance Factors

Resistance factors include intrapersonal dimensions, stress processing, and social–ecological factors. Assessment of the child's intrapersonal dimensions (temperament, competence, effectance motivation, social problem-solving ability) provides information about past stressors, coping strategies, psychological characteristics and responses, and ability to participate in and tolerate treatment.

The child's and family's individual cognitive appraisals of stressful situations and their attempts at coping or managing these stressors must be considered. The assessment of stress processing (cognitive appraisal and coping) conveys data regarding the child's and family's levels of comprehension and abilities to engage actively in the medical and psychological therapies. During this phase of the assessment, the therapist may want to gather information regarding the child's and family's locus of control, and attributions of causality and self-control.

Social–ecological factors (family environment, family member's adaptation, social support networks, utilitarian resources) describe the child's surroundings and resources. An active effort should be made to include all possible family members, whether or not biologically related and/or residing in the home. This identification of family members must include those often neglected (e.g., siblings, nonresident parents, grandparents, significant others). Another vital component is an understanding of the following aspects of the family environment (e.g., Carter & McGoldrick, 1988): (1) structure (hierarchy, alignments, power, and degree of cohesion versus disengagement), boundary quality, and resonance (sensitivity to the actions of individual members and tolerance for deviation from the family norm); (2) flexibility and capacity for change; (3) interactional patterns of the spousal, parental, and sibling subsystems; (4) role of the burned child and how his/her coping patterns maintain family homeostasis; (5) ecological context within which the child's adjustment develops and is maintained, emphasizing past family stressors and coping patterns; present level may not be indicative of the family's typical functioning; and (6) developmental stage of the family and its individual members.

Examination of family members' adaptation includes assessing parental mental health and marital satisfaction. This is important given the association between parental and child psychosocial functioning (for review see Hetherington & Martin, 1986), the fact that burn-injured children whose mothers evidence psychological difficulties may themselves have impaired adjustment (e.g., Browne *et al.*, 1985; Cahners & Bernstein, 1979), and the contention that children who reside in maritally discordant families have more difficulties coping with physical problems (e.g., Kazak & Nachman, 1991).

Medically ill children with high levels of both family and peer support evidence better adjustment than youth with high social support from only one group (Wallander & Varni, 1989). Further, medically ill children with minimal family or peer support networks evidence the highest levels of emotional and behavioral problems (Wallander & Varni, 1989). Similar patterns have been found with burn-injured children and adolescents (e.g., Blakeney *et al.*, 1990; Knudson-Cooper & Thomas, 1988). Part of the assessment needs to include the burn-injured child's family and peer social support networks, as well as ascertaining and mobilizing other support systems in the child's social environment. These individuals may help care for the child and child's siblings, and comfort and assist the parents.

One aspect of the evaluation of utilitarian resources that deserves particular attention is family SES, as children living in economically deprived environments are at high risk for incurring a burn injury (e.g., Tarnowski *et al.*, 1991), and these families tend to lack the financial resources and practical financial problem-solving abilities necessary to cope with the acute and chronic problems associated with the burn injury. Other important utilitarian resources include the number of caretakers, duration of marital relationship, and parents' education level and occupational status. Children with more utilitarian resources tend to adjust more positively to their burn injury, medical complications, and associated impairments.

Adaptation

Throughout the recovery process, it is imperative that the therapist continue to assess the child's and family's adjustment and adaptation to the effects of the burn injury. This includes gathering information regarding premorbid psychiatric and psychological functioning. Internalizing and externalizing emotional and behavioral problems that may present throughout the course of the treatment and rehabilitation also need to be assessed.

Feedback

Following the conclusion of this assessment, the therapist should provide feedback to the patient, family, and members of the burn team. These findings can guide the approach to and interactions between the burn unit staff, the child, and family. Additionally, results can direct the psychological interventions to be undertaken with the patient and family.

Family Classification Schema

Families can be classified as healthy, midrange, and dysfunctional (Beavers, 1982) based on how their risk and resistance factors affect adaptation. This classification may influence the intervention approach utilized. The classification schema and associated treatment recommendations should be viewed as a general guide, with the proviso that every family is unique and may require and/or be receptive to various types and intensities of interventions. For example, certain individuals, regardless of their family type, may require intensive psychiatric/psychological management, relating to premorbid psychopathology or emotional difficulties secondary to their child's burn injury (Cahners, 1988; Knudson-Cooper & Thomas, 1988). These interventions may be most important when the psychiatric symptoms of the burned child and/or the family negatively affect the staff or the child's care (Chedekel, 1983). Additionally, such interventions may be warranted in extremely stressful situations, such as death of the child, significant loss of property or other important individuals, and extensive impairment of the child.

Healthy Families

Children who reside in healthy families, typically those with a low risk–high resistance factor index, are likely to evidence the most adaptive functioning and generally require only supportive family contacts and psychoeducation. Characteristics of these families include: family cohesion, stability and flexibility in roles and dealing with change, adequate negotiation of tasks and conflicts, respect for individuality, and open and clear communication (Beavers, 1982; Olson *et al.*, 1983).

Dysfunctional Families

Children living in dysfunctional families tend to have a high risk–low resistance factor index, and to evidence marked adjustment difficulties. These families are either disengaged or enmeshed, chaotic or rigid in dealing with change or negotiating conflicts, manifest poor boundaries, and exhibit problematic communication (Beavers, 1982; Olson *et al.*, 1983). They possess few adaptive coping strategies and have difficulty mobilizing their support networks. Our clinical observations suggest that children whose burns are a result of abuse and/or neglect or whose burns reflect a self-destructive act most often have dysfunctional families. These families require intensive family intervention, yet often are resistant and/or inaccessible. Often there is significant psychopathology in individual family members, requiring extensive psychotherapeutic and pharmacological interventions.

Midrange Families

Children high or low on both the risk and resistance factor indices are likely to have families who evidence midrange levels of functioning. Midrange families, who constitute the bulk of families in the general population, fall on the continuum between healthy and dysfunctional families on a variety of variables, including family cohesion and adaptability (Olson *et al.*, 1983). At times, these families can evidence neglectful behavior toward their children that can be related to the burn injury. They frequently have unstable parental coalitions and conflicts regarding power and intimacy, communicate clearly but without taking responsibility for their own feelings and actions, and have difficulty adjusting to change (Beavers, 1982). Although these families initially may handle the crisis adequately, they can have increasing difficulties during the lengthy and stressful rehabilitation.

Intervention

Healthy Families

Healthy families are active collaborators in their child's medical care, respect the structure and boundaries of the inpatient unit, and attend to their own and their child's physical and emotional needs while promoting appropriate independence. They achieve a balance between caring for their child and maintaining their other familial and occupational obligations. These families may benefit most from supportive family contacts and psychoeducation. Supportive contacts provide emotional support and assistance to the family, attending to the parents' feelings of blame, guilt, despair, helplessness, and grief (e.g., Bernstein, Breslau, & Graham, 1988; Cahners & Bernstein, 1979; Chedekel, 1983; Knudson-Cooper & Thomas, 1988; Tucker, 1986). Family members are encouraged to share their feelings at a comfortable pace (Cahners & Bernstein, 1979), allowing them to adjust to the injury and its implications, and develop realistic expectations regarding recovery and rehabilitative outcomes (Chedekel, 1983).

Other possible concerns include: helping the family communicate with staff; educating them about burn care and medical and psychosocial sequelae of burns; promoting family cohesion; encouraging family members to address their own needs and reactions, as well as those of their child; enlisting family, peers, and other community support systems; and preparing for discharge and return to home and school (Blakeney *et al.*, 1988; Knudson-Cooper & Thomas, 1988; Mingledoff, 1988; Orr *et al.*, 1989; West & Shuck, 1978). A vital aspect of this work is to emphasize the importance of support and encouragement for age- and disease-appropriate autonomy and self-sufficiency for the child (Blakeney *et al.*, 1988, 1990; Bowden *et al.*, 1980). The family should be helped to utilize their own adaptive problem-solving and coping strategies to function effectively (Browne *et al.*, 1985).

R.S., a 22-month-old female, suffered second- and third-degree burns to the left side of her body (38% total body surface area burn) after leaning on the stove unit causing it to pivot forward (faulty installation). A pot of boiling water fell on R.S. The family consisted of R.S., her twin sister, a 5-year-old sister, and her biological parents who were in their 30s. Mother was college educated and cared for the children in the home. Father was an attorney.

On admission to the burn unit, both parents expressed appropriate anxiety, anger, confusion, and concern about R.S. and the situation. This family was able to mobilize successfully their resources; they had arranged for leave from work and for grandparents to care for the other children, contacted their pastor for spiritual support, and developed a system of alternate visitation so that one parent remained at the hospital, allowing the other to attend to family responsibilities and personal needs. This family previously had dealt successfully with another major stressor, as R.S. and her twin sister were born prematurely, with R.S. requiring extensive hospitalization and treatment. Initially, crisis intervention focused on providing education about the burn injury (physical and psychological sequelae), and the structure and function of the burn unit.

Once the acute period passed, R.S.'s parents expressed dissatisfaction and discomfort regarding the visitation policy and their level of involvement. R.S. was hospitalized at a regional burn unit that cared for both adults and children and was managed by the surgery service. Visitation was restricted and parents were not encouraged to be involved actively in the care of their child (i.e., tubbings, wound cares, rehabilitation protocols). Understandably, the family became increasingly frustrated, confused, and angry. They appropriately verbalized their concerns and worked with the family therapist to determine positive strategies so that they could participate more actively in R.S.'s care. Although R.S.'s parents had legitimate concerns about their daughter's management, they were able to listen to and understand the reasons for the unit's policies. Through negotiations, the burn staff and R.S.'s parents developed a mutually satisfactory approach that enhanced R.S.'s care.

As R.S.'s condition improved, it was realized that her language was delayed more severely than expected secondary to a burn injury. When her parents were informed of the need for further assessment and intervention, they were distressed but receptive to treatment recommendations. R.S. and her family were followed by the family therapist after discharge through coordinated visits with R.S.'s burn clinic appointments. She and her family continue to function well. Her parents seek information about the psychological sequelae of the burn as she matures and recommendations for strategies to promote optimal recovery and functioning in their daughter.

Additional services such as hospital-based parent groups can provide a much needed source of guidance and opportunity for sharing common concerns and obtaining peer support (Bernstein, Breslau, & Graham, 1988; Goodstein, 1985; Knudson-Cooper & Thomas, 1988; Miller *et al.*, 1988). These groups provide education, clarify procedures, reinforce the importance of compliance, and specify normal psychological reactions to burn injury. They also can aid in ameliorating family members' feelings of isolation and self-reproach, guilt and helplessness, and in encouraging empathic and supportive parental behavior. These groups may be useful during the rehabilitation phase and can help families deal with the stressors associated with the burn required care and changes in family structure and process that occur (Gonzalez, Steinglass, & Reiss, 1989).

Dysfunctional Families

In addition to receiving the interventions described above, dysfunctional families may require intensive family intervention. This intervention should be aimed at family restructuring to promote appropriate family interactions so that the family can adequately manage and support the injured child. It should be geared to decreasing controllable risk factors and helping the family develop and/or bolster their resistance factors.

These therapeutic pursuits are possible only when the therapist is able to form a working alliance with the family, a process that may entail using strategies effective in engaging resistant families (e.g., Weitzman, 1985). To secure a treatment alliance, the therapist needs to convey acceptance of the family system through sensitivity to their established rules with minimal emphasis on rapid change and communicate an empathic and supportive attitude, rather than focusing on interpretations and confrontation (Weitzman, 1985). The therapist must provide structure, set appropriate limits, and supervise interventions. Dysfunctional families are more likely to engage in treatment when the therapist helps the family anticipate the impact of a given intervention, modulate the expression of distressing affects, maintain an emphasis on the symptom, and reframe the symptom as reflecting family transition. Finally, it is important for the therapist and family to devise a treatment plan based on realistic goals for change.

For families with a burned child who are disengaged and noncompliant with recommended medical and psychological treatments, often the only recourse is involvement of previously uninvolved relatives and/or outside agencies (e.g., child protective services, religious leaders). In some cases, the most viable disposition is alternative placement for the child. This also may be the case for families who, despite participation in treatment, remain severely dysfunctional and are unable to provide the necessary support and care for their child. These families may elicit a negative, punitive, and blaming response from staff members. The family therapist may have to help the staff deal with their negative feelings and perceptions so that there is no interference with the provision of optimal medical care. For those disengaged families who ultimately are involved in treatment, a referral for outpatient family therapy often is indicated. This transition may be facilitated by involving the outpatient therapist while the child is hospitalized.

M.T., a 10-year-old boy, suffered 52% third-degree burns to his torso and upper extremities while burning leaves with gasoline without adult supervision. Several younger boys were present at the time; however, M.T. was the only child injured. M.T. was the second oldest child in a family consisting of the biological parents (in their 30s) and 11 children (ages 3 months to 11 years). Mother, a homemaker, had a high school education and father, also high school educated, was a mechanic.

M.T. required intensive medical care, including assisted ventilation and extensive excision and grafting. After signing the necessary consent forms, his mother left the hospital and did not return until requested to do so by the burn unit team. There was no family involvement or visitation while he was hospitalized, despite active outreach. Both parents promised to visit and to meet with the burn unit staff, but did not follow through. From the initial family assessment and telephone conversations with the parents, it was evident that this was an overwhelmed and chaotic family system. Parents evidenced few adaptive coping strategies and minimal ability to deal with the crisis. On numerous occasions, the therapist recommended that the parents take an active role in their son's care, suggesting multiple strategies and possible resources. The parents were unable to follow through. Unsuccessful attempts then were made to involve extended family members. Thus, the state child protective services agency (CPS) was contacted. Unfortunately, CPS judged this family to be adequate and allowed M.T. to be discharged home with continued CPS supervision.

Following discharge, M.T. was scheduled to attend daily physical therapy appointments. M.T. and his family only sporadically attended, and compliance with home exercises was problematic. M.T. developed a serious problem with contractures, severely limiting the use of his arms. CPS again was contacted regarding medical noncompliance; however, they did not feel there was sufficient reason for action. The burn team recognized the critical status of M.T.'s rehabilitation; the physical therapist and family therapist went to M.T.'s school, enlisting its support. A program was developed to incorporate M.T.'s required exercises into his daily school routine.

Throughout M.T.'s rehabilitation, multiple unsuccessful attempts were made to engage his family and provide family support. After M.T.'s discharge, his parents separated. M.T.'s attendance in clinic remains intermittent. His contractures and range of mobility have improved slightly, but he remains seriously impaired. The family therapist continues to be in contact with M.T. and his mother during any attended physical therapy or burn clinic appointments, and CPS remains involved.

Another type of dysfunctional family are those who are enmeshed. They will not leave the hospital, fail to take care of their own needs, neglect their other responsibilities, impede the child's gradual resumption of autonomy, and interfere with the delivery of care. They tend to be intrusive, overly demanding, and irritating to staff. The inpatient family therapist may serve as a buffer between the family and the staff, positively reframe the family's actions, and educate the staff about appropriate ways to interact with the family. In the midst of a medical crisis it is not advantageous to promote major structural changes in a family system. Thus, inpatient work with an enmeshed family should not attempt to address directly the overly involved parent–child bond. The therapist can encourage family members and the child to engage in separate, developmentally appropriate activities. This often entails involving other family members in the child's care and/or in helping the enmeshed family member(s) participate in activities not directly related to the child's care. These families typically benefit from a referral to an outpatient therapist skilled in medical family therapy (McDaniel, Hepworth, & Doherty, 1992).

C.C., a 16-year-old female, incurred second-degree burns (24%) to her arms and legs during a motor vehicle accident. C.C. lived with her biological mother, stepfather, 13-year-old brother, and 3-year-old half sister. Her biological father resided out-of-state, provided no financial support, but recently had initiated telephone contact with C.C. and her brother, promising to visit soon. C.C.'s mother was college-educated and employed as a secretary; her stepfather was a security guard.

C.C. arrived at the hospital accompanied by her mother and brother. Her stepfather remained home to care for the younger sibling. Although C.C.'s burns were not severe and the burn staff went to great lengths to explain and reassure her mother, the latter remained labile and anxious, with frequent demands for pain medication for C.C. and permission to remain in C.C.'s room. Once stabilized, C.C. appeared comfortable, was not interested in additional medication, and encouraged her mother to go home. C.C.'s biological father was notified of the accident and desired to visit; however, mother refused his requests. The morning after admission, C.C.'s mother quit her job, stating that she needed to remain at the hospital. She insisted that C.C.'s brother also remain, given the "gravity" of C.C.'s condition.

Initially, the family therapist worked with C.C. and her mother to reframe the structure and function of the burn unit in a more acceptable manner. Education was provided regarding pain management and treatment options. C.C. was made responsible for monitoring her pain; her mother had to consult C.C. before intervening with the nursing staff. The therapist helped coordinate a reasonable visitation schedule that met everyone's needs and responsibilities (e.g., school, rest, family time).

C.C.'s mother was engaged readily in family treatment and developed a strong working alliance. Throughout C.C.'s hospitalization the emphasis was on helping C.C. and her mother delineate appropriate boundaries and promote age-appropriate autonomy. The therapist encouraged the involvement of friends, extended family members, and biological father. An outpatient referral for family therapy was provided on discharge.

Those for whom the burn is the result of deliberate and self-injurious behavior in an attempt to harm or to kill themselves often have dysfunctional families. This is particularly true if the self-immolation reflects a manipulative or self-punitive act; it is less often the case if the burned individual has a psychotic illness (Walsh & Rosen, 1988). Thus, understanding the individual's motivation is crucial for psychiatric treatment planning and disposition. It is essential to understand what the child is attempting to communicate to others and their roles and reactions, to explore the feelings of the child and family regarding this behavior, and to develop mechanisms to protect the child from further attempts (Chedekel, 1983). These mechanisms typically include helping the family achieve a cohesive and flexible family structure, allowing for direct communication, expression of feelings, appropriate balance of power, and compromise between individual autonomy and intimacy. These mechanisms may be applicable to the treatment of all dysfunctional families with a burn-injured youth.

Midrange Families

Midrange families, who fall on the continuum between healthy and dysfunctional families, vary in their responses and ability to deal with the crisis engendered by having a burn-injured child. Given this variability, the therapeutic approach for these families must be based on their individual characteristics and consists of a combination of treatments. It may be necessary to actively assist them in identifying adaptive coping strategies and mobilizing their resources. More intensive contacts may be needed during the intermediate phase of the recovery process.

These families may need help in dealing with the frequently changing realities and limitations associated with the injury during rehabilitation (McDaniel *et al.*, 1992). Midrange families also may require support to maintain the "integrity of its relationships, rituals, and world view in the face of the demands" of the injury (McDaniel *et al.*, 1992, p. 226). Further, intervention with midrange families may need to focus on providing the child with developmentally appropriate responsibilities, with consideration of the realities and limitations of their condition.

K.H. was a 26-month-old female with 45% third-degree burns. Every portion of her body below the level of her navel was burned, with destruction of fascia and fat layers. She required extensive debridement, excision and grafting, intensive respiratory support, and therapy for systemic infections. K.H. remained in critical condition throughout her hospitalization.

K.H. was burned while taking a bath in a bathroom sink. Her mother left her in the basin to dispose of a soiled diaper. While outside, the mother engaged in a brief conversation with a neighbor. Despite previous instructions not to, K.H.'s 5-year-old sister turned on the water to start K.H.'s bath. The mother, finding K.H. sitting in scalding water, lifted her immediately from the sink, and saw that large patches of K.H.'s skin were blistering off. She contacted emergency services, and K.H. was transported to the regional burn unit.

K.H. lived with her biological mother and two older sisters. Her mother, age 19, had not finished high school, and was training to be a nursing assistant. Her biological father, age 21, had a high school education, and was unemployed. He maintained active contact with his children. The parents were not married and had never lived in the same home. The mother and her daughters resided in an apartment complex with one hot water heater that was set exceptionally high to provide adequate heat for the complex. The mother later learned that other children had been burned in a similar manner in the complex.

On admission, both mother and father accompanied K.H. The other two siblings were cared for by the maternal grandmother. The parents initially mobilized their support network and demonstrated reasonable coping strategies, asking appropriate questions, comforting one another and their other children, and communicating with the burn team regarding the needs of their child and necessary medical interventions. During this period, the therapist provided supportive contacts and education.

As K.H.'s medical status remained critical with the development of additional serious complications, her parents were informed of the possibility of K.H.'s death. Their coping strategies became less effective. In response to this news, K.H.'s mother initially demonstrated distress. She then suppressed these emotions, would not discuss the possibility of K.H.'s death, and focused on the lawsuit against the apartment complex. She refused to leave the hospital, remained in the waiting room when not allowed to visit K.H. She did not attend to her other children's needs, who remained with the grandmother. With the family therapist, the mother appeared superficial and guarded, and exclusively focused on K.H. and the pending lawsuit. She could not manage to bring her other children and their grandmother to the hospital for family meetings.

In response to the news that K.H. might die, her father wailed uncontrollably and was inconsolable. Later, he appeared affectively constricted, spent less time at the hospital, lessened his emotional support of K.H.'s mother while resisting her attempts to comfort him, avoided contacts with the family therapist, and decreased his involvement with his other children.

The family therapy work concentrated on supporting the mother, monitoring her denial, assisting her in dealing with her emotions, and underscoring the importance of resuming her other familial and personal responsibilities. It was reiterated that her other children and affected relatives required emotional assistance and interventions to minimize the long-term psychological effects on them. Nonintrusive efforts to engage K.H.'s father continued, and the family therapist's availability to him was underscored.

The family work also entailed liaison between the burn unit staff and the family. The burn staff became highly invested in K.H. and her outcome. They blamed the mother for being neglectful. The family therapist interceded by stressing the accidental nature of this injury.

CONCLUDING REMARKS

Children who evidence the most positive adjustment to their burn and associated difficulties tend to live in healthy families, with adequate utilitarian resources, cohesiveness, commitment to one another, effective communication and conflict resolution, and support of age-appropriate independence. These families typically have strong social support networks and realistic appraisals of their child's medical condition and the rehabilitation process and outcome. Conversely, children who demonstrate maladaptive patterns of psychological adjustment often come from environments with limited financial and social resources. Their families tend to be dysfunctional (enmeshed or disengaged). There is a lack of family cohesion and communication patterns are indirect and unclear. In many of these families, children are exposed to abuse and/or neglect, and individual members may demonstrate significant psychopathology. However, regardless of family type, all burn-injured children and their families require and can benefit from family intervention during all phases of the treatment and recovery process.

This chapter uses a disability-stress-coping model to guide assessment and intervention. In our clinical experience, this model provides a valuable framework for conceptualizing children and families who present with myriad psychological reactions to burns. The model encourages the consideration of the premorbid functioning of each family member and of the family system, as well as the identification of child and family risk factors associated with the injury and its treatment. Additionally, it attends to those positive family attributes that may assist the child and family in coping.

Hopefully, this synthesis, based on the disability-stress-coping model, will provide guidance for both clinical and research endeavors. More empirical data are needed regarding the interrelations between child variables, family factors, injury and treatment characteristics, and the child's and family's adjustment. Future studies should attempt to delineate which interventions are optimal for this population.

REFERENCES

Andreasen, N. J. C., Noyes, R., Jr., Hartford, C. E., & Proctor, S. (1972). Management of emotional reactions in seriously burned adults. *New England Journal of Medicine, 286,* 65–69.

Beard, S. A., Herndon, D. N., & Desai, M. (1989). Adaptation of self-image in burn disfigured children. *Journal of Burn Care and Rehabilitation, 10,* 550–554.

Beavers, W. R. (1982). Healthy, midrange, and severely dysfunctional families. In F. Walsh (Ed.), *Normal family processes* (pp. 45–66). New York: Guilford Press.

Bernstein, N. R. (1976). *Emotional care of the facially burned and disfigured child.* Boston: Little, Brown.

Bernstein, N. R., Breslau, A. J., & Graham, J. A. (Eds.). (1988). *Coping strategies for burn survivors and their families.* New York: Praeger.

Blakeney, P., Herndon, D. N., Desai, M. H., Beard, S., & Wales-Seale, P. (1988). Long-term psychosocial adjustment following burn injury. *Journal of Burn Care and Rehabilitation, 9,* 661–665.

Blakeney, P., Portman, S., & Rutan, R. (1990). Familial values as factors influencing long-term psychological adjustment of children after severe burn. *Journal of Burn Care and Rehabilitation, 11,* 472–475.

Blumenfield, M., & Reddish, P. M. (1987). Identification of psychologic impairment in patients with mild-moderate thermal injury: Small burn, big problem. *General Hospital Psychiatry, 9,* 142–146.

Bowden, M., & Feller, I. (1973). Family reaction to a severe burn. *American Journal of Nursing, 73,* 317–319.

Bowden, M. L., Feller, I., Tholen, D., Davidson, T. N., & James, M. H. (1980). Self-esteem of severely burned patients. *Archives of Physical Medicine and Rehabilitation, 61,* 449–452.

Browne, G., Byrne, C., Brown, B., Pennock, M., Streiner, D., Roberts, R., Eyles, P., Truscott, D., & Dabbs, R. (1985). Psychological adjustment of burn survivors. *Burns, 12,* 28–35.

Byrne, C., Love, B., Browne, G., Brown, B., Roberts, J., & Streiner, D. (1986). The social competence of children following burn injury: A study of resilience. *Journal of Burn Care, 7,* 247–252.

Cahners, S. S. (1979). Group meetings benefit families of burned children. *Scandinavian Journal of Plastic and Reconstructive Surgery, 13,* 169–171.

Cahners, S. S., & Bernstein, N. R. (1979). Rehabilitating families with burned children. *Scandinavian Journal of Plastic and Reconstructive Surgery, 13,* 173–175.

Carter, E., & McGoldrick, M. (1988). *The changing family life cycler: A framework* (2nd ed.). New York: Gardner.

Chedekel, D. S. (1983). The psychologist's role in comprehensive burn care. In N. R. Bernstein

& M. C. Robson (Eds.), *Comprehensive approaches to the burned person* (pp. 217–234). New York: Medical Examination Publishing Company.

Constable, J. D., & Bernstein, N. R. (1979). Public and professional reactions to the facially disfigured which interfere with rehabilitation. *Scandinavian Journal of Plastic and Reconstructive Surgery, 13*, 181–183.

Constable, J. D., Bernstein, N. R., & Sheehy, E. (1979). Unreasonable expectations of reconstructive patients affecting rehabilitation. *Scandinavian Journal of Plastic and Reconstructive Surgery, 13*, 177–179.

Fiese, B. H., & Sameroff, A. J. (1992). Family context in pediatric psychology: A transactional perspective. In M. C. Roberts & J. L. Wallander (Eds.), *Family issues in pediatric psychology* (pp. 239–260). Hillsdale, NJ: Lawrence Erlbaum Associates.

Gonzalez, S., Steinglass, P., & Reiss, D. (1989). Putting the illness in its place: Discussion groups for families with chronic medical illnesses. *Family Process, 28*, 69–87.

Goodstein, R. K. (1985). Burns: An overview of clinical consequences affecting patient, staff, and family. *Comprehensive Psychiatry, 26*, 43–57.

Hetherington, E. M., & Martin, B. (1986). Family factors and psychopathology in children. In H. C. Quay & J. S. Werry (Eds.), *Psychopathological disorders of childhood* (3rd ed., pp. 382–389). New York: Wiley.

Kazak, A. E., & Nachman, G. S. (1991). Family research on childhood chronic illness: Pediatric oncology as an example. *Journal of Family Psychology, 4*, 462–483.

Knudson-Cooper, M. S. (1981). Adjustment to the visible stigma: The case of the severely burned child. *Social Science in Medicine, 15*, 31–44.

Knudson-Cooper, M., & Thomas, C. M. (1988). Psychosocial care of the severely burned child. In H. F. Carvajal & D. H. Parks (Eds.), *Burns in children* (pp. 345–362). Chicago: Year Book Medical Publishers.

McDaniel, S. H., Hepworth, J., & Doherty, W. J. (1992). *Medical family therapy: A biopsychosocial approach to families with health problems*. New York: Basic Books.

Miller, M.D., Elliott, C. H., Funk, M., & Pruitt, S. D. (1988). Implications of children's burn injuries. In D. K. Routh (Ed.), *Handbook of pediatric psychology* (pp. 426–447). New York: Guilford Press.

Mingledoff, J. (1988). Parenting a burned baby. In R. N. Bernstein, A. J. Breslau, & J. A. Graham (Eds.), *Coping strategies for burn survivors and their families* (pp. 127–128). New York: Praeger.

Minuchin, S., & Fishman, H. C. (1981). *Family therapy techniques*. Cambridge, MA: Harvard University Press.

Molinaro, J. R. (1978). The social fate of children disfigured by burns. *American Journal of Psychiatry, 135*, 979–980.

Noyes, R., Jr., Frye, S. J., Slymeh, D. J., & Canter, A. (1979). Stressful life events and burn injuries. *Journal of Trauma,, 19*, 141–144.

Olson, D. H., McCubbin, H. I., Barnes, H., Larsen, A., Muxen, M., & Wilson, M. (1983). *Families: What makes them work*. Beverly Hills: Sage.

Orr, D. A., Reznikoff, M., & Smith, G. M. (1989). Body image, self-esteem, and depression in burn injured adolescents and young adults. *Journal of Burn Care and Rehabilitation, 10*, 454–461.

Rolland, J. S. (1987). Chronic illness and the life cycle: A conceptual framework. *Family Process, 26*, 203–221.

Shenkman, B., & Stechmiller, J. (1987). Patient and family perception of projected functioning after discharge from a burn unit. *Heart and Lung, 16*, 490–496.

Tarnowski, K. J., Rasnake, L. K., & Drabman, R. S. (1987). Behavioral assessment and treatment of pediatric burn injuries: A review. *Behavior Therapy, 18*, 417–441.

Tarnowski, K. J., Rasnake, L. K., Gavaghan-Jones, M. P., & Smith, L. (1991). Psychosocial sequelae of pediatric burn injuries: A review. *Clinical Psychology Review, 11,* 371–398.

Tucker, P. (1986). The burn victim—A review of the psychosocial issues. *Australian and New Zealand Journal of Psychiatry, 20,* 413–420.

Vanderplate, C. (1984). An adaptive coping model of intervention with the severely burn injured. *International Journal of Psychiatry in Medicine, 14,* 331–341.

Wallander, J. L., & Varni, J. W. (1989). Social support and adjustment in chronically ill and handicapped children. *American Journal of Community Psychology, 17,* 185–201.

Wallander, J. L., & Varni, J. W. (1992). Adjustment in children with chronic physical disorders: Programmatic research on a disability-stress-coping model. In A. M. LaGreca, L. J. Siegel, J. L. Wallander, & C. E. Walker (Eds.), *Stress and coping in child health* (pp. 279–298). New York: Guilford Press.

Wallander, J. L., Varni, J. W., Babani, L., Banis, H. T., & Wilcox, K. T. (1989). Family resources as resistance factors for psychological maladjustment in chronically ill and handicapped children. *Journal of Pediatric Psychology, 14,* 157–173.

Walsh, B. W., & Rosen, P. M. (1988). *Self-mutilation: Theory, research, and treatment.* New York: Guilford Press.

Weitzman, J. (1985). Engaging the severely dysfunctional family in treatment: Basic considerations. *Family Process, 24,* 473–485.

West, D. A., & Shuck, J. M. (1978). Emotional problems of the severely burned patient. *Surgical Clinics of North America, 58,* 1189–1204.

Wisely, D. W., Masur, F. T., & Morgan, S. B. (1983). Psychological aspects of severe burn injuries in children. *Health Psychology, 2,* 45–72.

9

School Reintegration

PATRICIA BLAKENEY

INTRODUCTION

Preparation for the pediatric burn patient to reenter society begins almost as soon as the child is admitted for acute care, intensifying as discharge becomes imminent. The specter of returning home and resuming life outside the hospital can be frightening for the pediatric burn survivor, especially if that injury renders the child visibly changed and different from other children in appearance and/or in mobility (Harrison, 1985; Knudson-Cooper, 1982; Luther & Price 1981). Children as young as 3 years old have been observed to attend to physical appearance as a factor in social acceptance (Barden, 1990; Langlois & Downs, 1979). Clinical observations indicate that preschool children, as well as older children and adolescents, who have been burned almost invariably express negative feelings on viewing their burn scars. Their verbal expressions of their own reactions to their changed appearances frequently include a reference to fear of rejection by others. "I look like a monster" is a frequent statement summing up the child's predictions that other people will be rejecting or demeaning.

Depending on the child's developmental status and premorbid psychological functioning, the expression of separation anxiety varies. While one child withdraws and appears sad, another child rages against fear, striking out at all caretakers; another actively resists rehabilitation exer-

PATRICIA BLAKENEY • Shriners Burns Institute, Galveston, Texas 77550.

Behavioral Aspects of Pediatric Burns, edited by Kenneth J. Tarnowski. Plenum Press, New York, 1994.

cises and refuses to eat. Occasionally, the older child or adolescent may say clearly, "I don't want to get well and leave the hospital. I'm scared." More often, however, to give voice to the fears is in itself frightening, and the child relies on sensitive and knowledgeable adults to detect the fear and to help in the expression of ambivalence. Fears most often relate to how others will react to the child's changed body. Caring family members share the child's fears of rejection and ridicule. Wanting to protect the child from hurt, they worry about the child's return to society where disfigurement is shunned or denounced. "Children can be so cruel," parents often say. Indeed children—and adults—can be rude and mean. Patients and families returning to the burn center for follow-up typically provide reports of social cruelty. Strangers stare at the burned child; friends and relatives withdraw and are no longer available as they had been prior to the injury. Friends, relatives, and strangers alike often make hurtful remarks (Knudson-Cooper, 1981; Riis, Anderson, Pedersen, & Hall, 1992).

Such "cruelty" most often stems from the general public's lack of familiarity with burn injuries, curiosity at seeing something novel, and anxiety at not knowing what to say or how to behave in this unfamiliar situation. Persons viewing an injured and disfigured individual may be expected to experience not only awkwardness but also anxiety. The sight of a child who is visibly disfigured challenges the commonly held assumption of a fair and benevolent world, thus threatening the viewers' beliefs in their own security. People so threatened may attempt to defend against their feelings of vulnerability by creating psychological distance between themselves and the injured person. Defensive behaviors, such as social withdrawal or blaming the victim, can be perceived as negative reactions to, and rejection of, the injured person (Janoff-Bullman, 1992).

PSYCHOSOCIAL ADJUSTMENT OF THE BURNED CHILD

Outcome studies indicate that many, if not the majority of, children who are burned achieve satisfactory psychological and social adjustment, at least insofar as being relatively free of significant psychopathology (Blakeney, Herndon, Desai, Beard, & Wales-Seale, 1988; Blakeney *et al.*, 1993; Browne, Byrne, & Brown, 1985; Byrne *et al.*, 1986; DeWet, Cywes, Davies, & Van der Riet, 1979; Knudson-Cooper, 1981, 1984; Koon *et al.*, 1992; Meyer *et al.*, in press; Ries *et al.*, 1992; Stoddard, Norman, & Murphy, 1989; Stoddard, Norman, Murphy, & Beardslee, 1989; Tarnowski, Rasnake, Linscheid, & Mulick, 1989; Wright & Fulwiler, 1974). However, the findings of these studies also reveal a segment of the population that does not fare well and suggest that disturbed social relationships are an important factor related to adjustment. Byrne *et al.* (1986) found that over 30% of a large ($N = 125$) sample of burned children were rated by their parents as having impaired social competence, i.e., were not well integrated socially within school and peer groups. Tarnowski *et al.* (1989) found clinically significant behavioral problems, measured by parental ratings, for 13% of a sample of children ($N = 68$) 1 to 5 years postburn; all of the "deviant" children were rated to have exacerbated social withdrawal. Knudson-Cooper (1984) found perceived social support to be an important contributor to the self-esteem of pediatric burn survivors. The personality characteristics of extroversion and social boldness were found to correlate with good psychological adjustment in another study of burned children (Moore *et al.*, 1993). Assuming that social support depends on both intra- and interpersonal characteristics, it seems likely that the children who were more extroverted would also have engendered greater perceived social support among their acquaintances.

Even those children who are apparently adjusting well are frequently noted to have difficulties in interpersonal relationships. Blakeney *et al.* (1993) found a sample of 60 children (1–5 years postburn), as assessed by self, parent, and teacher, to be within the normal range of behavioral functioning. However, parents did note that their children experienced increased social problems and decreased social competence relative to nonclinical reference groups. The injured children themselves reported significantly more social problems than did those in the reference group. Within a somewhat larger sample ($N = 72$), the same measures yielded similar results (Meyer *et al.*, in press). Further analyses of the responses to standardized checklists revealed significant differences between endorsements by parents of the burned children and parents of a nonclinical reference sample. Parents of burned children more often endorsed items describing their female children as "sulking" and "more withdrawn," their male children as "shy," their teenage sons as "lonely," their younger daughters as "crying a lot," and their younger sons as "sad." Parents of burned children also more often endorsed items attributing aggressive behaviors to their children. Teachers of the burned children also more often endorsed items reflecting aggressive behaviors and social problems than did teachers of the reference group. All observers—parents, teachers, and the children themselves—agreed in describing the burned children significantly more often as "not liked by other children."

Obviously, disturbed social relationships are not necessarily a consequence of a child's burn injuries and disfigurement. However, a large body of evidence supports the conclusion that attractiveness is an important variable in social interactions, influencing both interpersonal and intrapersonal processes that play a vital role in the development of the individual's concept of self and others (Lerner & Jovanovic, 1990). Even for very young children, physical attractiveness has been noted to relate to friendship patterns and peer acceptance (Langlois & Downs, 1979). Not only children but adults, including medical staff and teachers, appear to attend more often, attribute less blame, and react more positively to attractive children (Bordlieri, Solodky, & Mikos, 1985; Cash, 1990).

Enhanced self-esteem and diminished anxiety have also been linked to greater physical attractiveness (Jovanovic, Lerner, & Lerner, 1989; Lefebvre & Arndt, 1988). A number of studies have explored the impact of the perceived unattractiveness of visibly disfigured individuals on psychological development (see review by Barden, 1990). Findings suggest that children with visible disfigurement resulting from burn injuries are hindered in social transactions important for the development of self-efficacy and social competence. Most studies of the psychological adjustment of pediatric burn survivors have attempted to examine the relationship between disfigurement and adjustment. Goldberg (1974) found children with facial burns to be significantly less well adjusted than a comparable group of children with congenital heart disease on a number of measures related to adjustment; the groups did not differ, however, on social adjustment. In another study, visible scars were related to low self-esteem for boys, but not for girls (Abdullah *et al.*, 1992). Visible disfigurement has been found to differentiate poor from good psychological adjustment among a group of adults who had suffered childhood burn injuries (Love, Byrne, Roberts, Browne, & Brown, 1987).

Methodological flaws in the existing outcome studies of burn children may obscure the relationship between disfigurement, social acceptance, and psychological adjustment, if such a relationship does exist (Eyles, Browne, Byrne, Brown, & Pennock, 1984; Tarnowski, Rasnake, & Drabman, 1987). Concerning disfigurement, a particular flaw may be that most researchers have judged visible disfigurement by external criteria, such as number of visible scars (Abdullah *et al.*, 1992), or ratings of others (Love *et al.*, 1987) or, even less directly, by size of the burn injury (Blakeney *et al.*, 1988). The crucial variable may be the individual's own perception of his or her attractiveness and disfigurement which may differ dramatically from the perception of others (Jovanovic *et al.*, 1989).

TRANSITION TO THE COMMUNITY OF SCHOOL

Armed with anecdotal information about the perceived social rejection that burned children often experience and empirical data about the potentially damaging effects of physical unattractiveness and social rejection, the burn care staff can intervene to ease the patient's transition from hospital to home. Interventions should begin early in the child's hospitalization with three primary targets: the patient, family, and community (Adriaenssens *et al.*, 1987). The primary "community" that influences a child's life outside the family is school. School is a critical domain in providing a context for the development of academic skills, social skills, and a sense of self-worth (Barbarin, 1990; Katz, 1980; Katz, Dolgin, & Varni, 1990; Luther & Price, 1981).

Yet, it is quite likely that school personnel have little or no information about or experience with burn injury and recovery; and they are susceptible to all of the fears, anxieties, and failings of the general public. Teachers' concerns about having a burned child enter their classes are similar to those identified for teachers of children with cancer (Henning & Fritz, 1983; Ross, 1984). Major concerns are that a burned child will require too much specialized attention and that school personnel may be unable to meet the child's needs. Teachers also fear that the other students will be insensitive to the burned child and will be frightened by the child's appearance. To address the concern of patients, parents, and school personnel, burn treatment programs have developed formal, organized programs for school reentry and reintegration.

SCHOOL REENTRY OR REINTEGRATION PROGRAMS: GUIDING PRINCIPLES

Programs to ease the transition from hospital to home and school have been developed for patients with several conditions treated in different types of hospitals, located in diverse geographical areas, who are returning to a variety of community settings. Despite such demographic and patient differences, program strategies are remarkably similar. They share the common goal of preparing the ill or injured child, the child's family, school personnel, and peers for the patient's transition back into the normal routine of attending school (Davis, 1989; Katz *et al.*, 1990; Lefebvre & Arndt, 1988). The underlying premises are that: education about burn treatment and about needs and limitations of the burned child will diminish anxiety related to the unknown; enhancing the students' identification with the burned child and assisting the unburned students prepare for their injured classmate's arrival can diminish anxiety and awkwardness; as anxiety decreases, the need for defensive behaviors such as withdrawal and ridicule will also decrease, and the burned child's peers will be more accepting and supportive. A few central guiding principles are reiterated throughout the scant literature on school reintegration (Cahners, 1979; Davis, 1989; Doctor, 1987; Katz *et al.*, 1990; Walls Rosenstein, 1987).

Principle 1: Planning for School Reentry Begins as Soon as Possible

From the time of the child's acute admission to the hospital, return to school is part of the treatment and discharge plans. A member of the burn team, with parental permission, contacts the child's home school to notify personnel of the child's status, obtain information about the child's academic and social functioning, and elicit any concerns from the school's perspective. The reintegration process begins with that first contact.

School status is also discussed with the parent(s) of the child during an early interview. As soon as the child can communicate, school is an area frequently discussed as the team becomes acquainted with their patient. School instruction in some form is incorporated into the child's daily inpatient treatment as early as the medical condition allows. Ideally, the hospital has a school program; but if not, schoolwork can be forwarded from the home school, and a parent or staff member can function as the "teacher." School is an integral component of a child's life, and the burn team wants to convey to the children that they are expected to resume normal lives.

Principle 2: Parents or Guardians of the Child Should Be Empowered to Actively Participate as Advocates for Their Child

Families that value autonomy and encourage individual expression within the context of family cohesion seem to provide an environment that is most conducive to the positive psychosocial adjustment of children (Blakeney *et al.*, 1988; Blakeney, Portman, & Rutan, 1990; Tyc, 1992). Work with the burned child requires family involvement in the child's treatment so that the parents or guardians feel competent to care for the child outside of the hospital setting. Work with the families must include training not only in wound care, but also in providing a supportive and positive psychological milieu. A part of the family's work is to focus on the importance of supporting the child in returning to school as soon as possible—usually within a few days of discharge from the hospital.

Parents may be reluctant to allow the injured child to return to school. They want to protect their child from potential hurt, ridicule, and/or rejection by other children. They may also want to keep the child at home and physically close for fear that some other catastrophe may occur while the parent is not physically available to protect the child. For parents there are a multitude of emotional demands. The child voices fears of rejection and ridicule. The child may be physically unable to be fully independent. The child's very appearance reminds the parents of the trauma their "baby" has endured. The burn team must consistently strive to include parents in the treatment, discharge, and school reentry plans. Understanding the importance of the child's reintegration, parents can provide support by contacting the child's school, keeping teachers and classmates informed of the child's progress, and encouraging mutual communication between the injured child and his or her school peers (Adriaenssens *et al.*, 1987; Davis, 1989; Lefebvre & Arndt, 1988).

Principle 3: Plans for Each Child Should Be Individualized

Age and developmental level of the child, visibility of the burn scars, degree of physical impairment, the child's previous level of psychological and social functioning, the composition of the community in which the child lives, school size, school distance from the hospital—all must be considered in designing the reentry program for the child. Ideally, a multidisciplinary team integrates information about the child, family, and discipline-specific concerns. Based on these data, the child's individual needs can be assessed and assigned priority in terms of their potential impact on the child's recovery. Based on this assessment, a plan for the child's reentry can be developed.

Several important decisions must be made: whether the situation demands a visit to the school by members of the burn team; which member(s) should visit the school; whether such a visit is affordable; which teaching aids should be utilized; whether a videotape showing the child's changed image is required; and which audience should be targeted for presentation. These considerations are given detailed attention in a later section of the chapter.

Principle 4: Each Child Is Treated with the Expectation of Returning to School on Discharge

The burn team wants to convey to the child and family that the burn injury is only a temporary disruption to life. A burned child may have to learn new ways of performing some activities, and may have to move at a slower pace than in preburn days; but the child will resume former activities and, with time and practice, in most instances will be able to fully participate.

Even adolescents who dropped out of school prior to injury should be expected to become involved in some structured educational or vocational program. Most importantly, the child cannot be allowed to withdraw into the safety of isolation, receiving no new information or feedback from others. The child who is allowed to withdraw may experience each day of isolation as confirmation that he or she is, in fact, incompetent, without value, and repulsive to others.

Principle 5: Continued Availability of Burn Team Professionals for School Consultation

A part of the school reintegration program is to identify for school personnel the person(s) on the burn team who will act as liaison for the child, family, school, and hospital. Teachers are more likely to report difficulties or ask questions if they have some acquaintance—even if only by phone or letter—with a specific team member. In addition, continued communication between school and hospital is important, given the amount of school a child will typically miss in order to return to the hospital for follow-up assessment and treatment (Katz *et al.*, 1990).

ELEMENTS OF SCHOOL REINTEGRATION PROGRAMS

Although school reintegration programs are available through many regional burn centers, few have been described in the literature or at professional meetings. One of the first program descriptions was authored by Cahners at the Boston Unit of the Shriners Burns Institute. Cahners asserted that teachers, "like the vast majority of people untouched by fire, do not understand the problem, are afraid to approach the problem, and feel threatened by the need to deal with it" (Cahners, 1979). Cahners centered the Boston Shriners Burns Institute reentry program around visits to each child's school where one or more burn consultants provided teachers with support and information. With the assistance of the reentry team, teachers learned to recognize their own reactions that might impede their ability to work effectively with a burned child. The team also worked with the child's peers to provide information about burn injuries and about the injured classmate who would be returning to school, as well as to assist children in processing their reactions.

Similar reintegration programs were developed in other burn centers as staff recognized the needs of their young patients. Although programs developed unique intervention approaches, most utilized multiple strategies to provide information and address the discomforts of a school community unaccustomed to burn scars and pressure garments. At the North Carolina Jaycee Burn Center, allied health representatives who were involved in the child's inpatient care accompany the child to an on-site school visit where the child actively participates in presenting information about burn injury and treatment, demonstrating any splint or special garment the child wears (Walls Rosenstein, 1987). At Children's Hospital in Denver, Doctor has advocated school visits by a team of medical and psychosocial staff (Doctor, 1987). Typically, the visit includes a meeting with school personnel followed by an assembly for the entire student body and/or the patient's classroom; the patient and the patient's family participate in both the preparation and the on-site presentation (Doctor, 1987, 1992). The Shriners Burns Institute in Cincinnati and in Galveston developed reentry programs for populations who were often at great geographical distances from the regional burn centers. Because the cost of travel and the time required for staff to be away from the hospital prohibited school visits for every child, these two centers rely heavily on written materials, phone calls, photographs, slides, and videos. School visits have, of necessity, been reserved for those patients with the greatest social/physical needs.

In general, the school reentry programs that have been described to date include the same core elements: (1) address the diverse needs of the school administration, classroom teacher(s), children, and ancillary school personnel such as librarians, cafeteria workers, or bus drivers; (2) include the patient and family in planning and, to some extent, presentation; (3) present generic burn educational information; (4) present specific information about the individual child who is returning; (5) direct the presentations at both the intellectual and emotional issues surrounding the return of the burned child; (6) consider physical adaptations which may be required in the school environment or in the patient's daily schedule; and (7) present material in a developmentally sensitive format.

PRESENTATION OF GENERIC BURN INFORMATION

Written Materials

Written materials are efficient in conveying basic information. Booklets mailed to the school early in the child's hospitalization provide personnel with salient information about the nature of burn injuries and the rehabilitation process. One excellent example is the "Back to School" booklet used by both the Galveston and Cincinnati units of Shriners Burns Institute. This booklet was originally developed primarily by Knudson-Cooper who is a behavioral scientist and burn survivor. The booklet highlights the perspective of burned children interfacing with the unburned community. The booklet contains information about burn injuries including a glossary of terms commonly encountered; typical physical, emotional, and social problems; and advice on how to assist a burned child's return to school. It addresses questions frequently asked by teachers such as, "Why not a homebound program?" This booklet has been modified several times over the years to reflect changes in burn management and rehabilitation methods. The most recent modification of the booklet was undertaken by Washam and the reentry team at the Cincinnati Unit of Shriners Burns Institute (Shriners Burns Institute, 1993a). Washam and the Cincinnati team emphasize the involvement of parents in their child's reintegration and have developed an additional booklet that provides guidelines for parents as they plan for their child's return to school (Shriners Burns Institute, 1993b).

Audiovisual Materials

It is impossible to describe with words alone the nature of disfigurement simultaneously with a description of the attractive qualities of a child. Scars, amputations, prostheses, pressure garments, splints, and masks may combine to create a visual image that is strange and frightening to the naive observer. Photographs and slides have been very useful in reentry programs and serve to both provide information and assist the audience in becoming accustomed to viewing these unfamiliar and potentially disturbing sights.

In the last decade, the popular use of videotapes has provided an informational format of potential importance for reentry programs. The viewer can hear the voices, see the children move, and observe the children's affect as they express their concerns and experiences. At the Galveston Unit of Shriners Burns Institute, we have relied heavily on the use of video both with and without a school visit. In fact, the videos are particularly valuable when a visit is not possible.

Four recent videos provide excellent examples of the use of this medium to address generic issues related to burned children. "Brandon" (Blakeney, Washam, Cahners, & Driscoll, 1993a) features a 6-year-old boy with significant cosmetic and functional difficulties following a severe burn. The video follows him through typical activities in school and at play. The child, as well as his family members and best friend, tell others that he can be a good friend and provide advice about how to relate to a burned child. "Megan" (Blakeney, Washam, Cahners, & Driscoll, 1993b) is available on video or in its original form as a slide–audio tape show. This presentation was developed for reentry with early school-age children (K–4). It features a 7-year-old girl who describes peer teasing and how it affects her. In addition, the video provides a visual overview of the rehabilitation process of several patients. Splints, pressure garments, masks, and prostheses are presented and described in detail. "Going Home" (Bains, 1993) is a short video developed for pediatric burn survivors to enhance compliance with the wearing of pressure garments. The video is compiled of interviews with several burned children who describe their injuries and their experiences in wearing pressure garments. The video can also be useful with nonburned age-mates of burn survivors by helping them understand the importance as well as the discomfort of wearing the garments. "Through the Eyes of a Child: Burn Recovery" (Doctor, Burne, & Jarecke, 1993) also features burned children talking about themselves, their coping strategies, and how they are able to participate in life in spite of "disability." The tape illustrates clearly that burned children can resume normal social and physical activity. Counselors also describe their feelings on meeting the burned children initially.

Photographs, slides, and home-made videos are used not only for generic education but also to educate the target audience specifically about the individual patient. The "Megan" slide series allows space to insert slides of the individual child who is the focus of the reentry program. When a school visit is impossible, the slide–tape show can be sent with slides and a brief script tailored to the burned child who will be joining the school. Individually made videotapes featuring the specific patient are very effective in introducing or reintroducing the children to their peers. At the Galveston Shriners unit, we make frequent use of this relatively inexpensive method of introducing a child and providing information to classmates. This includes a demonstration of any special devices such as splints and garments. Patients and their parents help plan what is included in their tapes. Patients are encouraged, but not pressured, to verbalize on videotape whatever they feel comfortable sharing. A tape may also demonstrate a child's prescribed exercises for the family and local physical or occupational therapist. Individualized videotapes are typically used concurrently with a generic video, written materials, and phone follow-up.

Other Teaching Aids

In conjunction with school visits, there are many creative ways to use materials to graphically portray aspects of burn treatment, rehabilitation, and recovery. Every effort should be made to ensure that children are actively involved in the educational process. Dolls can be used to illustrate the application of splints or a face mask or garments; dolls can also be outfitted with a "graft" and a "donor site" attached by tape. Encouraging the unburned children to try on a face mask or a splint or a pressure garment can enhance their ability to empathize with the burned child. Taping fingers together to simulate an injured and limited hand or, if the burned child has had amputations, involving the class in ordinary activities using only one hand or one arm or one leg and then asking them to reflect on the difficulties involved in those ordinary activities helps them to appreciate the extra effort, time, and patience their injured classmate may need. The materials and activities used to facilitate empathy are limited only by the imaginations of the burn unit staff.

CONTENT OF SCHOOL PRESENTATION

Whatever the presentation format, there are specific content areas that must be addressed. The words and methods used to communicate will vary with the targeted audience but the content remains the same.

Injury Etiology

Explaining the cause of the burn is important with older children and adult audiences. It is also important to include the injured child and that child's parents in deciding what type and how much information to provide. Explanations should emphasize that accidents happen despite our best efforts to prevent them, and that the child is not to be blamed for the injury. For young children, a limited explanation that is not too frightening is sufficient and preferable. For example, young children may need to know only that the house caught fire—which is frightening enough—but not that it was started by a spark of electricity that ignited a leak in a gas line. When the cause of injury lends itself to a lecture on burn prevention, it is important to remember that the goal is to facilitate the burned child's return to normality and not to use that child as an example of what happens when one makes a mistake. Burn prevention can be addressed without blaming the child.

Those instances in which the burn injury occurred as a result of child abuse present an apparent dilemma but can be explained by relaying information about the agent of injury without divulging specific circumstances. For example, an injury resulting from abuse by hot water scald can be explained by stating that the child was burned by very hot water without saying anything to indicate that the child was purposefully hurt by another.

Hospital Care

Although there is little need for detailed descriptions of burn treatment, it is helpful to relate information about the hospital to reassure the audience who often are as anxious about hospitalization as they are by the notion of a burn accident. Without being dishonest about procedures that are frightening or painful, one emphasizes that a team of health care professionals provided comprehensive care for the child, the child's parents were present, and the child had friends and toys to play with during hospitalization.

Scarring

Age-appropriate explanations of scarring demystify the burned child's skin appearance and provide the rationale for the wearing of special appliances and garments. In discussing scarring, it is important to acknowledge explicitly that the scarred area has a different color and texture from unscarred skin and to provide a positive way of viewing these differences. For example, one can say, "The skin here is red and bumpy because it is the new skin" subtly suggesting ways of referring to such areas other than with negative descriptors. If the burned child is comfortable with the idea, it is usually helpful to suggest that he or she invite others to touch the scars. Once children have experienced touching the scars they may feel more comfortable with viewing such areas.

Splints, Masks, Pressure Garments, and Other Appliances

Knowing that the burned child wears these unusual-looking and uncomfortable devices to continue their physical recovery can facilitate the nonburned classmates' acceptance of the strange garb. Educated peers often can be recruited to support the injured child by reminding him or her to wear the mask or glove. The more familiar the class becomes with how it feels to wear a mask (or a splint or a pressure suit), the more empathetic they can be.

Patient Limitations

Most children who have been burned will attempt, on at least one occasion, to gain special dispensation by claiming that "Burned children can't. . . ." It is of paramount importance that the child's capabilities be made clear and emphasized during reentry presentations. When communicating about any restrictions or special concerns, suggestions can be made about positive ways to cope. For example, in the context of emphasizing what the child can do, the burn team might say, "She can sit at her desk and keep her legs elevated with this chair and pillow."

Peer Support

Classmates and teachers alike are usually grateful for directions about what to say or how to assist an injured child. In consultation with the burned child, the burn team can provide concrete suggestions to the class about what questions are appropriate to pursue with their injured classmate. Most children and adults want to be supportive but, if they have little idea about what to say or how to relate, they will likely withdraw from the discomfort of an awkward situation.

Physical Appearance

"The burned child looks different on the outside, but is the same on the inside." Not only is this statement made explicitly in every school reentry presentation of a burned child, it is an implicit theme throughout the presentation. Empirical evidence suggests that children as young as 6 can comprehend the emotional responses of others and imagine themselves to feel as others do (Gove & Keating, 1979). Every aspect of the presentation is designed to guide peers toward imagining how they might feel if they had been so injured, thus enhancing empathy and peer support.

SPECIAL CONSIDERATIONS

Faculty

Teachers and school administrators are usually concerned that they will be inadequate in meeting the needs of the burned child. It is especially important to provide them with information about the child's functional capabilities and specific details about rehabilitation needs as related to participation in the school curriculum. School personnel must be assured that, except for the school nurse, they are not expected to provide medical care; and the nurse is not expected to be an expert in burn care. All concerned must be assured that the burn team staff remain available for assistance.

Burned Child

Regardless of how much planning and preparation work has been done to facilitate the child's transition back to school, most children will still be worried about the initial return. Bland reassurance is typically not helpful, and it is not reasonable to expect that the child will cease being anxious. Often children are asked to maintain a log (written for older children and for younger, by informing their parents) of critical events at school that are problematic. The children are told that an identified expert will review the log with them to plan ways of coping with such events in the future. Providing children with problem-solving skills is often helpful clinically in enhancing self-efficacy and alleviating anxiety. Given that all children are teased at some time, parents and children need practice in problem solving how to handle teasing.

Preschool and Early Elementary School Classmates (Grades K–2)

Young children are curious and involved in learning about everything. They also can be remarkably accepting of other children regardless of marked differences. When their questions are answered, children can feel more secure and focus on their commonalities (Davis, 1989). The introduction of an injured child and discussion about that child's accident may elicit unexpected fears in a child. It is important to word explanations to this age group in a way that makes what happened seem more acceptable, reassuring the children that their classmate's injuries can be healed and their friend can play with them (Bibace & Walsh, 1980; Billingham, 1982).

Older Elementary School Classmates (Grades 3–6)

Older children become more aware of their social liaisons and form social groups which, by definition, exclude others (Davis, 1989). Teasing and nicknaming are prime modes of defining the boundaries of the group, and physical appearance is an easy way to differentiate among peers. Fortunately, the group boundaries at this age are fairly fluid, and a child who is excluded on one day may find acceptance the next (Billingham, 1982). Children in this age group are often highly motivated to gain adult approval and can be motivated to be supportive of each other. Activities that facilitate empathy with the injured child are especially useful in this age group.

Adolescents

This age group has the most difficulty in dealing with intragroup differences. Healthy adolescents often are insecure about their changing bodies. With rapid change and insecurity, adolescents cling to peers for reassurance. Any child who may detract from the perceived attractiveness of the group is a threat to each individual in the group and therefore likely to be excluded (Barden, 1990; Davis, 1989). A teenager who has been burned has many complex body image issues to resolve (see chapter by Pruzinsky and Doctor). In addition, disfiguring scars put a teenager at high risk for social exclusion during a psychologically tumultuous period.

Individually, and in small groups, adolescents are more accepting of peers who look different (Davis, 1989). With this age group, reintegration efforts may be directed not only to the school but also to the specific groups with whom the student identifies, such as a church group or an athletic team or drama class.

PRACTICAL ISSUES

Scheduling

The presentation of audiovisual materials and/or a school visit should be scheduled for a time immediately preceding the child's return. It is important that information about the child and his or her capabilities be accurate and current. If presented too early, information may create a false picture of the child that will have to be modified.

There have been occasions when, for logistical reasons, reentry presentations occurred several days after the child had returned to school. The results of these experiences suggest that, if it is impossible to prepare the school before the child's return, it is still valuable to proceed with the presentation following the child's return. Reports from both children and teachers in these instances often indicate that, prior to the presentation, the burned child had been the target of some teasing and name calling that was eliminated following the intervention.

Patient Participation

Whether the injured child is present during the reentry presentation is a decision that needs to be made on an individual basis in consultation with the patient and parents. In general, our preference is to conduct the initial presentation in the child's absence. Peers and faculty tend to ask more questions and become more actively involved in the learning process when they are not anxious about hurting the injured child's feelings or concerned about bringing up issues that might induce sadness or discomfort.

There are children who are eager to be present during the meetings with their peers and who can function as effective advocates for themselves. Some centers regularly include the child in the reentry presentation

(Walls Rosenstein, 1987). Unfortunately, no objective data exist to guide decision making in this regard.

Including the child's parents in the presentation to the students may be helpful. Teachers report that parental participation in relaying information can be useful whether or not the parent is physically present during the presentation. The more parents can actively and appropriately participate in assisting their burned child, the more competent and confident the parents are likely to feel. Such self-efficacy can have a positive impact on the entire family, including the burned child.

Burn Team Representation

There are several factors that influence the choice of which burn team professionals should visit the school. In general, the tasks to be accomplished guide this decision within the parameters of budget and time limitations.

Ideally, a reentry visitation team should be comprised of two or three members. There are likely to be many concerns about physical limitations, rehabilitation exercises, applying splints, and other issues requiring the expertise of occupational or physical therapists. There are also many psychosocial issues that are best addressed by an expert in this area. Inevitably, there are concerns from school administrators and faculty about the burned student's attendance, flexible scheduling, and need for modification of the academic curriculum. When these concerns are paramount, the hospital teacher, an expert not only in student instruction but also in working within diverse school systems, can be an invaluable resource for establishing pragmatic solutions to these potential problems.

Practical constraints often do not allow the luxury of several team members visiting the school. One person may have to act as the communicator for the other specialists. When psychological difficulties are the predominant issue, a psychologist or social worker may attend as the lone representative of the team. The psychosocial expert typically spends time with the school psychologist or local psychotherapist to acquaint them with specific psychological needs to be addressed. Occasionally, the nurse case manager or the physical therapist is the most appropriate staff member to make the visit. The nurse case manager can visit the school and teach wound care to family members who were unable to be at the hospital to learn detailed care procedures. The physical therapist can teach the exercises and splint application methods to the local therapist who will work with the patient. Clearly written guidelines and checklists for what should be accomplished during a visit can serve as a "script" that any team member can follow to ensure that all general issues are competently addressed. This allows the team flexibility in deciding who will conduct the presentation.

Program Audience

In planning the program, child, parents, and the school contact person can participate in designating the target audience. The audience for the visit may be limited by the time constraints posed to the burn team by their own scheduling demands. However, other audiences can be targeted for presentation of the audiovisual materials. Inexpensive home-made videotapes can be shown to extended family, neighbors, church groups, or whomever is important in contributing to the child's successful return. This is an elaboration of the concept of "school reintegration" but can be critical to the success of the child's overall community reintegration.

Administrators, teachers, and counselors who will be working with the child should be included. If there is a visit by the burn team, it should include a separate meeting with these staff. If possible, this meeting should occur before the student presentation. Staff often require privacy to fully voice their concerns and questions and, hopefully, be reassured before meeting with the students.

Which students to target for inclusion depends on the school situation. If possible, an attempt is made to include the entire student body because all students are likely to see the child before or after school or in the cafeteria, and their questions need to be addressed. Whether or not all students are included, the class or classes in which the injured child is enrolled must have their own special time to process information and plan for the entry of the student.

Some school-affiliated employees do not fall into the categories of faculty or student, but may need to be included. For example, cafeteria workers, office secretaries, janitors, and bus drivers may have a great deal of informal interaction with the students. Another important group are parents of other students. Parents are often uncomfortable with the idea of their children interacting with an ill, handicapped, or disfigured child, and their influence is obviously very strong. Whether invited to attend the program with the students or to have a separate meeting in which to receive information and address their concerns, their inclusion should be considered as a potentially influential part of the reintegration program.

Child/Parent Program Compliance

Sometimes a child or parent is concerned about inordinate attention being devoted to the child. They fear that calling attention to the child's injuries will create or exacerbate problems. Parents who are provided with a detailed description of the presentation and how such programs have been helpful to others typically agree to participate fully, contingent on the child's endorsement of the program. Predictably there are times when the child is extremely resistant. Arguing and cajoling are useless in these situations. Adolescents, insecure about being perceived as different from others, are especially apt to argue that they do not need a special presentation to the school, sometimes making very dramatic and unrealistic plans to appear "normal." One boy who had lost a hand insisted that he would just keep his prosthetic hand in his pocket at all times so no one would know about his loss.

In such a situation, it is important for the burn team to retreat from the power struggle, maintain support of the child and family, and develop alternative plans for aiding the patient in the reintegration process. Every child and adolescent can have a school reentry program. As with any psychological intervention, the formal content and timing of the program must be negotiated based on the needs and willingness of all participants. Sometimes a program may be altered to include a period of homebound instruction while the child and family gather energy and establish their own recovery rhythm. The burn team continues involvement with the goal of helping the child reintegrate socially beyond the limits of family and home.

Alternatives to "standard" reintegration programs can be offered to patients. One adolescent refused to allow a videotape to be made of him but did agree to make one of himself in private. The team advised him of frequently asked questions he might want to answer and issues he might want to address. He was then given a blank videotape. Alone, he talked into the camera, voicing his ideas and feelings to his classmates. In the end, he produced an excellent reentry video which he allowed to be shown at his school in conjunction with a school visit.

Usually parents and children agree to comply with the team's suggestions. When they do not or when they resist one particular aspect of a plan, it is important to remember that our role is to use our expertise to assist them in their recovery, not to dominate their decision making.

ASSESSMENT OF SCHOOL REINTEGRATION PROGRAMS

Unfortunately, there are no reports of objective data gathered by experimental design to support the conclusion that current variants of school reintegration programs are, in fact, helpful. We do have teachers' evaluations and unsolicited positive anecdotal data. At our burn center, we have collected follow-up questionnaires ($N = 84$) from schools that have received either reentry videotapes or videotapes plus an on-site visit. The responses have been overwhelming positive. All respondents indicated the program to be valuable, and all but one respondent described the program as beneficial to the burned child. Unsolicited comments appeared on 80% of the questionnaires, and all were positive. There were no significant differences in comparisons of evaluative responses toward videotapes alone versus videotapes plus on-site visits.

The data also suggest that parents perceived the school reintegration program to play a central role in facilitating their children's postinjury adjustment. In interviews with parents ($N = 44$) of a randomly selected group of our patients, 1–5 years postburn, we asked what had been the most difficult aspect of adjustment for the child and whether there had been certain experiences that were particularly helpful. Although 32% of the parents named reactions of other people as being most difficult, only 11% named school return as most difficult. Though not conclusive, these data suggest that social difficulties occurred more frequently with persons outside of school than within the school environment. The parents cited the school reentry program most frequently as the experience most important to their child's adjustment.

Likewise, similar questions were posed to the child participants with consistent results. Forty percent of the children indicated that the reactions of other people present the greatest adjustment challenges, but only 3% cited the return to school as the most difficult.

Anecdotal responses from the program participants support the idea that social shunning was diminished by the school reentry program. One teacher writes of a student who returned to school before her video arrived, "the video relieved the tension and anxiety . . . ;" another says, "The students have become protective of [her] and don't allow others to make fun of her." Another said, "It's helped him wear his mask—all the kids agree he has to wear it!" A principle writes, "The program allowed one tough old teacher to get her tears out of the way before meeting the child."

We can tentatively conclude that, although insults, teasing, and staring remain major problems for children who are burned and who have participated in reentry programs, these problems appear to occur more frequently outside of the school environment.

Few attempts to empirically assess the effectiveness of school reintegration programs for *any* groups of ill or injured children have been documented. The majority of studies in this small body of literature report anecdotal information supporting the conclusion that such programs are important and effective (Cahners, 1979; Henning & Fritz, 1983; Manger & Speed, 1986; McCormick, 1986). Ross (1984) reported results of a questionnaire mailed to participants 3 weeks following an educational program for teachers of children with cancer. Results indicated that the teachers believed they had an increased understanding of the illness, enhanced self-confidence, and greater optimism about the futures of their ill students following exposure to the educational program. However, there were relatively few who believed the program had been helpful in their roles with either the ill or the healthy students; many participants said they had not yet experienced an opportunity to observe changes in their roles with students.

Empirical data have been reported suggesting the positive effects of a school reintegration program for pediatric cancer patients (Katz, Rubenstein, Hubert, & Blew, 1988). These authors compared a group of children who had received a reintegration program with another group who had not received such intervention. The intervention group was rated by their parents to have experienced significant gains in social competence following the intervention. In addition, the group appeared to be significantly higher in social competence than the nonintervention group as measured by parental ratings. Children in the treatment group perceived themselves to have significantly gained in social acceptance following the school program. Furthermore, their self-perceptions of social acceptance were also higher than those of the children who had not received the program. The latter group was not actually a formally established control group, having been diagnosed up to 3 years earlier than the intervention group. Thus, the difference between the groups may reflect the effect of time or other uncontrolled variables. Nevertheless, these data support anecdotal reports that school reintegration programs can be effective in ameliorating the potentially negative impact of social rejection.

Anecdotal and empirical reports, although limited, suggest that school reintegration programs have been helpful in easing the process of social adjustment for the ill or injured child. Because of these positive reports, controlled investigations comparing the adjustment of burned children who have received a reentry intervention with a control group are made difficult by the ethical concerns regarding withholding treatment. One possible procedure would be to contrast outcome for children treated in hospitals where such programs are not offered with those children treated in hospitals where school reentry programs are offered. Difficulties are apparent with this proposal; for example, the varying approaches to medical/surgical treatment of burns that characterize different institutions may impact outcome in a variety of ways. A first step toward this end, however, would be to survey burn centers to identify those that offer school reintegration programs, to examine the content and format of such programs as well as the evaluation process used by each center to determine program effectiveness, and to report the results of the evaluations.

Another approach to program assessment would be to compare the outcomes of existing programs which serve comparable patient populations to determine whether there are identifiable elements that seem to be critical in achieving positive results. Within the same institution, elements of reentry programs could be modified to assess the importance of each element in effectiveness. For example, comparisons of written materials with and without a school visit or a visit with and without a videotape could be made using a randomized sample of patients assigned to different program formats.

Choosing appropriate outcome measures remains a challenge. A multifaceted assessment of social adjustment appears to be an obvious choice; however, even utilizing the approach of gathering data from parents, teachers, and the burned children themselves fails to answer the question of whose perception is the most accurate (Meyer *et al.*, in press). Broad-spectrum measurement utilizing a multitrait–multimethod approach is warranted.

Additionally, there are no known sociometric studies that have assessed the acceptance and friendship patterns of burned children versus those of their uninjured peers. The assumption that burned and disfigured children risk rejection by their peers is based primarily on anecdotal information and ratings by parents, teachers, and burned children. Although this assumption appears to be supported by the literature on physical attractiveness and chronic or terminal illness in pediatric patients, it is an assumption yet to be demonstrated empirically and explored. Social acceptance and social adjustment are based on complex, dynamic transactions that involve the belief systems of the burned child, peers, parents, and other adult authority figures. For example, a child believing that he or she will be rejected may behave toward others in ways that prompt rejection, thus affirming the child's belief. Further elucidation of the processes by which the burned child can gain social acceptance as well as the impact of such acceptance on affective and behavioral adjustment would be important contributions to those who attempt to intervene with this population.

SUMMARY

School reintegration programs may appear to represent a simple intervention which can be readily implemented. However, the process by which an injured child reenters the school community and become reintegrated into that social milieu is a complex, multilevel process. Further empirical elucidation of all aspects of this process comprises an important goal for those involved in expanding our current body of knowledge concerning pediatric burn survivors. Following a pattern reflected in the literature on pediatric cancer (Walco & Varni, 1991), the psychological foci for children surviving burn injuries should be expanded from concern with the prevention of severe psychopathology to facilitating adaptation and improving the quality of life for burned children and their families.

REFERENCES

Abdullah, A., Blakeney, P., Koon, K., McCauley, R., Robson, M., & Herndon, D. (1992). Visible scars and self-esteem in pediatric burn survivors. *Proceedings of the American Burn Association, 24,* Abstract No. 111.

Adriaenssens, P., Boeckx, W., Gilles, B., Mertens, S., Nijs, P., & Pyck, K. (1987). Impact of facial burns on the family. *Scandinavian Journal of Plastic and Reconstructive Surgery, 21,* 303–305.

Bains, P. (1993). *Going home* [videotape]. Sacramento: University of California at Davis Regional Burn Center.

Barbarin, O. A. (1990). Adjustment to serious childhood illness. In B. B. Lahey & A. E. Kazdin (Eds.), *Advances in clinical child psychology* (Vol. 13, pp. 377–403). New York: Plenum Press.

Barden, R. C. (1990). The effects of cranio-facial deformity, chronic illness, and physical handicaps on patients and familial adjustment: Research and clinical perspectives. In B. B. Lahey & A. E. Kazdin (Eds.), *Advances in clinical child psychology* (Vol. 13, pp. 343–375). New York: Plenum Press.

Bibace, R., & Walsh, M. E. (1980). Development of children's concepts of illness. *Pediatrics, 66,* 912–917.

Billingham, K. A. (1982). *Developmental psychology for the health care professions (Part 1—Prenatal through adolescent development).* Boulder, CO: Westview Press.

Blakeney, P., Herndon, D., Desai, M., Beard, S., & Wales-Sears, P. (1988). Long-term psychological adjustment following burn injury. *Journal of Burn Care and Rehabilitation, 9,* 661–665.

Blakeney, P., Portman, S., & Rutan, R. (1990). Familial values as factors influencing long-term psychosocial adjustment of children after severe burn injury. *Journal of Burn Care and Rehabilitation, 11,* 472–475.

Blakeney, P., Meyer, W., Moore, P., Broemeling, L., Hunt, R., Robson, M., & Herndon, D. (1993). Social competence and behavioral problems of pediatric survivors of burns. *Journal of Burn Care and Rehabilitation, 14,* 65–72.

Blakeney, P., Washam, K., Cahners, S., & Driscoll, E. (1993a). *Brandon* [videotape]. Tampa, FL: Shriners Hospitals for Crippled Children.

Blakeney, P., Washam, K., Cahners, S., & Driscoll, E. (1993b). *Megan* [videotape]. Tampa, FL: Shriners Hospitals for Crippled Children.

Bordlieri, J. E., Solodky, M. L., & Mikos, K. A. (1985). Physical attractiveness and nurses' perceptions of pediatric patients. *Nursing Research, 34,* 24–26.

Browne, G., Byrne, C., & Brown, B. (1985). Psychological adjustment of burn survivors. *Burns, 12,* 28–35.

Byrne, C., Love, B., Browne, G., Brown, B., Roberts, J., & Steiner, D. (1986). The social competence of children following burn injury: A study of resilience. *Journal of Burn Care and Rehabilitation, 7,* 247–252.

Cahners, S. (1979). A strong hospital–school liaison: A necessity for good rehabilitation planning for disfigured children. *Scandinavian Journal of Plastic and Reconstructive Surgery, 13*, 167–168.

Cash, T. F. (1990). The psychological of physical appearance: Aesthetics, attributes, and images. In T. F. Cash & T. Pruzinsky (Eds.), *Body images: Development, deviance, and change* (pp. 51–79). New York: Guilford Press.

Davis, K. G. (1989). Educational needs of the terminally ill student. *Issues in Comprehensive Pediatric Nursing*, 12, 235–245.

DeWet, B., Cywes, S., Davies, M. R. Q., & Van der Riet, L. (1979). Some aspects of post-treatment adjustment in severely burned children. *Burns, 5*, 979–980.

Doctor, M. E. (1987). Returning to school after a severe burn. In J. A. Boswick, Jr. (Ed.), *The art and science of burn care* (pp. 323–328). Rochelle, MD: Aspen Press.

Doctor, M. E. (1992). Burn camps and community aspects of burn care. *Journal of Burn Care and Rehabilitation, 13*, 68–76.

Doctor, M. E., Burne, B., & Jarecke, D. (1993). *Through the eyes of a child: Burn recovery* [videotape]. Denver, CO: Children's Hospital.

Eyles, P., Browne, G., Byrne, C., Brown, B., & Pennock, M. (1984). Methodological problems in studies of burn survivors and their psychosocial prognosis. *Burns, 10*, 427–433.

Goldberg, R. T. (1974). Adjustment of children with invisible and visible handicaps: Congenital heart disease and facial burns. *Journal of Counseling Psychology, 21*, 428–432.

Gove, F., & Keating, D. (1979). Empathic role-taking precursors. *Developmental Psychology, 14*, 594–600.

Harrison, A. (1985). Body image and self-esteem. In J. Mack & M. Abalon (Eds.), *The development and sustenance of self-esteem* (pp. 90–183). New York: International Universities Press.

Henning, J., & Fritz, G. K. (1983). School reentry in childhood cancer. *Psychosomatics, 24*, 261–269.

Janoff-Bullman, R. (1992). *Shattered assumptions: Toward a new psychology of trauma*. New York: Free Press.

Jovanovic, J., Lerner, R. M., & Lerner, J. V. (1989). Objective and subjective attractiveness and early adolescent adjustment. *Journal of Adolescence, 12*, 225–229.

Katz, E. R. (1980). Illness impact and social reintegration. In J. Kellerman (Ed.), *Psychological aspects of childhood cancer* (pp. 14–45). Springfield, IL: Charles C. Thomas.

Katz, E. R., Rubenstein, C. L., Hubert, N. C., & Blew, A. (1988). School and social reintegration of children with cancer. *Journal of Psychosocial Oncology, 6*, 123–140.

Katz, E. R., Dolgin, M. J., & Varni, J. W. (1990). Cancer in children and adolescents. In A. M. Gross & R. S. Drabman (Eds.), *Handbook of clinical behavioral pediatrics* (pp. 129–146). New York: Plenum Press.

Knudson-Cooper, M. S. (1981). Adjustment to visible stigma: The case of the severely burned. *Social Sciences Medicine, 15*, 31–44.

Knudson-Cooper, M. S. (1982). Emotional care of the hospitalized burned child. *Journal of Burn Care and Rehabilitation, 3*, 109–116.

Knudson-Cooper, M. S. (1984). The antecedents and consequences of children's burn injuries. *Advances in Developmental and Behavioral Pediatrics, 5*, 33–74.

Koon, K., Blakeney, P., Broemeling, L., Moore, P., Robson, M., & Herndon, D. (1992). Self-esteem in pediatric burn patients. *Proceedings of the American Burn Association, 24*, Abstract No. 112.

Langlois, J. H., & Downs, A. C. (1979). Peer relations as a function of physical attractiveness: The eye of the beholder or behavioral reality? *Child Development, 50*, 409–418.

Lefebvre, A. M., & Arndt, E. M. (1988). Working with facially disfigured children: A challenge in prevention. *Canadian Journal of Psychiatry, 33*, 453–458.

Lerner, R. M., & Jovanovic, J. (1990). The role of body images in psychosocial development across the life span: A developmental contextual perspective. In T. F. Cash & T. Pruzinsky (Eds.), *Body images: Development, deviance, and change* (pp. 110–130). New York: Guilford Press.

Love, B., Byrne, C., Roberts, J., Browne, G., & Brown, B. (1987). Adult psychological adjustment following childhood injury: The effect of disfigurement. *Journal of Burn Care and Rehabilitation, 8,* 280–285.

Luther, S. L., & Price, J. H. (1981). Burns and their psychological effects on children. *Journal of School Health, 51,* 419–422.

McCormick, D. (1986). School reentry program for oncology patients. *Journal of the Association of Pediatric Oncology, 3,* 13–17.

Manger, G., & Speed, E. (1986). A coordinated approach to the discharge of burned children. *Journal of Burn Care and Rehabilitation, 7,* 127–129.

Meyer, W., Blakeney, P., Holzer, C., Moore, P., Murphy, L., Robson, M., & Herndon, D. (in press). Inconsistencies in psychosocial assessment of children post major burn. *Journal of Burn Care and Rehabilitation.*

Moore, P., Blakeney, P., Broemeling, L., Portman, S., Herndon, D., & Robson, M. (1993). Psychologic adjustment after childhood burn injuries as predicted by personality traits. *Journal of Burn Care and Rehabilitation, 14,* 80–82.

Riis, A., Anderson, M., Pedersen, M. B., & Hall, K. W. (1992). Long-term psychosocial adjustment in patients with severe burn injuries: A follow-up study. *Burns, 18,* 121–126.

Ross, J. W. (1984). Resolving non-medical obstacles to successful school reentry for children with cancer. *Journal of School Health, 54,* 84–86.

Shriners Burns Institute. (1993a). *Back to school.* Cincinnati, OH: Shriners Hospitals for Crippled Children.

Shriners Burns Institute. (1993b). *Back to school guidelines for parents.* Cincinnati, OH: Shriners Hospitals for Crippled Children.

Stoddard, F., Norman, D., & Murphy, M. (1989). A diagnosis outcome study of children and adolescents with severe burns. *Journal of Trauma, 29,* 471–477.

Stoddard, F., Norman, D., Murphy, M., & Beardslee, W. R. (1989). Psychiatric outcome of burned children and adolescents. *Journal of the American Academy of Child and Adolescent Psychiatry, 28,* 589–595.

Tarnowski, K. J., Rasnake, L. K., & Drabman, R. S. (1987). Behavioral assessment and treatment of pediatric burn injuries: A review. *Behavior Therapy, 18,* 417–441.

Tarnowski, K. J., Rasnake, L. K., Linscheid, T. R., & Mulick, J. A. (1989). Behavioral adjustment of pediatric burn victims. *Journal of Pediatric Psychology, 14,* 607–615.

Tyc, V. L. (1992). Psychosocial adaptation of children and adolescents with limb deficiencies: A review. *Clinical Psychology Review, 12,* 275–291.

Walco, G. A., & Varni, J. W. (1991). Cognitive behavioral interventions for children with chronic illnesses. In P. C. Kendall (Ed.), *Child and adolescent therapy: Cognitive behavioral approaches* (pp. 209–244). New York: Guilford Press.

Walls Rosenstein, D. L. (1987). A school reentry program for burned children: Part I: Development and implementation of a school reentry program. *Journal of Burn Care and Rehabilitation, 8,* 319–322.

Wright, L., & Fulwiler, R. (1974). Long range emotional sequelae of burns: Effects on children and their mothers. *Pediatric Research, 8,* 931–934.

10

Prevention

RUSSELL T. JONES and
VASILIKI ZAHAROPOULOS

INTRODUCTION

Accidents are the leading cause of death among children. While there exist a variety of causes of accidents ranging from automobiles to playground equipment, a major source of accidents is fire. More specifically, burn injuries account for 15% of all accidental injuries among individuals admitted to hospitals for burns and scalds (Accident Facts, National Safety Council, 1987). Most fire-related deaths and injuries occur in the home; sources frequently are matches, stoves, and heaters. Hot beverages such as coffee are responsible for many of the reported scalds (Baker, O'Neill, & Kerpf, 1984). Younger children and children who lack parental supervision are at greatest risk for injury (Jones, McDonald, & Shinske, 1990). Most importantly, authorities on burns agree that 75% of all burn injuries can be prevented (Lalor, 1981).

The goals of this chapter are to: (1) provide a brief description of major conceptual models that may be used to target the prevention of fire-related injuries; (2) present a review of the literature on passive and active strategies, employed to reduce or prevent the occurrence and incidence of untoward consequences resulting from fire emergencies; and (3) discuss the implications for future efforts stemming from both methods of inter-

RUSSELL T. JONES and VASILIKI ZAHAROPOULOS • Department of Psychology, Virginia Polytechnic Institute and State University, Blacksburg, Virginia 24060.

Behavioral Aspects of Pediatric Burns, edited by Kenneth J. Tarnowski. Plenum Press, New York, 1994.

vention. It should be noted that a variety of injuries have been investigated. However, only unintentional fire-related injuries will be discussed.

MODELS

Traditionally, it was believed that injuries were totally unavoidable, unpredictable, and, therefore, unpreventable. However, more enlightened thinking has dispelled this notion as reflected in the following quote: "An injury is the outcome of a behavior environment interaction that leads to death or damage. Perhaps the most effective mode of injury control is prevention. Prevention can be directed toward changes in behavior or environment, or in the complex interaction of the two" (Finney *et al.*, 1993). Given the increased awareness of the psychological and behavioral relationships in health promotion and physical disorder prevention, several major conceptual models have been employed to guide intervention efforts. A brief presentation of major models follows.

In contemporary pediatric psychology the treatment of existing physical and psychological problems has received the most attention (Roberts, 1986). However, according to Roberts, pediatric psychology has recently intensified its basic orientation toward health promotion and illness and injury prevention. Both goals have included the application of psychology to the prevention and remediation of behavioral disorders, and the prevention of childhood injuries and illness (Roberts & Peterson, 1984). Strategies stemming from this model embrace a behavioral framework. Research efforts reflecting this approach have gained encouraging results.

A second model for conceptualizing children's injury prevention strategies emerged from the public health perspective of injury control (Margolis & Runyan, 1983). The identification of host (e.g., the child), agent (e.g., mechanical, electrical, thermal, or chemical), environment (i.e., home, playground, school), and vehicle (i.e., person, object) has been extremely useful for describing causative factors categorization, and estimating injury incidence, and prevalence of injuries. A major advantage of this approach is the ability to apply empirically derived strategies to large groups of individuals. However, its use of education and mass media procedures has often led to equivocal changes in behavioral functioning (Peterson & Mori, 1985). Overall effectiveness for these strategies has been wanting, and the breadth and scope for such strategies has been restricted.

A third model proposed by Peterson and Mori (1985) advocates a preventive intervention conceptualization. This model invokes three factors. The first factor is the target of intervention, which is usually the harmful agent (i.e., the child or caretaker). The second factor involves the methods of intervention which typically fall into one of two categories: mandated/legislated or educational/persuasive. Both passive and active methods are invoked. The third factor identifies tactics through which methods can contact the targets. Included in these strategies are widespread population prevention, milestone preventions, and high-risk group prevention. This model borrows heavily from the discipline of psychology. It has great potential for the treatment of child injury in general, and fire safety more particularly.

An integrative effort has produced a complementary intervention model. This model embraces a number of cardinal features of the previously mentioned models, and underpins an increasing number of effective empirical studies targeting injury prevention. It should be noted that this model may be applied to a variety of intentional and unintentional injuries. However, only fire-related injuries will be discussed in this chapter. This prevention model (Jones & McDonald, 1986) draws from three related frameworks: prevention, behavioral, and community. More specifically, the prevention framework provides the timing (primary, secondary, and tertiary), and goals of the intervention efforts (Bloom, 1977). The behavioral framework ensures objective identification of target responses, specification of behavior change strategies, and the methodology for assessment and evaluation procedures (Mahoney, Kazdin, & Lesswing, 1974). The community psychology perspective facilitates widespread usage of empirically derived intervention (Glenwick & Jason, 1980). (For more specific details, see Jones & McDonald, 1986.) This integrative prevention model provides several advantages over above-mentioned approaches, including consideration of developmental factors when attempting to optimally effect change in child and adolescent behavior and cognitions as well as specific components to guide efforts to enhance appropriate functioning. There are six components of this prevention model which are used to document the need for intervention, ascertain and validate needed skills, provide methods to teach skills as well as the timing of skills, document the most appropriate trainers of skills and the benefits of community involvement. In that this model has been successfully applied to the development of fire safety skills (see Figure 1) in the context of our ongoing program of research, we will discuss each component under the training of fire emergency responding section provided later in this chapter.

REVIEW OF LITERATURE

In an attempt to meaningfully classify intervention efforts, we have selected two categories, namely active and passive, as have previous investigators. Definitions of each category as well as accompanying research will be discussed in the following sections. It should be recognized that treatment components within strategies may fall into both categories and therefore may not always conform to our classification system.

Active Strategies

Active intervention focuses on individuals and their behavior (Finney *et al.*, 1993). Repeated action is often required in order to reduce risk (Frank, Bouman, Cain, & Watts, 1992). An important aspect of this perspective is that safety is only achieved when the individual responds appropriately (Frank *et al.*, 1992). This section will discuss active strategies for reducing the occurrence of burn-related injuries and promoting proper behavioral and cognitive functioning in a fire emergency situation. Although a number of these studies stem from the Jones and McDonald (1986) model mentioned earlier, several are not related to any of the previously described models (the interested reader is referred to Jones & McDonald, 1986). Each study will be discussed under only one target area (responding prior to fire, responding during fire, or responding after fire), although they may target multiple areas of responding.

Training of Prefire Emergency Responding

In the first area, training of responding prior to fire, intervention efforts have focused on preventing fires from occurring. An intervention program that targeted the prevention of burn injuries in two Massachusetts communities employed mass media versus school-based instructions (McLaughlin, Vince, Lee, & Crawford, 1982). The mass media campaign included television announcements, posters, free booklets, and news coverage of the project. The school-based program included presentations, filmstrips, an audio cassette, a game, and other lecture materials. Control communities received no intervention. A modified Solomon four-group design was used to evaluate the effectiveness of the intervention.

The school-based instruction produced an increase in knowledge, while the community-based instruction did not. However, it seemed that neither school nor media campaigns minimized the occurrence of severe burns. The community intervention may have had a moderate, temporary effect on burn occurrence and severity, but it appeared that this effect was more likely related to random variation (Mackay & Rothman, 1982). The enormous amount of information disseminated, the brevity of intervention, and absence of a combined treatment package may have lessened the effectiveness of this program.

Strengths of this study include the obtainment of pre, post, and follow-up data. Additionally, the use of a control group was an important component. Obviously, additional research is needed regarding issues related to social validation and treatment acceptability.

Training of Fire Emergency Responding

In the second area of intervention, attention has focused on two behaviors: evacuation and obtainment of assistance. The primary focus of the first authors' program of research has been these two areas. As alluded to earlier, the Jones and McDonald (1986) prevention model was employed to guide these efforts. Before discussing a sample of these empirical studies, the six components of this model will be provided.*

1. *Document the need for intervention.* After selecting the target geographic area, relevant information may be obtained from a variety of sources at the local and national levels regarding the incidence and prevalence of injury. In our research program targeting fire-related injuries, we contacted the National Fire Protection Association and the National Commission of Fire Prevention and Control to obtain such information (Jones, Kazdin, & Haney, 1981).

2. *Decide what skills to teach and validate them.* A crucial component of this model is determining what skills to teach. Information for this may be obtained from existing materials, federal and national agencies, mental health professionals, teachers, parents, and children. Objective evaluation by "experts" in the particular area is essential in ensuring that the appropriate skills and cognitions will be appropriately taught. Following this, a pilot study should be carried out to ensure that the target population can learn and perform the desired responses. Special considerations concerning children's developmental levels should be noted. Fire skills were selected based on existing materials from the National Fire Protection Association (NFPA). Identified skills were socially validated by expert fire fighters (Jones *et al.*, 1981a).

3. *How to teach skills.* A variety of methods exist on how to teach target skills including mandated/legislated or educational/persuasive and passive or active depending on factors including the type of target response, the child's developmental level, and the availability of the change agent (i.e., caregiver, parent, or teacher). However, from our perspective, the model adopted to teach skills need not be based on a single conceptualization (e.g., educational or behavioral). For example, although the behavioral

*Adopted from the Jones & McDonald (1986) model.

approach served as the primary model used to enhance a variety of personal safety skills (Peterson, 1981; Poche, Brouwer, & Swearington, 1981; Rivera-Tovar & Jones, 1988; Wurtele, Marrs, & Miller-Perrin, 1986), recent efforts in the area of fire safety have combined cognitive and "memorial" conceptualizations to enhance the desired behavioral and cognitive skills as well as lessen reported fear levels (Jones, McDonald, Foire, Arrington, & Randall, 1990; Jones, Ollendick, McLaughlin, & Williams, 1989; Jones, Ollendick, & Shinske, 1989; Jones & Randall, 1989; Williams & Jones, 1989).

4. *When to teach skills*. Determining when to teach skills and cognitions may be as important as the decision as to how to teach such competencies. For example, investigators have pointed out limitations associated with specific developmental variables that prevent certain groups of children from mastering certain skills (i.e., Robertson, 1983). Timing of instruction deserves consideration here as well (i.e., primary, secondary, or tertiary). The primary prevention conceptualization has been adopted to guide our thinking in the teaching of fire evacuation skills. Timing of training has been based on ideas stemming from this model. The consultant can decide whether to prevent a behavior from occurring and/or teach individuals to cope with stressful events that have occurred. By training competencies to enhance functioning in fire emergencies, we can further reduce or prevent the occurrence and incidence of untoward consequences.

5. *Selection of change agents and training setting*. Who are the best trainers of various skills? The response to this question has crucial implications for skill acquisition and generalization. For example, the ability to transfer acquired skills to a setting other than the one in which they were originally acquired (i.e., classroom, home, community center) is often directly related to the change agent (i.e., teacher, parent), as well as conditions where training took place. The continuation of acquired behavior after treatment has been terminated (response maintenance) is frequently correlated with these variables. Although several exhortations have been made advocating the use of parents to enhance both types of generalization, few investigations have actually implemented such procedures (Karoly, 1980).

6. *Community involvement*. The extent to which community involvement is maintained may have significant implications for the development and generalization of desired skills. Lack of involvement by the community limits overall effectiveness of treatment programs. Caplan's notion of populationwide prevention is certainly an appropriate approach to enhance overall effectiveness of a given program (Caplan, 1964). A combination of active and passive methods may be employed, depending on the type of skills to be trained as well as the target population (child or parent).

In addition to its legislative action, educational messages may enhance children's awareness and ability to cope with various threatening situations. Given the success of these and related methods, one can seen an obvious need of complementary approaches stemming from clinical and behavioral psychology. For instance, although children's awareness levels have increased from television spots providing important educational safety messages, improvements in skill functioning have more often been correlated with behavioral interventions, at least in simulated situations (Jones, Ollendick, & Shinske, 1989).

Emergency Training: Evacuation. In an initial investigation, Jones *et al.* (1981a) examined a behavioral procedure to train fire emergency evacuation skills. Fire fighters validated a series of behavioral steps deemed appropriate to evacuate a burning house (see Figure 1). Training of third graders took place in a simulated bedroom setting. Behavioral techniques used were instruction, shaping, modeling, feedback, and external and self-reinforcement. Training resulted in a substantial improvement in skill acquisition as evaluated with a multiple baseline design. Presenting the level of gains to fire fighters indicated that the improvement was likely to result in safety, in the event of an actual fire. A 2-week follow-up indicated that these gains were maintained.

In a second investigation by Jones *et al.* (1981b), children from the above-mentioned investigation were assessed for response maintenance 5 months after the original training had been terminated. Because only moderate levels of maintenance were obtained, brief retraining sessions were conducted. Four months after termination of retraining, assessment again showed a decline in responding, although to a lesser extent.

A third study by Haney and Jones (1982) was designed to enhance maintenance and transfer of training. Maintenance was programmed through: (1) isolated followed by simultaneous presentation of situations; (2) fading of reinforcement; and (3) alteration from external to self-reinforcement. Additionally, transfer was conducted through fading of the reinforcement schedule, self-reinforcement, and training in a third setting (separate from other training or transfer assessment rooms). A multiple baseline design across subjects (four mentally retarded individuals) showed a correlation between training and improvement (correct responding rose from 0.9% during baseline to 72.1% during training). Social validation indicated that gains were likely to lead to desired level of functioning in the event of an actual emergency. Both the maintenance and transfer procedure proved successful. A mean score of 79.9% was attained for the 6-month maintenance period. Generalization training was also shown to be effective.

In an attempt to ascertain factors that mediate response maintenance

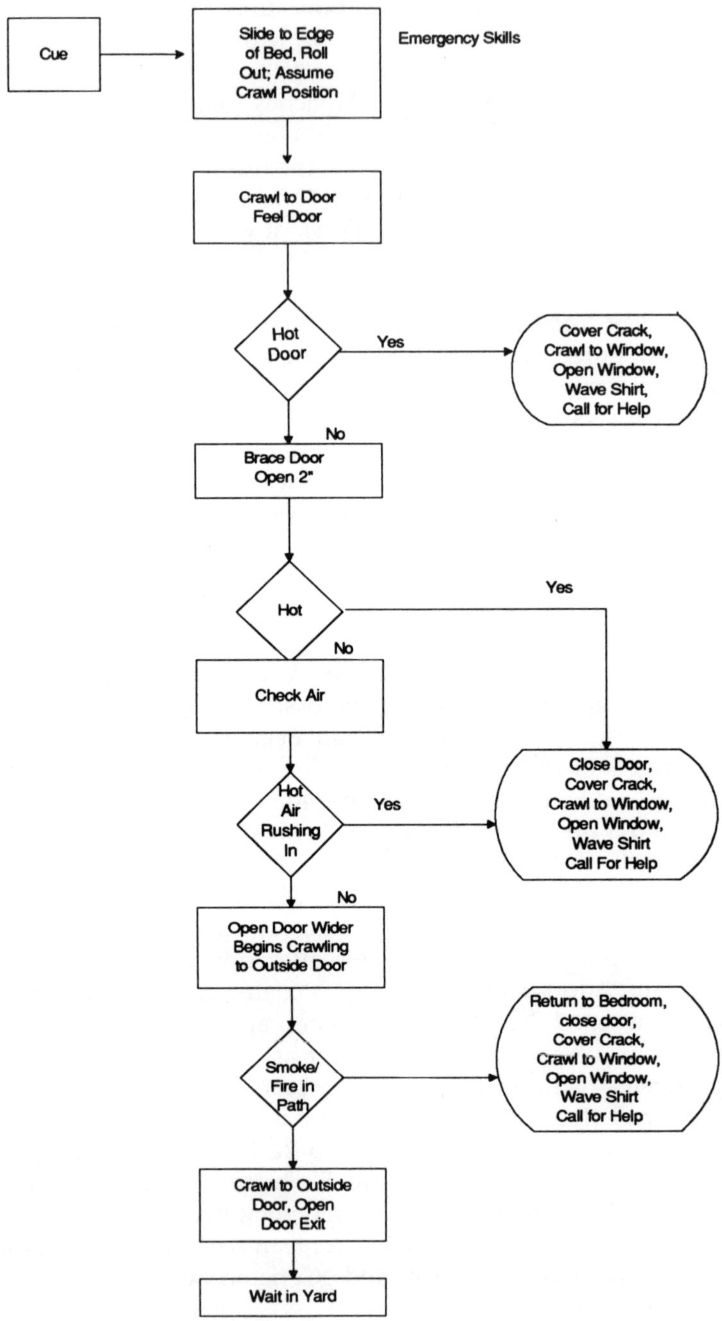
Cue
Slide to Edge of Bed, Roll Out; Assume Crawl Position
Emergency Skills
Crawl to Door Feel Door
Hot Door
Yes
Cover Crack, Crawl to Window, Open Window, Wave Shirt, Call for Help
No
Brace Door Open 2"
Hot
Yes
No
Check Air
Close Door, Cover Crack, Crawl to Window, Open Window, Wave Shirt Call For Help
Hot Air Rushing In
Yes
No
Open Door Wider Begins Crawling to Outside Door
Smoke/ Fire in Path
Return to Bedroom, close door, Cover Crack, Crawl to Window, Open Window, Wave Shirt Call for Help
Crawl to Outside Door, Open Door Exit
Wait in Yard

of evacuation skills, both external and self-regulatory methods were examined (Jones & Haney, 1984). Children in the external regulation groups were monitored externally, evaluated, and reinforced, while the self-regulation group was trained to use self-monitoring, self-evaluation, and self-reinforcement. Both groups attained equally high levels of acquisition (99% as opposed to a 1% gain for the control group). Responding dropped substantially at the 8-month postcheck for both treatment groups. However, rates of decline varied across the two groups. The external regulation subjects' performance declined 4.36 percentage points during the first 4 months where frequent assessments were conducted. Under conditions where the intervals between assessment were longer, performance declined 43.7 percentage points. The self-regulation subjects maintained a constant performance level with a decline of 14.2 and 19.4 percentage points during the first and second 4-month periods, respectively. An important implication from these data is that self-regulatory procedures (self-monitoring, self-evaluation, and self-reinforcement) may enhance maintenance over more externally focused procedures.

A more recent study (Jones, Ollendick, McLaughlin, & Williams, 1989) aimed at fire safety skills acquisition and fear reduction assessed two training procedures, behavioral rehearsal and elaborative rehearsal. Both groups were compared with untrained controls. Behavioral performance and fear level for all subjects in all conditions were measured before and immediately after training. Significant performance gains were found only in the trained groups. Elaborative rehearsal produced significantly more fear reduction than behavioral rehearsal which did not surpass that of controls. These results affirmed the value of elaborative rehearsal in improving performance in fire emergencies and in reducing children's fear of responding.

A follow-up study assessed three training procedures (behavioral, elaborative, and elaborative–behavioral) to determine the relative effectiveness in the acquisition of fire emergency skills and attainment of knowledge (Jones, Ollendick, & Shinske, 1989). Each of these training groups was compared with attention and nontreatment control groups. Sixty-four second and third graders were randomly assigned to conditions. Performance on dependent measures was assessed before and immediately after training. Regarding skill acquisition, elaborative–behavioral and behavioral groups showed significantly higher levels of achievement. But a higher level of knowledge was evidenced by the

←

Figure 1. A flowchart analysis of emergency escape skills in the home and at night. The diamonds represent the decision points, the rectangles represent the responses, and the ovals represent the termination points.

elaborative–behavioral and elaborative groups. The study demonstrated the importance of elaborative–behavioral training in producing changes on behavioral and cognitive components.

An investigation by Randall and Jones (1993) examined the effectiveness of three training procedures (elaborative rehearsal, rehearsal-plus, and behavioral rehearsal) in producing children's acquisition and maintenance of fire safety skills, as well as knowledge regarding these skills (for a description of each group, see Table 1). In addition, the study also targeted reduction of fire-related fears. Fifty-two randomly assigned subjects (second and third graders) were assessed prior to, immediately after, as well as 3 months after training. At posttest checks, performance gains were significantly greater for all groups except the untrained control. At the 3-month follow-up, elaborative rehearsal and rehearsal-plus groups reported significantly more knowledge of skills than the two remaining groups. No differences were found among groups concerning fear at posttest and follow-up.

More recently, computer technology has been employed to enhance acquisition of behavioral skills and knowledge (see Holmes & Jones, 1992). The primary implications from these studies are that overall elaborative procedures appear to facilitate knowledge of skills and some fear reduction. Obviously, the need for continued research in this area is warranted.

Emergency Training: Obtaining Assistance. In a related area of functioning, Jones (1980) examined the effectiveness of a behavioral procedure versus a teacher-devised method for training children enrolled in a Head Start Program to make emergency calls. Consultation with telephone officials, fire officials, child development specialists, and parents assisted

Table 1. Brief Description of Training Groups

Behavioral rehearsal	Elaborative rehearsal	Rehearsal-Plus
1. Teaching fire safety skills via instructions, modeling, and reinforcement.	1. Teaching fire safety skills via instructions, modeling, and reinforcement.	1. Teaching fire safety skills via instructions, modeling, and reinforcement.
2. Reciting the steps aloud, first as a group, then individually.	2. Giving children reasons for the importance of each step; having children repeat the reasons; and allowing them to ask questions about the material.	2. Teaching children how to pair self-instructional statements with fire-related stimuli to show them how to reduce their fire-related fears.

in the content validation of a component analysis of emergency dialing (see Table 2). The behavioral group demonstrated significant gains in their ability to identify their names, addresses, and telephone numbers as well as engage in emergency assisted dialing. These subjects performed significantly better than did subjects in the teacher-devised and control groups. Testing of one-third of the children in the behavioral group at 6 and 12 months following termination of training indicated that all were able to dial the operator and provide information with minimal prompting.

A follow-up study by Jones and Kazdin (1980) targeting not only emergency dialing but also discriminations of how and when to request assistance was carried out. In the first phase of this investigation, 18 children received behavioral training, 23 children received teacher-devised training, and 19 children received assessment only. It was found that the behavioral group performed significantly better than both the control and teacher-devised groups at posttesting. In the second phase, six children received discrimination training. The effectiveness of intervention was determined by multiple baseline designs. The three children who

Table 2. Checklist of Dialing Skills

Dials		
1. Picks up the receiver (Pushes dial tone)	Yes	No
2. Places receiver on ear	Yes	No
3. Dials 0 (zero)	Yes	No
"Let's pretend I am the operator. 'Operator.'"		
Reports Fire		
4. There is a fire at my house.	Yes	No
Gives Name		
5. First name	Yes	No
6. Last name	Yes	No
Gives Address		
7. House number	Yes	No
8. Street name	Yes	No
9. City	Yes	No
Tell the child to put the receiver down.		
Tell the child to pick up the receiver and put it to his ear.		
"Let's make believe the operator is listening."		
"Tell the operator what your full name is." (TIME)		
10. My name is ____________ (first, last).	Yes	No
"Tell the operator to send the fire truck to your house."		
11. Send the firetruck to my house.	Yes	No
12. House number	Yes	No
13. Street name	Yes	No
14. City	Yes	No
"Put the receiver down. Thank you."		

received training of fire emergency scenes improved in responding following the introduction of training.

A related study by Rosenbaum, Creedon, and Drabman (1981) trained twenty-seven 4- and 5-year-old children in emergency dialing. Training consisted of instructions, discussion, practice, praise, feedback, and modeling. Multiple baseline designs were employed to evaluate the intervention. Training resulted in high levels of performance (94 to 100%) on emergency–nonemergency discriminations as well as the provision of appropriate rationale for these discriminations. Regarding actual phone calls, children learned to dial 911, correctly provide their names, and correctly identify the type of emergency. Correct responses concerning the number of people injured, the need for an ambulance, phone numbers, and addresses all increased substantially before the end of training. Generalization to four untrained scenes was noted. The rate of response reported for posttraining was maintained at a 3-month follow-up.

In addition to teaching how to respond to fire emergencies, it is important that they know when to make an emergency call. A study by Rivera-Tovar and Jones (1988) showed that children could be trained to discriminate among fire emergencies, nonemergencies, and neutral scenes. These data added to this vitally important data base highlighting children's mastery of fire-related skills.

Training of Postfire Emergency Responding

Investigations carried out in this last area focused on decreasing emotional problems resulting from fire emergencies. Unfortunately, there is a dearth of theoretical models and actual investigations targeting fire victims.

Documentation of the psychological impact of fire on children's and adolescent's functioning argues strongly for intervention efforts (Jones & Haney, 1984; Jones & Ribbe, 1991). Until recently, assessment of posttraumatic stress disorder (PTSD) symptoms in children has been rare. However, several investigations have suggested that children are susceptible to developing PTSD symptoms following traumatic events (Applebaum & Burns, 1991; Earls, Smith, Reich, & Jung, 1988; Malmquist, 1986; McFarlane, Policansky, & Irwin, 1987; Pynoos, Nader, Frederick, Gonda, & Stuber, 1988). Similar symptoms have resulted from residential fire in children and adolescents (Jones & Ribbe, 1991; Jones, Ribbe, & Cunningham, 1994).

The vast array of negative consequences resulting from fire-related disasters with adults provides additional justification for intervention efforts targeting victims. For example, among adults, consequences of fire include threat to life or bodily integrity (Green, Grace, & Gleser, 1985; Maida, Gordon, Steinberg, & Gordon, 1989; McFarlane *et al.*, 1987), severe physical harm or injury (Green *et al.*, 1985), and sudden loss of a loved one (Green *et al.*, 1985; Green, Lindy, Grace, & Gleser, 1989). The impact of parents' reactions on a child's functioning provides further justification for exploring children's reactions. As stated earlier, few theoretical models exists for guiding intervention efforts of fire victims. While several studies have targeted individuals actually burned during fire-related accidents (Roberts & Gordon, 1979; Weinstein, 1976), few have focused specifically on nonburned individuals.

A cognitive behavioral strategy devised by the first author (see Jones & Randall, 1989) entitled Rehearsal-Plus (R+) has recently been applied to a child and an adolescent victim of fire, neither of whom were physically injured. Briefly, the R+ strategy consists of teaching specific behavioral steps accompanied by their rationale. Based on behavioral and cognitive conceptualizations, behavioral techniques are employed to foster skill acquisition, and elaborative rehearsal is engaged to enhance learning, retention, and appreciation of such skills (Craik & Watkins, 1973). While similar to other stress-reducing strategies including stress inoculation (Meichenbaum & Cameron, 1973), R+ differs in that it focuses on specific stimuli (chains of behavioral responses), employs elaborative rehearsal, and integrates both behavioral and cognitive components throughout training. Several investigations stemming from this framework have shown various aspects of this strategy to be effective (Jones *et al.*, 1989; Jones *et al.*, 1990).

A recent application of R+ was employed with a 7-year-old girl and an 11-year-old boy who experienced a residential fire. A major portion of their home was severely damaged, forcing them to relocate for several months (Jones, 1993). Prior to the implementation of the R+ strategy, a thorough multimethod assessment procedure was carried out. Significant decrease of symptoms was obtained. One explanation for the relative effectiveness of the R+ strategy was the targeting of specific symptoms (i.e., behavior and cognitions). The need for further application and refinement of the R+ strategy is warranted. However, current findings are encouraging.

In conclusion, although subjects exposed to behavioral and cognitive behavioral interventions often show some decline in performance of safety behaviors, these behaviors can return to higher levels with booster sessions or retraining (Finney *et al.*, 1993). Shortcomings for active strategies include repeated effort on the part of individuals, the fact that strategies may be inappropriate for some injuries (Rivera & Mueller, 1987; Wilson & Baker, 1987), and the potential for side effects. An example of a side effect of active interventions is related to the pervasiveness of warnings and reminders about potential hazards in the environment and the need for prevention measures. Etzioni (1978) noted that too many warnings about health and safety may cause individuals to discount each new warning.

Passive Strategies

Passive prevention or environmental intervention consists of limited or no individual action. It is directed toward a population- or communitywide level (Finney *et al.*, 1993). Passive interventions provide automatic protection for the individual without any cooperation or action on their part (Williams & Lund, 1992; Frank *et al.*, 1992). Although there have been numerous suggestions and solutions for promoting fire safety and reducing burn injuries, success in obtaining needed legislation has been limited. Two relative successes include the production of flame-resistant sleepwear and the widespread use of smoke detectors. Beginning in 1973, the Department of Commerce required the use of triphosphate coating on all pajamas. This law has resulted in less frequent sleepwear burns. For example, treatment results for the Shriners Burns Institute in Boston showed that prior to the enactment of this law, 25% of the Institute's flame burns involved sleepwear (O'Shea, Collins, & Butler, 1982).

Regarding smoke detectors, there has been an increase in usage as a result of the passage of state smoke detector ordinances. A significant correlation has been demonstrated between increased smoke detector usage and reduced fire-related deaths and injuries (Fire Safety Hearing, 1993). Unfortunately, the following nine states have not passed smoke detector ordinances: Colorado, Idaho, Kansas, Mississippi, Missouri, Oklahoma, Pennsylvania, South Carolina, and South Dakota (Fire Safety Hearing, 1993).

The National SAFE KIDS Campaign is working with several other U.S. organizations to provide every state with a thorough fire prevention policy. This is the first and only nationwide childhood injury and prevention program. It has three main goals: (1) to change the notion that "accidents just happen"; (2) to change or reduce dangerous products in the environment so as to passively reduce the causes of injury; and (3) to work to make childhood injury prevention a public priority for all levels of the government (Fire Safety Hearing, 1993). Additionally, this group is working toward two goals on the federal level, namely to increase the use and maintenance of smoke detectors by pairing with the United States Consumer Product Safety Commission, and to meet standards of the Federal Fire Safety Act (H.R. 3360). This act requires all federally assisted housing to contain smoke detectors, and all new multifamily high-rise housing subsidized by the federal government to contain mandatory automatic sprinkler systems.

Another successful passive fire prevention program for children, "Project GET ALARMED: A Residential Fire Detection Strategy," has existed since October, 1990, resulting from efforts of the National SAFE KIDS Campaign. The four goals of Project GET ALARMED are to: (1) increase the number of working smoke detectors in use in low-income homes with young children; (2) raise awareness about the need to install, test, and maintain smoke detectors; (3) inform parents about the importance of home escape plans; and (4) mobilize individuals to strengthen smoke detector ordinances across the country (Fire Safety Hearing, 1993, p. 35).

Activities for the second year of the project include a battery replacement campaign in addition to the distribution of smoke detectors. A coalition is urging utility companies to provide reminders of smoke detector maintenance on customers' utility bills (Fire Safety Hearing, 1993). In addition to that effort, the National SAFE KIDS Campaign urges educational programs to include the following list of both passive and active instructions that will better prepare caregivers and their children in fire emergency situations (Fire Safety Hearing, 1993):

1. Teach children to recognize and distinguish the sound of a smoke detector alarm.
2. Families should plan two escape routes out of their home. These escape routes should be simple enough so that children can follow them if an adult is absent. The significance of a second route is to provide an alternate path for escape should the initial path be blocked.
3. To conduct fire drills, especially at night since most fires occur between midnight and 6 a.m. This allows for practice of escape routes (try to make the drills spontaneous so members of the family react instinctively to the alarm).
4. Children should learn how and why it is important to crawl under smoke during a fire and to touch all doors to see if they are hot before opening them.
5. The family should have an outside meeting place that is familiar to all family members.
6. There is no reason to reenter a burning building at all.
7. Parents should make sure children know what a fireman looks like in all of their gear so the child will not be frightened or mistake him for a monster.

Additional passive strategies for future consideration might include change of electric plugs to reduce mouth burns in young children and reduction of home water heating temperature set points in order to reduce the incidence of burns caused by scalds.

The most common type of electrical burn injury seen in young children is oral contact with outlets, electrical cords, or contact with wall sockets that is either direct or through a conductive object (Baker & Chiavello, 1989). One preventive method proposed for this type of injury is the use of a new wall outlet cover. This new type of socket cover is hypothesized to be much safer than the currently used outlet plugs (Baker & Chiavello, 1989).

There are three main advantages to this newly proposed type of cover. First, it is a permanent device, and therefore will not be misplaced. Second, the effort required to replace the cover is minimized since the cover closes automatically. Thus, there is no chance of a parent forgetting to cover the outlet. Third, the effort required to open the device is too complicated for a young child, which prevents them from coming in contact with the outlet altogether (Baker & Chiavello, 1989).

Another area where passive strategies may be beneficial is tap water burns. Although most adults are aware of the potential danger of tap water burns, little has been done to deal with this problem. A survey regarding hot water temperature was conducted with 100 adults, ages 18 to 83. The results showed that the majority of subjects were well aware of the possibility of being burned by tap water, but took no special precautions to regulate the tap water temperature. Even those who had been burned at one time had not lowered the settings on their thermostats. Children are frequent victims of tap water burns. For example, data on patients admitted to Parkland Memorial Hospital in Dallas, Texas, from 1982 through 1989 showed that 83.4% of tap water burns involved children under 9 years old. Nearly 40% of these cases were a result of accidental injury (Adams, Purdue, & Hunt, 1991). Similarly a study conducted at a Mt. Vernon hospital showed that one-third of the patients admitted for burns over a 4-year period were under the age of 3 (Murray, 1988). Next, the survey required physicians going to respondents' homes to do two things: measure their hot water temperature, and have them fill out questionnaires. Respondents were asked to fill a bathtub with water at the same temperature they allow their children to bathe in. Then a minimum intolerable temperature was determined by having subjects add more hot water to what they considered a comfortable bath until the water was hot enough to prevent them from putting their child into it.

According to the results, the average comfortable temperature was 37°C, ranging from 32 to 41°C, and the average minimum intolerable temperature was only 3–4°C higher than the comfortable temperature (Murray, 1988). It seems that in the case of hot tap water, scald burn passive prevention is the most effective method to minimize accidents. The passive approach would be to lower the temperature of the hot water to a safer level. However, there are several factors that need to be considered in determining a safe hot water temperature.

To begin with, there is no completely safe temperature that would prevent all burns, but the problem could be decreased significantly by lowering the temperature. Many studies recommend 60°C in the storage vessel as the best temperature to avoid scalding of the water container and to avoid energy loss. The hottest water that actually runs out of the tap should be set at 43°C (Murray, 1988).

There have been guidelines proposed to effectively regulate water temperature according to the different types of heating device. The previous study concluded that 70% of the families studied who had toddlers owned a gas boiler and 23% an immersion heater. The mean temperature of the water in the houses with gas boilers was 57.1°C with a range from 42 to 78°C. The mean temperature for those with immersion tanks was 62.1°C with a range from 48.5 to 82°C. Fifty percent of immersion heaters and twenty-five percent of gas boilers have a water temperature at or above 60°C, even the ones that contain thermostats (Murray, 1988). Why are they so hot?

One reason is that the hot water stored rises to the top and forms a hot layer, whereas the rest of the vessel contains colder water. Therefore, plumbers tend to set thermostats higher to give more hot water. A new high-performance Economy 7 cylinder has been invented which provides a much better arrangement for heating the water. Its low side-entry heating element causes rapid circulation of the water in the vessel which results in a more equal temperature distribution from top to bottom. It contains two side-entry heating elements, one for day and one for night. The night element automatically turns on for 7 hours every night at a much lower rate (Murray, 1988).

For those who have gas boiler central heating systems, the most common type of heating cylinder that regulates the water also regulates the radiators at the same temperature, usually 80–85°C. A wiser system would be to have full control over the thermostat and to be able to regulate the temperatures of the water and the radiator separately. When heat is not required for the radiator, the cylinder thermostat is set at 60°C. To do this, a two-port valve is used. This would enable the radiator and the hot water to be used at the same time but at different temperatures. The results of recent surveys show that campaigning to update the two heating devices would be effective but it would still be possible to receive a subcutaneous burn (Murray, 1988).

The best solution to the problem seems to be thermoscopic mixing valves which can only be used in high-usage areas such as hospitals. Among other things, the device consists of a temperature-sensitive polycutectic compound and a spring-loaded mechanism called an "actuator." The polycutectic compound expands or contracts depending on the temperature of the water. This causes the actuator to move forward or backward, allowing the right proportions of hot and cold water to enter the valve for the desired temperature. The temperature is controlled within 1°C of the desired temperature, and if the cold water supply fails, complete shutoff occurs in less than 2 seconds. Installation of this valve into water outlets completely eliminates the problem of tap water burns. Unfortunately, it is too expensive to install in every household (Murray, 1988).

Notwithstanding problematic solutions concerning tap water, the use of passive strategies to reduce burn injuries has been relatively effective. Passive intervention measures in general have been shown to be effective once implemented and enforced (Wagenaar & Webster, 1986; Wagenaar, Webster, & Maybee, 1987). Passive approaches eliminate the need for repeated individual action so that safety is achieved by design or one-time changing of the environment (Finney *et al.*, 1993). However, the need for continued attention to shortcomings of this method, including the restricted range and implementation of passive intervention (Cataldo *et al.*, 1986), obtaining approval of passive strategies (Roberts, 1987), and the possibility of such strategies creating new problems and hazards is obvious. For example, certain flame retardants used in children's sleepwear have been shown to be carcinogenic (Blum & Ames, 1977).

SUMMARY

In summary, it is clear that fire-related injury is a major problem, particularly in the United States. Fortunately, many of these injuries are preventable. Although previous views of such injuries have provided limited insight into etiology and treatment, the prevention model espoused by Jones and McDonald (1986) provides useful guidelines for intervention. Although both active and passive methods of intervention have been found to be quite effective, active methods may prove expensive. Future research is warranted to improve the cost-effectiveness of such methods. Although a review of the literature revealed that the bulk of research attention has targeted primary prevention, the need for additional attention to secondary and tertiary prevention appears essential. The Rehearsal-Plus strategy employed to lessen elevated levels of symptomatology may be a good starting point for victims of fire and related injuries. Future research should examine the negative impact of fire and fire-related injury on individuals across the life span. Both cross-sectional and longitudinal investigations should be carried out to determine the precise impact of such occurrences on psychosocial functioning. Funding from both private and governmental agencies should be increased to systematically and comprehensively examine the causes, assessment, and treatment of fire-related injuries. Although much progress has been made in this area, we still have a long way to go. Hopefully, this chapter has provided some insight into the magnitude of fire-related injuries and efforts to lessen such injuries. Future research is indeed warranted to add to these efforts.

REFERENCES

Accident Facts, National Safety Council. (1987).

Adams, L. E., Purdue, G. F., & Hunt, J. L. (1991). Tap-water scald burns: Awareness is not the problem. *Journal of Burn Care and Rehabilitation, 12,* 93–95.

Applebaum, D. R., & Burns, G. L. (1991). Unexpected childhood death: Post traumatic stress disorder in surviving siblings and parents. *Journal of Clinical Child Psychology, 20,* 114–120.

Baker, M. D., & Chiavello, C. (1989). Household electrical injuries in children. *Epidemiology and Identification of Avoidable Hazards,143,* 62.

Baker, S., O'Neill, B., & Kerpf, R. (1984). *The inquiry fact book.* Boston: Heath.

Bloom, B. L. (1977). *Community mental health: A general introduction.* Monterey, CA: Brooks–Cole.

Blum, A., & Ames, B. N. (1977). Flame retardant additives as possible cancer hazards: The main flame retardant in children's pajamas is a mutagen and should not be used. *Science, 195,* 17–22.

Caplan, G. (1964). *Principles of preventive psychiatry.* New York: Basic Books.

Cataldo, M. F., Derschewitz, R. A., Wilson, M., Christopherson, E. R., Finney, J. W., Fawcett, S. B., & Seekins, T. (1986). Childhood injury control. In N. A. Krasnegor, J. D. Arasrh, & M. E. Cataldo (Eds.), *Child health behavior: A behavioral pediatric perspective* (pp. 217–253). New York: Wiley.

Craik, F. J. M., & Watkins, M. J. (1973). The role of rehearsal in short-term memory. *Journal of Verbal Learning and Verbal Behavior, 12,* 599–607.

Earls, F., Smith, E., Reich, W., & Jung, K. G. (1988). Investigating psychopathological consequences of a disaster in children: A pilot study incorporating a structured diagnostic interview. *Journal of the American Academy of Child and Adolescent Psychiatry, 27,* 90–95.

Etzioni, A. (1978). Caution: Too many health warnings could be counterproductive. *Psychology Today, December,* 20–22.

Finney, J. W., Christopherson, E. R., Friman, P. C., Kalnins, I. V., Maddux, J. E., Peterson, L., Roberts, M. C., & Wolraich, M. (1993). Society of Pediatric Psychology Task Force Report: Pediatric psychology and injury control. *Journal of Pediatric Psychology, 18*(4), 499–526.

Fire safety: Protecting our children and families. Hearing presentation in Washington, DC, August 11, 1993.

Frank, R. G., Bouman, D. E., Cain, K., & Watts, C. (1992). Primary prevention of catastrophic injury. *American Psychologist, 47,* 1045–1049.

Glenwick, P., & Jason, L. (Eds.). (1980). *Behavioral community psychology*. New York: Praeger.

Green, B. L., Grace, M. C., & Gleser, G. C. (1985). Identifying survivors at risk for long-term impairment following the Beverly Hills Supper Club fire. *Journal of Consulting and Clinical Psychology, 53*, 672–678.

Green, B. L., Lindy, J. D., Grace, M. C., & Gleser, G. C. (1989). Multiple diagnosis in post-traumatic stress disorder: The role of war stressors. *Journal of Nervous and Mental Disease, 177*, 329–355.

Haney, J. I., & Jones, R. T. (1982). Programming maintenance as a major component of a community-centered preventive effort: Escape from fire. *Behavior Therapy, 13*, 47–62.

Holmes, G. A., & Jones, R. T. (1992). *The role of computer-assisted instructions on the acquisition and maintenance of fire safety skills*. Paper presented at the 99th annual convention of the American Psychological Association, Boston.

Jones, R. T. (1980). Teaching children to make emergency calls. *The Journal of Black Psychology, 6*(2), 81–93.

Jones, R. T. (1993). *Components of a conceptually-based strategy for children and adolescents experiencing trauma*. Paper presented in symposium entitled: Natural disasters and mental health implications of research for prevention. Presented at the 101st Annual American Psychological Association Convention, Toronto, Ontario, Canada.

Jones, R. T., & Haney, J. I. (1984). A primary preventive approach to the acquisition and maintenance of an adaptive community behavior: Fire emergency responding. *Journal of Community Psychology, 12*, 180–191.

Jones, R. T., & Kazdin, A. E. (1980). Teaching children how and when to make emergency telephone calls. *Behavior Therapy, 11*, 509–521.

Jones, R. T., & Randall, J. (1989). *Role of rehearsal-plus on children's coping with stressful events*. Paper presented at the 23rd annual convention of the Association for Advancement of Behavior Therapy, Washington, DC.

Jones, R. T., & Ribbe, D. P. (1991). Child, adolescent, and adult victims of residential fire. *Behavior Modification, 139*, 560–580.

Jones, R. T., & McDonald, D., III (1986). Childhood injury: A prevention model for intervention. *Education and Treatment of Children, 9*, 307–319.

Jones, R. T., Kazdin, A. E., & Haney, J. I. (1981a). A follow-up to training emergency skills. *Behavior Therapy, 12*, 716–722.

Jones, R. T., Kazdin, A. E., & Haney, J. I. (1981b). Social validation and training of emergency fire safety skills for potential injury prevention and life saving. *Journal of Applied Behavior Analysis, 14*, 249–260.

Jones, R. T., Ollendick, T. H., McLaughlin, K. J., & Williams, C. E. (1989). Elaborative and behavioral rehearsal in the acquisition of fire emergency skills and the reduction of fear of fire. *Behavior Therapy, 20*, 93–101.

Jones, R. T., Ollendick, T. H., & Shinske, F. K. (1989). The role of behavioral versus cognitive variables in skill acquisition. *Behavior Therapy, 20*, 293–302.

Jones, R. T., McDonald, D. W., III, Fiore, M. F., Arrington, T., & Randall, J. (1990). A primary preventive approach to children's drug refusal behavior: The impact of rehearsal-plus. *Journal of Pediatric Psychology, 25*, 211–223.

Jones, R. T., McDonald, D., III, & Shinske, F. (1990). Accident prevention: Overview and reconceptualization. In A. M. Gross & R. S. Drabman (Eds.), *Handbook of clinical behavioral pediatrics* (pp. 383–401). New York: Plenum Press.

Jones, R. T., Ribbe, D. P., & Cunningham, P. B. (1994). Psychosocial correlates of fire disaster among children and adolescents. *Journal of Traumatic Stress, 7*, 117–122.

Karoly, P. (1980). Person variables in therapeutic change and development. In P. Karoly & J. J. Steffen (Eds.), *Improving the long-term effects of psychotherapy: Models of durable outcome* (pp. 195–262). New York: Gardner.

Lalor, W. R. (1981). Development of a preventive fire education program based on a profile of the hospitalized burn victim. *Journal of School Health,51*, 80–84.

McFarlane, A. C., Policansky, S. K., & Irwin, C. (1987). A longitudinal study of the psychological morbidity in children due to a natural disaster. *Psychological Medicine, 17*, 727–730.

Mackay, A. M., & Rothman, K. J. (1982). The incidence and severity of burn injuries following Project Burn Prevention. *American Journal of Public Health, 72*, 248–252.

McLaughlin, E., Vince, C. J., Lee, A. M., & Crawford, J. D. (1982). Project Burn Prevention: Outcome and implications. *American Journal of Public Health, 72*, 241–247.

Mahoney, M. J., Kazdin, A. E., & Lesswing, W. J. (1974). Behavior modification: Delusion or deliverance? In C. M. Franks & G. T. Wilson (Eds.), *Annual review of behavior therapy: Theory and practice* (Vol. 2, pp. 11–33). New York: Brunner/Mazel.

Maida, C. A., Gordon, N. S., Steinberg, A., & Gordon, G. (1989). Psychosocial impact of disasters: Victims of the Baldwin Hills fire. *Journal of Traumatic Stress, 2*, 37–47.

Malmquist, C. P. (1986). Children who witness parental murder: Posttraumatic aspects. *Journal of the American Academy of Child Psychiatry, 25*, 320–325.

Margolis, L. H., & Runyan, C. W. (1983). Accidental policy: An analysis of the problem of unintended injuries of childhood. *American Journal of Orthopedic Psychiatry, 53*, 629–644.

Meichenbaum, D. M., & Cameron, R. (1973). *Stress inoculation: A skills training approach to anxiety management*. Unpublished manuscript, University of Minnesota, Minneapolis.

Murray, J. P. (1988). A study of the prevention of hot tap water burns. *Burns, 14*(3), 185–193.

O'Shea, J. S., Collins, E. W., & Butler, C. B. (1982). Pediatric accident prevention. *Clinical Pediatrics, 21*(5), 290–297.

Peterson, L. (1981). *The importance of comparative research in psychological preparation of children* (ERIC Document Reproduction Service No. PS012502). Columbia: University of Missouri.

Peterson, L., & Mori, L. (1985). Prevention of child injury: An overview of targets, methods, and tactics for psychologists. *Journal of Consulting and Clinical Psychology, 53*, 586–595.

Poche, C., Brouwer, R., & Swearington, M. (1981). Teaching self-protection to young children. *Journal of Applied Behavior Analysis, 14*, 169–176.

Pynoos, R. S., Nader, K., Frederick, C., Gonda, L., & Stuber, M. (1988). Grief reactions in school-age children following a sniper attack at school. In E. Chigler (Ed.), *Grief and bereavement in contemporary society* (Vol. 1, pp. 29–41). London: Freund Publishing House.

Randall, J., & Jones, R. T. (1993). Teaching children fire safety skills. *Fire Technology, 29*, 268–280.

Rivera, F. P., & Mueller, B. A. (1987). The epidemiology and causes of childhood injuries. *Journal of Social Issues, 43*, 13–31.

Rivera-Tovar, L. A., & Jones, R. T. (1988). An extension and refinement of telephone emergency skills training: A comparison of training methods. *Behavior Modification, 12*, 445–465.

Roberts, M. C. (1986). The future of child's health care: What do we do? *Journal of Pediatric Psychology, 11*, 3–14.

Roberts, M. C. (1987). Public health and health psychology: Two cats of Kilkeny? *Professional Psychology Research and Practice, 18*, 145–149.

Roberts, M. C. & Peterson, L. (Eds.). (1984). *Prevention of problems in childhood: Psychological research and applications*. New York: Wiley–Interscience.

Roberts, R. N., & Gordon, S. B. (1979). Reducing childhood nightmares subsequent to a burn trauma. *Child Behavior Therapy, 1*, 373–381.

Robertson, L. S. (1983). *Injuries: Causes, control strategies, and public policy*. Lexington, MA: Lexington Books.

Rosenbaum, M. S., Creedon, D. I., & Drabman, R. S. (1981). Training preschool children to identify emergency situations and make emergency phone calls. *Behavior Therapy, 12,* 425–435.

Wagenaar, A. C., & Webster, D. W. (1986). Preventing injuries to children through compulsory automobile safety use. *Pediatrics, 78,* 662–672.

Wagenaar, A. C., Webster, D. W., & Maybee, R. G. (1987). Effects of child restraint laws on traffic fatalities in eleven states. *Journal of Trauma,27,* 726–731.

Weinstein, D. J. (1976). Imagery and relaxation with a burn patient. *Behaviour Research and Therapy, 14,* 481.

Williams, A. F., & Lund, A. K. (1992). Injury control: What psychologists can contribute. *American Psychologist, 47,* 1036–1039.

Williams, C. E., & Jones, R. T. (1989). Impact of self-instructions on response maintenance and children's fear of fire. *Journal of Clinical Child Psychology, 18,* 84–89.

Wilson, M., & Baker, S. (1987). Structural approach to injury control. *Journal of Social Issues, 43,* 73–86.

Wurtele, S. K., Marrs, S. R., & Miller-Perrin, C. L. (1986). Practice makes perfect? The role of participant modeling in sexual abuse prevention programs. *Journal of Consulting and Clinical Psychology, 54,* 688–692.

11

Future Directions

KENNETH J. TARNOWSKI
and RONALD T. BROWN

INTRODUCTION

Given the breadth and complexity of the issues discussed in the preceding chapters, the tasks of deriving general conclusions and outlining a prospectus for future research are challenging. As we have seen, in many ways burns are a unique type of injury. However, we have also demonstrated that burns share some of the characteristics exhibited in other forms of acute trauma and in chronic illness. Although the previous chapters have emphasized the importance of being well versed with the medical, surgical, developmental, cognitive, emotional, behavioral, social, and preventive considerations associated with pediatric burns, it also may be beneficial to incorporate these findings with those in the broader injury, chronic illness, and rehabilitation literature. A summary comment by Dell Orto (1991) approximates the intent. In discussing the psychological and social impact of disability, Dell Orto noted that:

—No one is completely prepared for illness or disability
—Illness changes a family and challenges its resources
—The illness process brings out the best and worst in people
—Disability can deplete resources as well as create them

KENNETH J. TARNOWSKI • Department of Psychology, University of South Florida, Fort Myers, Florida 33919. **RONALD T. BROWN** • Departments of Psychiatry and Behavioral Sciences and Pediatrics, Emory University School of Medicine, Atlanta, Georgia 30322.

Behavioral Aspects of Pediatric Burns, edited by Kenneth J. Tarnowski. Plenum Press, New York, 1994.

—Often the only support is the family
—All people do not have families they can rely on
—Not all family members are capable of responding to the illness and disability of a family member
—New skills are needed to meet the new challenges created by illness
—Coping with chronic disability is an ongoing developmental process
—Existing health care resources can help as well as hinder adjustment [p. 333]

Although these observations were made in the context of the general adult rehabilitation literature, the empirical findings cited in the present volume support the validity of these comments as applied to pediatric burns.

In this concluding chapter, we offer some additional general observations specific to burn-injured children. Specifically, the central conclusions of the preceding chapters are highlighted, their interrelatedness considered, and implications for future directions discussed.

GENERAL CONCLUSIONS AND COMMENTARY

Medical and Surgical Advances Will Continue to Decrease Mortality and Contribute to Reduced Psychosocial Morbidity

In discussing the etiology and epidemiology of pediatric burns in Chapters 1 and 2, we noted that burn injuries almost invariably occur suddenly and unexpectedly, and, in this sense, share properties with other natural and human-made disasters (Rubonis & Bickman, 1991). The physical devastation caused by thermal injuries makes patient survival the foremost initial consideration. As detailed in Chapter 2, advances in our understanding of burn physiology have been translated into improved patient care procedures. Specifically, recent developments in fluid resuscitation, pulmonary care, nutritional support, infection control, and surgical interventions have markedly reduced patient mortality even in the case of massive (e.g., > 80% TBSA) burns. Importantly, in many instances, children now survive injuries which would have proven fatal even a decade ago.

From a psychosocial perspective, we have seen that issues of survival anxiety and blame, including those relevant to abuse and neglect, are ubiquitous; consequently, much of the early inpatient effort needs to be oriented to crisis management. Unfortunately, we know very little about the effectiveness of our efforts in this regard. Although it is reasonable to assume that all burn units strive to establish a compassionate and supportive environment, as is the case with most psychosocial treatments, these are likely necessary but insufficient conditions to bring about the effective resolution of emergent problems.

As emphasized in Chapters 3–9, the mental health consultant must possess a fairly sophisticated understanding of burn physiology, and medical and surgical interventions to put into perspective the unusual, but often predictable, patterns of patient responding (e.g., delirium, acute psychotic symptoms). As we have seen, various forms of physiological compromise are directly responsible for certain types of mental status changes. These changes may be particularly problematic to assess accurately in young children. Furthermore, the biologic etiology of these symptoms does not preclude the implementation of psychological means to improve patient functioning. Finally, given the significant patient mortality associated with burns and smoke inhalation, consultants are advised to be well acquainted with grief and bereavement issues so as to provide optimal support for families in need.

In light of recent advances in infection control and emergent technology aimed at the development of cultured skin, there is every expectation that mortality will decrease further. In addition, surgical refinements coupled with advances in dermatologic research (e.g., keratinocyte cultures) hold considerable promise to reduce the most salient causes of burn-related social stigma—physical deformation and scarring. How such advancements may impact children's body image, social functioning, and general adaptation constitutes a critical area for future research. Finally, pharmacologic advances coupled with refinements in the methods used to administer drugs (e.g., patient-controlled analgesia) will likely result in improvements in the treatment of burn-related pain and associated distress.

Recent and impending advances should translate into: (1) a less deleterious impact on body image development as a function of reductions in cosmetic and functional physical disability, (2) less traumatic social reentry including school reintegration, (3) reduced negative reactions associated with inadequate pain control, and (4) anticipated decreases in other commonly observed acute behavioral problems (e.g., procedural nonadherence).

In spite of these substantial advances and continuing research, it is apparent that the utility of injury and medical rehabilitation variables in understanding patient and family psychosocial adaptation is quite limited. In general, a variety of injury parameters have been shown to be predictive of recovery (acute medical response and requisite care). These parameters include burn etiology, type, and extent of injury. However, such variables have been of more restricted value in predicting acute psychosocial response and are especially poor predictors of long-term sequelae. Finally, we know very little of the interaction of specific developmental and injury/rehabilitation variables.

The Acute Phase Functioning of Pediatric Burn Victims Is Characterized by Common and Often Predictable Forms of Behavioral Disturbance and Emotional Distress

Given the devastating injuries caused by burns, it is understandable that most observers predict a negative psychosocial outcome for burned children. Indeed, given the life-threatening nature of these injuries combined with the highly visible cosmetic insult, patient suffering, and seemingly crude and unrefined medical treatment procedures (e.g., debridement, grafting), it may seem highly unlikely that patients will survive physically or recover psychosocially. Herein lies the importance of distinguishing between predictable, acute problems (e.g., anxiety, depression) and long-term adjustment prognostications. As previously noted, children endure immense physical suffering and psychological distress during the acute phase of treatment. The point is that *all* pediatric burn victims exhibit considerable distress. However, considerable care must be taken not to generalize inappropriately from observations based on acute patient functioning in the interest of making judgments concerning long-term sequelae. An exception to this involves the documentation of patient symptoms that reflect continuity of premorbid functioning. This issue is discussed in more detail below. As evidenced throughout this volume, it is apparent that the quality of the medical and psychosocial treatment made available to children and families during the acute phase holds considerable potential to effect long-term well-being. Unfortunately, we know very little of the acute phase–postdischarge adjustment relationship. Prospective longitudinal investigations are needed that relate various parameters of acute care and patient response to intermediate and long-term child and family functioning.

The spectrum of acute reactions commonly observed in pediatric burn victims is generally known and, for the most part, readily identifiable (e.g., disruption of sleep, treatment nonadherence, self-excoriation, body image disturbance, intractable pain). In general, approaches to managing these difficulties are typically adapted from the general clinical child and pediatric psychology literature. For some problems (e.g., nonadherence), interventions require little modification. However, this is not true for all techniques. For example, common methods of pediatric pain management have proven to be of limited use in treating burn-injured youth. The literature on pediatric pain assessment and treatment has focused on the management of acute procedural-related distress (e.g., bone marrow aspiration). Unfortunately, methods found to be useful in the context of such brief procedural-related distress appear to be limited in mitigating discomfort associated with the intensity and duration of procedural treatments required for burn victims. In addition, repeated aversive treatment procedures are implemented concurrent with the constant distress associated with the acute healing process. Similar difficulties become apparent with social reintegration and body image interventions, which are also adapted from the existing literature.

In general, although there has been expansion of the literature on the assessment and treatment of acute problems, for the most part, the data base is a composite of controlled single case and uncontrolled small-sample designs. Expanding knowledge of the spectrum of acute symptomatology and promising intervention alternatives justify controlled treatment trials. However, the limited samples available at most centers will likely require a coordinated multicenter research effort.

Efforts to Enhance Acute-Phase Patient Adjustment Are Constrained by Limitations in the Consultation–Liaison Literature, Which Remains at a Descriptive Level

The specialty area of pediatric burn consultation–liaison is an exciting and challenging area with significant professional training demands. Moreover, this area offers an extensive research agenda. Children's initial responses to burn injuries and associated medical care may contribute importantly in predicting long-term outcome. Unfortunately, there remains considerable uncertainty about the variables that predict a positive hospital course. It is apparent that the consultation literature remains primarily at the descriptive level of development. However, as we have documented, the empirical data base has evolved to the point where behavioral consultation–liaison is a viable clinical enterprise likely to be accepted and valued by most burn team staff. In particular, recent advances in the behavioral assessment and treatment of pain have added new dimensions to the range of practical activities in which consultants may productively engage.

Although the assessment and management of common acute patient problems form the core of consultation requests, typical patient needs demand expansion of the scope of these activities. Such problems include procedural distress, affective disturbance, transient organic syndromes, consummatory responses, sleep-related problems, general family concerns, and issues related to patient/family premorbid psychopathology. In particular, issues related to social reentry and body image require closer scrutiny by consultants.

Unfortunately, with the exception of childhood cancer, few programs of research have been devoted to the investigation of the reentry process for children with serious medical conditions. We have provided anecdotal and empirical support for the development of community-based programs which have as their ultimate goal the school reintegration of the burned child. Several principles that are echoed throughout this scant literature are applied to children who have sustained burn injuries; they include: (1) planning for school reentry during the acute phase of injury; (2) empowering the family to actively participate as advocates for their child; (3) individualizing a unique plan for school reintegration that emphasizes an appropriate match between the child and the intervention, including consideration of developmental level, degree of physical impairment, premorbid functioning, and school size; (4) treating pediatric burn survivors with the expectation that they will return to school; and (5) having burn team professionals available for ongoing consultation. Of central importance to the consultant working with these children is the availability of pragmatic curricula to provide teachers and classmates with detailed age-appropriate information regarding the burn injury. Also important to the consultant is a summary of particular concerns shared by classmates at various developmental levels, and other practical issues including appropriate scheduling of a school-based intervention, patient participation, and burn team representation. Written and videotaped materials specific to the burn-injured child have been developed to assist in school integration and have been described in detail.

Similar issues arise when considering consultation requests that involve body image concerns. A compelling argument is presented for the development and evaluation of psychometrically sound methods to assess pediatric body image constructs. Given the primacy of family, patient, staff, and societal concerns with patient physical appearance, it is surprising how little is known on this topic. Consultants frequently struggle and equivocate when faced with these issues. However, clinical experience suggests that the press for action and intervention is considerable. Pruzinsky and Doctor have been sensitive to this dilemma and have extrapolated some tentative clinical intervention guidelines from diverse but related adult and child literature.

In essence, although effective consultation efforts depend largely on the development of the general pediatric burn data base (e.g., acute problems, long-term sequelae, social reentry), research efforts on the consultation process itself are needed. There are numerous complexities involved in implementing services within the broader medical treatment system context. Unfortunately, pediatric consultation process variables have received little empirical attention. The importance of such variables deserves increased recognition as a research focus in their own right. This apparent need exists not only for pediatric burn consultation but for the entire field of pediatric health consultation in general.

The Majority of Pediatric Patients Do Not Appear to Suffer Negative Long-Term Psychosocial Sequelae

One of the more intensively studied psychosocial aspects of pediatric burns it that of long-term adjustment. Early studies dramatically over-reported the prevalence of poor adjustment for childhood burn victims. Although most existing studies have been found to be methodologically lacking to varying degrees, the literature supports the conclusion that the majority of children do not evidence maladjustment at extended follow-up. A similar conclusion has been established for adult burn survivors (Patterson *et al.*, 1993).

Although considerable emphasis has been placed on the contribution of injury variables to psychological adjustment, such factors have typically not been found to account for much variance in patient outcome. However, continued attention to specific injury and rehabilitation variables appears important as some recent medical and surgical developments described previously may contribute significantly to outcome (e.g., new cosmetic rehabilitation methods).

Concerns about the long-term psychosocial fate of children are central to most parents and health care providers. The impressive medical and surgical advances discussed earlier have dramatically improved the prospects for patient survival. Clearly, more children who sustain extensive injuries now survive this trauma. One may find some comfort in the data which indicate that only a minority of children appear to be doing poorly at follow-up. However, most families are not readily consoled by such generalities. Unfortunately, as we have seen, the interacting complexities of treatment, injury variables, developmental factors, family variables, and premorbid competence make individual prognostications extremely difficult, if not inaccurate.

The methodological challenges of conducting research on the long-term issue are daunting. In part, the area has stagnated because of a lack of an integrative theoretical framework. However, current risk and resource models have helped to refocus attention to this area. With the establishment of a more secure theoretical foothold, progress in this area should be forthcoming.

One outstanding issue that continues to resurface when discussing this area is the problem of estimating children's premorbid competence. This issue is critical to progress yet has proven so problematic that most investigators simply choose to ignore it. Clearly, this line of research will require considerable developmental and methodologic sophistication to produce useful results. However, if forthcoming, such advancements will: (1) help to quickly resolve several of the outstanding unanswered questions concerning children's long-term outcome and (2) become an integral component of more sophisticated longitudinal studies.

Theoretical Advances Offer Conceptual Linkages among Etiologic, Contextual, Acute, Long-Term, and Prevention Considerations

As noted above, progress in understanding child and family adjustment to burn trauma has been hindered by a lack of theoretical framework. Some recent work has examined adjustment issues within a general stress-resiliency framework that has been used profitably with a variety of other pediatric and adult mental and physical disorders. Chapter 8 expands the scope of this framework model by drawing on the conceptual model described recently by Wallander and associates (e.g., Wallander & Varni, 1992). This model identifies risk and resistance factors that predict familial adjustment and maladjustment for children and adolescents with burn injuries. Because research involving the psychosocial adjustment of pediatric burn victims is still in the descriptive or intuitive phase, such a model paves the way for a theoretical basis for understanding child and family adjustment. Although the study of families as they mediate coping and adjustment in acutely and chronically ill children is a recent endeavor, it appears that children's adjustment to burn injuries will be most profitably studied within a systemic framework.

According to Kaslow *et al.*, children who evidence the most positive adjustment to their burn injuries tend to come from families characterized by adequate utilitarian resources, social support networks, cohesiveness, and effective communication and conflict resolution. Such families support age-appropriate autonomy of their children while, at the same time, they have more realistic appraisals of their child's medical conditions and the rehabilitation process. These families also maintain informed expectations for injury outcome. Not surprisingly, children who tend to evidence a less favorable pattern of adjustment frequently come from families with limited financial resources and social support. The dysfunctional pattern of these children's families tends to be characterized by enmeshment and overprotectiveness, and the families support a coping style in their children typified by disengagement and passivity. Finally, children whose burn injuries are the result of abuse or neglect often come from families in which individual family members demonstrate significant psychopathology.

As we have stressed, the disability-stress-coping model for conceptualizing family functioning is important because it facilitates the identification of child and family risk factors associated with burn injury. This model is also useful in providing a theoretical foundation for future research endeavors. Such a model provides an infrastructure for examining how risk and resource variables may combine differentially to predict adjustment. Thus, programmatic research that examines stress and resiliency in children as mediated by family functioning is an important step in transforming this literature from a descriptive phase to a clear theoretical basis. In particular, more empirical study is needed pertaining to the relationship of family factors, child variables, injury severity, and the mechanism by which the family promotes child adjustment and maladjustment. Additionally, grater research efforts must be mounted to assess the contribution of premorbid family functioning to the child's adjustment to injury. More importantly from a prevention framework, the relationship of premorbid family functioning to injury risk is a fertile area for research. Finally, the family psychotherapy literature has demonstrated considerable clinical promise for adults with chronic illness as well as for children and families characterized by numerous stressors. However, few studies have tested the efficacy of family interventions for children with protracted illness.

The Majority of Pediatric Burn Injuries Are Preventable

Prevention efforts remain a high-priority area for pediatric researchers as they participate in the new health care reform (Finney *et al.*, 1993). As noted in the introduction, burns remain the third leading cause of death for children. Research efforts in prevention of burn injuries have primarily focused on behavioral–environmental interactions that have resulted in injury and death. Environmental causes of burns include hot tap water sources, hair dryers, oil and grease burns, electrical injuries, and gasoline accidents. Behavioral safeguards include close parental supervision of toddlers, community intervention designed to educate parents about the spectrum of home hazards, and policy initiatives designed to regulate sources of possible injury. It will also be important to specify developmental factors that designate children of particular age groups at risk for various types of burn injuries (Finney *et al.*, 1993). There also exists an accumulating body of evidence to suggest that specific premorbid child characteristics may place children at significant risk for accidental injuries (Langley, McGee, Silva, & Williams, 1983). Such research programs will make a viable contribution to primary prevention efforts, particularly in the identification of preexisting competencies and behavioral deficits and excesses. Finally, the model prevention programs that currently exist are encouraging, although their efficacy in comparison with control groups awaits empirical support.

Large-scale epidemiologic investigation is needed to identify children and adolescents at risk for burn injuries and appropriate intervention efforts need to be activated based on these epidemiologic results. Jones and Zaharopoulos have discussed in detail the components of a skills-based competency model that appears to hold considerable promise in assisting children and youth to take appropriate actions to prevent injury and seek assistance. Although passive prevention strategies may be preferred, inadequate attention has been devoted to active prevention tactics. Such approaches appear to hold considerable promise and should be exploited on a larger scale.

Prevention efforts targeted at children who have sustained burn injuries are also important in preventing subsequent injuries associated with environmental risks or premorbid adjustment difficulties. There is a need for increased activity in community-based intervention programs that seek to educate families regarding environmental hazards that place children at risk for injury. Coupled with such programs, it will be important for professionals to advocate for children on the policy level through state and federal legislation. Finally, the development, implementation, and evaluation of intervention programs that target primary and secondary prevention efforts will be an important agenda for the next decade.

Another important area concerning prevention is the deterrence of negative psychosocial sequelae for children who have already sustained burn injuries. An important program of research will be the identification of factors that designate children and their families at risk for future psychological adjustment difficulties. Intervention programs are needed that are designed to target at-risk children and their families by strengthening coping resources and providing the necessary support services to sustain them throughout the difficult rehabilitation period. As we have noted, frequently psychosocial support services are provided to children during hospitalization, although programs that foster coping and ameliorate stressors are often lacking during the rehabilitation phase, particularly following discharge from the hospital. Finally, careful evaluation of such programs will be needed as well to demonstrate their efficacy.

School integration interventions appear to hold considerable promise for preventing adjustment difficulties and for enhancing quality of life for these children. The salient stressors for burn-injured youth frequently revolve around body image and compliance with treatment demands. In this regard, teachers and peers play an important role in terms of enhancing competence and providing social support. An exciting program of research regarding school reentry involves the area of sociometry and how acceptance and friendship patterns of burned children compare with those of their healthy peers. This research would also have the potential for expanding the literature on body image and sociometry. Those factors that predict adequate adjustment, acceptance, and socialization patterns require careful study. More importantly, the mechanism by which adequate socialization and school reintegration is attained needs systematic investigation. Further, ongoing intervention efforts that carefully evaluate various programs of school reintegration with burn-injured youth are sorely needed. Finally, the development of research programs that compare the outcomes associated with various school reentry programs will be a long-term goal which, if brought to fruition, will likely have relevance for children recovering from other illnesses and disability.

CONCLUDING COMMENT

In all areas of clinical practice, we strive to develop and place a premium on a well-defined and methodologically sound literature that provides definitive answers to our most pressing questions. Unfortunately, there are few topics for which the existing data base can provide such assurances. Indeed, the literature on the behavioral aspects of pediatric burn injuries is not among these. Those responsible for the psychological care of pediatric burn victims and their families often express frustration with the lack of an integrated resource on the topic. This problem has been ameliorated, in part, by the empirical summaries provided in the preceding chapters. However, in the process of enhancing our understanding of the medical and psychosocial management of the pediatric burn survivor, the contributing authors have also made apparent the multiple deficiencies of this literature.

In part, the relative dearth of information in the area reflects the highly specialized nature of burn treatment and the relatively limited number of professionals who devote attention to this population. Moreover, as evidenced by the studies reviewed, there exists a set of unique and particularly thorny methodological problems associated with the psychological study of pediatric burn victims and their families.

Alternatively, there is ample documentation that the field has not been stagnant and noteworthy strides have been made in the medical and psychosocial management of burn-injured youth. In essence, the contributors to this volume have conducted a baseline assessment of the status of the field. In the process, they have also charted directions for future clinical and research activities which hold promise to be immensely challenging and rewarding.

REFERENCES

Dell Orto, A. E. (1991). Coping with the enormity of illness and disability. In R. P. Marinelli & A. E. Dell Orto (Eds.), *The psychological and social impact of disability* (3rd ed., pp. 333–335). Berlin: Springer.

Finney, J. W., Christopherson, E. R., Friman, P. C., Kalins, I. V., Maddux, J. E., Peterson, L., Roberts, M. C., & Wolraich, M. (1993). Society of Pediatric Psychology Task Force Report: Pediatric psychology and injury control. *Journal of Pediatric Psychology, 18,* 499–526.

Langley, J., McGee, R., Silva, P., & Williams, S. (1983). Child behavior and accidents. *Journal of Pediatric Psychology, 8,* 181–189.

Patterson, D. R., Everett, J. J., Bombardier, C. H., Questad, K. A., Lee, V. K., & Marvin, J. A. (1993). Psychological effects of severe burn injuries. *Psychological Bulletin, 113,* 362–378.

Rubonis, A. V., & Bickman, L. (1991). Psychological impairment in the wake of disaster: The disaster–psychopathology relationship. *Psychological Bulletin, 109,* 384–399.

Wallander, J. L., & Varni, J. W. (1992). Adjustment of children with chronic physical disorders: Programmatic research on a disability-stress-coping model. In A. M. LaGreca, L. J. Siegel, J. L. Wallander, & C. E. Walker (Eds.), *Stress and coping in child health* (pp. 279–298). New York: Guilford Press.

Index